LABORATORY PROCEDURES

FOR

VETERINARY TECHNICIANS

LABORATORY PROCEDURES

FOR

VETERINARY TECHNICIANS

FOURTH EDITION

Edited by

Charles M. Hendrix, DVM, PhD

Professor of Parasitology
Department of Pathobiology
Auburn University College of Veterinary Medicine
Auburn University, Alabama

With 307 illustrations

An Affiliate of Elsevier

An Affiliate of Elsevier

Publishing Director: Linda L. Duncan
Senior Editor: Elizabeth M. Fathman
Senior Developmental Editor: Teri Merchant
Project Manager: Linda McKinley
Production Editor: Julie Eddy
Designer: Julia Dummitt

Fourth EDITION
Copyright © 2002 by Mosby, Inc.

Previous editions copyrighted 1985, 1992, 1997

Permissions may be sought directly from Elsevier's Health Sciences Rights Department in Philadelphia, USA: phone: (+1)215-238-7869, fax: (+1)215-238-2239, email: healthpermissions@elsevier.com. You may also complete your request on-line via the Elsevier Science homepage (http://www.elsevier.com), by selecting 'Customer Support' and then 'Obtaining Permissions'.

Mosby, Inc.
An Affiliate of Elsevier
11830 Westline Industrial Drive
St. Louis, Missouri 63146

Printed in the United States of America

Library of Congress Cataloging-in-Publication Data

Laboratory procedures for veterinary technicians / edited by Charles M. Hendrix.—4th ed.
    p. cm.
    Includes bibliographical references (p.).
    ISBN 0-323-01396-1
    1. Veterinary clinical pathology—Laboratory manuals. 2. Veterinary
    medicine—Laboratory manuals. I. Hendrix, Charles M. (Charles Mackey)

SF772.6 .L32 2002
636.089′60756—dc21   2002024434

04 05 06 GW/QF 9 8 7 6 5 4

Contributors

Joann Colville, DVM
Fargo, North Dakota

Rick L. Cowell, DVM, MS, Dipl ACVP
Professor, Veterinary Clinical Pathology
Director, Clinical Pathology Laboratory
Department of Veterinary Pathobiology
College of Veterinary Medicine
Oklahoma State University, Stillwater, Oklahoma

Bernard F. Feldman, DVM, PhD
Department of Pathobiology
Virginia-Maryland Regional College of Veterinary Medicine
Virginia Polytechnic Institute
Blacksburg, Virginia

Rafael Ruiz de Gopegui, DVM, PhD
Department of Pathology and Animal Production
Veterinary Faculty
Autonomous University of Barcelona
Barcelona, Spain

Charles M. Hendrix, DVM, PhD
Professor of Parasitology
Department of Pathobiology
Auburn University College of Veterinary Medicine
Auburn University, Alabama

Eloyes Hill, MT (ASCP)
Department of Veterinary and Microbiological Sciences
North Dakota State University
Fargo, North Dakota

Peter J. Ihrke, VMD, Dipl ACVD
Professor of Dermatology
Department of Medicine and Epidemiology
School of Veterinary Medicine
University of California
Davis, California

Muhammed Ikram, DVM, MSc, PhD
Animal Health Technology Program
Fairview College
Fairview, Alberta, Canada

Bruce W. Parry, BVSc, PhD
Department of Veterinary Paraclinical Sciences
University of Melbourne
Werribee, Victoria, Australia

Mary Anna Thrall, DVM, MS, Dipl ACVP
Professor, Department of Pathology
College of Veterinary Medicine
Colorado State University
Fort Collins, Colorado

M. Glade Weiser, DVM, Dipl ACVP
Professor, Department of Pathology
College of Veterinary Medicine
Colorado State University
Fort Collins, Colorado

Joseph G. Zinkl, DVM, PhD, Dipl ACVP
Professor of Clinical Pathology
Department of Pathology, Microbiology, and Immunology
School of Veterinary Medicine
University of California
Davis, California

To my wife, Becky, and my daughter, Charlotte.

Contents

LABORATORY
PROCEDURES
FOR
VETERINARY TECHNICIANS

The Veterinary Practice Laboratory

1

JOANN COLVILLE

Comprehension of the information gained from laboratory tests has increased dramatically over the last few decades. Veterinarians depend on laboratory results to help establish diagnoses, track the course of diseases, and offer prognoses to clients. Many veterinarians routinely request presurgical laboratory screening tests to help identify "at risk" patients before general anesthesia.

Even with the availability of large commercial veterinary reference laboratories, some practices must still wait 2 or 3 days for results. Sometimes, especially when dealing with a critically ill animal, the veterinarian needs immediate laboratory test results. In other circumstances, only one value is sought and sending the sample to a reference laboratory for a single test is not practical. Reference laboratories offer panels or batteries of tests that are useful as screening tests, but these typically are not readily available for immediate or emergency analyses. Tests such as complete blood counts (CBCs), fecal examinations, skin scrapings, and urinalyses are more economically performed in house than sending them to a commercial laboratory. For these reasons, many veterinarians have purchased or leased analytic instruments for routine in-house laboratory testing.

Veterinary practice laboratories are more common and sophisticated than those of 15 years ago. The availability of educated veterinary technicians to set up and operate the laboratories has played a major role in the development of in-house diagnostic systems. Increased availability of affordable analytic instrumentation has made the purchase of these instruments economically feasible for veterinary technicians. As practice laboratories become more sophisticated, the list of assays performed by veterinary technicians becomes longer, and veterinary technicians become more indispensable in the practice.

ROLE OF THE VETERINARY TECHNICIAN

The veterinary technician/veterinarian team approach works efficiently in a laboratory situation. A veterinarian is trained to interpret test results, whereas a veterinary technician is trained to generate these results. Consistent generation of reliable laboratory results requires an educated veterinary technician. A veterinary technician must understand the value of quality control in the laboratory. A person without the proper educational background may easily follow "cookbook" instructions, but a veterinary technician is prepared to make educated decisions if something goes wrong or to recognize an unusual test result.

GENERAL CONSIDERATIONS

Although each veterinary practice is unique, every practice laboratory must meet five criteria: a dedicated area, a sink, storage space, electrical outlets, and Internet access.

◆ Dedicated Area

A specific area should be designated as the laboratory and may range in size from a dedicated space on a counter to an entire room, depending on the layout of the facility. The area should be out of the main flow of traffic in the practice but easily accessible when needed. Room temperature controls should provide a consistent environment, which in turn provides for optimal quality control. A draft-free area is preferable to one with open windows or with air conditioning or heating ducts blowing air on the area. Drafts can carry dust, which may contaminate specimens and interfere with test results. Signs should be posted that notify employees that eating, drinking, applying cosmetics, and adjusting contact lenses in the laboratory is prohibited.

◆ Sink

The laboratory area needs a sink and a source of running water to provide a place to rinse, drain, or stain specimens and reagents and to discard fluids. In every veterinary practice, caution should be paramount; handling and disposing hazardous laboratory materials bears legal and ethical responsibilities that have increased substantially over the last 2 decades. Certain basic laboratory practices are essential for protection of workers and the environment. Some of these practices are simply good laboratory hygiene, whereas federal, state, and local regulations have mandated others. A thorough understanding of the laws is at the foundation of proper laboratory practices regarding hazardous chemicals and specimens. When in doubt, the veterinary technician should never dispose of unknown reagents or chemicals down any sink drain.

◆ Storage Space

Adequate storage space must be available for reagents and supplies to avoid clutter on the laboratory counter space. Some reagents and specimens must be kept refrigerated or frozen. A refrigerator/freezer should be readily available. A compact countertop refrigerator is sufficient for most practice laboratories. Frost-free freezers remove fluid from frozen samples, making them more concentrated if they are left in the freezer too long. For long-term storage of fluid samples (serum, plasma, etc.), a chest freezer or freezer that is not self-defrosting should be used.

◆ Electrical Outlets

Placement of electrical equipment requires careful consideration. Sufficient electrical outlets and circuit breakers must be available. Circuits must not be overloaded with ungrounded three-prong adapters or extension cords. Veterinary technicians should avoid working with fluids around electric wires or instruments.

◆ Internet Access

The diagnostic laboratory of the twenty first century veterinary clinic should have Internet access (in the laboratory or at another location within the veterinary clinic). Many reference laboratories use e-mail (or fax) to report the critical results of submitted diagnostic tests. In a veterinary clinic that has access to a digital camera attachment for the compound microscope, the veterinarian and the veterinary technician should use the Internet as a diagnostic aid. Photographic images such as scanned microscopic images of blood smears, urine sediments, and fecal flotations may be sent as attachments in JPG or JPEG format to an e-mail address to an outside reference laboratory for diagnostic assistance.

The Internet also may be a valuable resource for veterinary medical information. However, information on the Internet may be overly simplified, incomplete, or even inaccurate. The veterinary technician should use Internet sources for additional information, along with consultation with the veterinarian. Together, the veterinarian and the technician should examine all Internet resources carefully to determine the quality of the website.

Two basic determinants are used to assess website quality. First, high-quality Internet sites are unbiased—the group providing the information should not have a vested interest (such as selling a product) in slanting the information a certain way. Second, sources should be staffed by recognized experts in the field, such as the staff of a government agency, college or university diagnostic laboratory, or the American Veterinary Medical Association.

Other signs of quality in a website are as follows:
- Funding and sponsorship are clearly shown.
- Timeliness (date of posting, revising, and updating) are clear and easy to locate.
- Information about the source (e.g., the organization's mission statement) is clear and easy to find.
- Authors or contributors to references on the site are clearly identified.
- References and sources for information are listed on the website.
- Experts have reviewed the website's content for accuracy and completeness.

◉ EQUIPMENT AND INSTRUMENTATION

The size of the veterinary practice and the tests routinely performed in the laboratory determine the equipment and instrumentation needed. Minimal equipment includes a microscope, refractometer, microhematocrit centrifuge, microcapillary reader, and tabletop centrifuge. Additional instrumentation needed, including blood chemistry analyzers, cell counters, incubators, and microbiology and parasitology equipment, depends on the type and size of the practice, geographic locale of the practice, and the special interests of practice personnel.

◆ Microscope

A good compound light microscope is essential, even in the smallest laboratory (Procedure 1-1). It may be used to evaluate blood, urine, semen, exudates, and transudates; other body fluids; feces; and other miscellaneous specimens. It also may be used to detect internal and external parasites and to initially characterize bacteria.

A compound light microscope consists of two separate lens systems: the ocular system and the objective system. The *ocular lenses* are located in the eyepieces and most often have a magnification of 10×. This means that the ocular lens magnifies an object 10 times. A monocular microscope has one eyepiece, whereas a binocular microscope, the most commonly used type today, has two eyepieces.

PROCEDURE **1-1**

Microscope operating procedures

1. Lower the stage to its lowest point.
2. Turn on the light.
3. Inspect the eyepieces, objectives, and condenser lens and clean as necessary. (Consult the manufacturer's operating manual for any special cleaning instructions.)
4. Place the slide or counting chamber on the stage, appropriate side up.
5. Move the 10× objective into position by turning the turret, not the objective lens.
6. Looking through the eyepieces, adjust the distance between them so that each field appears nearly identical and the two fields can be viewed as one.
7. Using the coarse and fine focus knobs, bring the image into focus.
8. Adjust the condenser and diaphragms according to the manufacturer's instructions. This allows you to take full advantage of the microscope's resolving power.
9. When using the *40× (high-dry) objective:*
   • Look for a suitable examination area using the 10× (low-power) objective.
   • Swing the high-dry objective into place.
   • Do not use oil on the slide when using the high-dry objective.
10. When using the *100× (oil-immersion) objective:*
    • Locate a suitable examination area using the 10× (low-power) objective.
    • Place a drop of oil on the slide.
    • Swing the oil-immersion objective into place.
11. When finished:
    • Turn the light off.
    • Lower the stage completely.
    • Swing the 4× or 10× objective into place.
    • Remove the slide or counting chamber.
    • Clean the oil-immersion lens, if necessary.

Most compound light microscopes have three or four objective lenses, each with a different magnification power. The most common objective lenses are 4× (scanning), 10× (low power), 40× (high dry), and 100× (oil immersion). The scanning lens is not found on all microscopes. An optional fifth lens, a 50× (low oil immersion), is found on some microscopes.

Total magnification of the object being viewed is calculated as the ocular power × objective power. For example, an object viewed under the 40× objective is 400 times larger in diameter than the unmagnified object:

10× (ocular lens) × 40× (objective lens) = 400× (total magnification)

When viewed through a compound light microscope, an object appears upside down and reversed. The actual right side of an image is seen as its left side, and the actual left side is seen as its right side. Movement of the slide by the mechanical stage also is reversed. Travel knobs are used to move the glass slide and thus the object (or portion of the object) to be moved. When the stage is moved to the left, the object appears to move to the right.

Compound light microscopes have many components and a light path (Figure 1-1). The optical tube length is the distance between the objective lens and the

Figure 1-1
Components of and light path through a compound microscope.

eyepiece. In most microscopes this distance is 160 mm. The mechanical stage holds a glass slide to be evaluated. It contains an assembly to move the slide smoothly, which allows evaluation of numerous sections of the slide. Coarse and fine focus knobs are used to focus the image of the object being viewed.

The substage condenser consists of two lenses that focus light from the light source on the object being viewed. Light is focused by raising or lowering the condenser. Without a substage condenser, haloes and fuzzy rings appear around the object. The iris (aperture) diaphragm consists of a number of leaves that are opened or closed to control the amount of light illuminating the object.

In modern microscopes, the light source is contained within the microscope (Figure 1-2). A transformer controlled by a rheostat controls the intensity of the light entering the condenser. If a field diaphragm is contained in the light source, it may be used to focus the light entering the condenser. Older microscopes used an external light source and a mirror to project rays of light from the light source to the condenser system.

The initial price of the microscope is important as is the quality of the microscope. The financial investment in a good-quality compound light microscope is offset by the potential income-generating analyses the practice can perform with the aid of the microscope.

Figure 1-2
Modern binocular microscope. (Courtesy Swift Instruments.)

A poor-quality microscope may sit unused on the laboratory bench because of inferior performance and frequent down time for repairs. Durability and the availability of repair service with replacement or loaner microscopes must be considered. A microscope that must be sent away for repair is of no value to the practice while it is gone.

Microscope prices vary, depending on quality and accessories included. The best microscope for an average practice is most often neither the most expensive nor the least expensive one. The quality of the microscope purchased depends partly on the special interests of practice personnel. For example, if a veterinarian has a special interest in cytology, the practice should purchase a better-quality microscope than a practice that sends all of its hematologic and cytologic samples to a reference laboratory. Accessories such as dual viewing, phase-contrast or darkfield capabilities, digital cameras, and lighted pointers add to the price but also increase the versatility of the microscope (and the diagnostic laboratory). Reconditioned microscopes are sometimes available through medical or optical equipment suppliers and are an economical alternative to purchasing a new microscope.

Care and Maintenance

Only lens paper or a soft brush should be used to clean the lenses and eyepieces. Lens paper is designed for this purpose and does not scratch the lenses.

Dust, smudges, marks, or fingerprints are removed with gauze, lens paper, or a soft brush.

Oil is removed from the oil-immersion objective with lens paper each time the objective is used. Any oil left on the objective can seep into the inside of the lens, damaging the lens.

Veterinary technicians should use xylene, methanol, ethanol, or commercial lens cleaner sparingly. Because of the solvent qualities of the solutions, with time they may loosen the adhesive that holds the lens in place. Xylene is a carcinogen and ethanol is a controlled substance. Furthermore, methanol, ethanol, and xylene are flammable and toxic.

Extra light bulbs should be available. Changing a light bulb requires turning off the power and unplugging the microscope. When the defective bulb has cooled, it should be removed and replaced with a new bulb, following the manufacturer's instructions. Replacement bulbs should be identical to those they are replacing.

A dirty field of study may be caused by debris on the eyepiece. The eyepieces should be rotated one at a time while the technician looks through them. If the debris also rotates, it is located on the eyepiece. The eyepiece is cleaned with lens paper or a soft brush.

The microscope should be placed in an area where it can not be moved frequently, jarred by vibrations from centrifuges or slamming doors, or splashed with liquids. It must be kept away from sunlight and drafts and should be covered with a plastic cover when not in use to prevent accumulation of dust on the lenses. The microscope is carried using both hands, one hand securely under the base and the other holding the supporting arm.

If the microscope is used frequently throughout the day, some people prefer leaving the microscope light on all day. This saves the wear and tear that occurs when the light is constantly turned on and off and may extend the life of the bulb.

Calibration of the Microscope

The size of various stages of parasites is often important for correct identification. Some examples are eggs of *Trichuris vulpis* versus eggs of *Capillaria* species and microfilariae of *Dirofilaria immitis* versus microfilariae of *Dipetalonema reconditum*. Accurate measurements are easily obtained by using a calibrated eyepiece within the microscope. Calibration should be performed on every microscope that is used in the laboratory. Each objective lens (4×, 10×, and 40×) must be individually calibrated.

Instruments for Calibration

The stage micrometer is a microscope slide etched with a 2-mm line marked in 0.01-mm (10-m) divisions (Figure 1-3); 1 micron (m) equals 0.001 mm. The stage micrometer is used only once to calibrate the objectives of the microscope. Once the ocular micrometer within the compound microscope has been calibrated at 4×, 10×, and 40×, it is calibrated for the service life of the microscope; the stage micrometer is never used again. Therefore it is a good idea not to purchase the stage micrometer,* but rather borrow one from a university or some other diagnostic laboratory.

The eyepiece scale (or ocular micrometer)† is a glass disc that fits into and remains in one of the microscope eyepieces. The disc is etched with 30 hatch marks spaced at equal intervals (see Figure 1-3). The number of hatch marks on the disc may vary, but the calibration procedure does not change.

---

*Item number CE-59-1430, Carolina Biological Supply Company, Burlington, NC, 27215, 1-800-334-5551, http://www.carolina.com.
†Item number CE-59-1423 or CE-59-1425, Carolina Biological Supply Company, Burlington, NC, 27215, 1-800-334-5551, http://www.carolina.com.

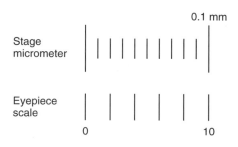

Figure 1-3
Stage micrometer *(upper scale)* and eyepiece scale *(lower scale)* used to calibrate the microscope.

The stage micrometer is used to determine the distance in microns between the hatch marks on the ocular micrometer for each objective lens of the microscope being calibrated (Procedure 1-2). This information is recorded and labeled on the base of the microscope for future reference.

◆ Centrifuge

Another vital instrument in the veterinary practice laboratory is the tabletop centrifuge. It is used to separate cells and particulate matter from the fluids in which they are suspended. The centrifuged fluid (supernatant), such as plasma or serum from a blood sample, can be removed from the particulate matter (sediment) and stored, shipped, or analyzed. Centrifuges also concentrate cells or other sediment material for analysis, such as in preparation of urine or fecal sediment for analysis.

Most centrifuges used in veterinary laboratories are one of two types, depending on the style of the centrifuge head. A horizontal centrifuge head, also known as the *swinging-arm type*, has specimen cups that hang vertically when the centrifuge is at rest (Figure 1-4). During centrifugation, the cups swing out to the horizontal position.

PROCEDURE **1-2**

Instructions for calibration procedures

1. Start at low power (10×) and focus on the 2-mm line if using the stage micrometer. The 2-mm equals 2000 μm.
2. Rotate the ocular micrometer within the eyepiece so that its hatch-mark scale is horizontal and parallel to the stage micrometer (see Figure 1-3).
3. Align the 0 points on both scales.
4. Determine the point on the stage micrometer aligned with the 10 hatch mark on the ocular micrometer. (In Figure 1-3, this point is at 0.100 mm on the stage micrometer.)
5. Multiply this number by 100. In this example, 0.100 × 100 = 10 μm. This means that at this power (10×), the distance between each hatch mark on the ocular micrometer is 10 μm. Any object may be measured with the ocular micrometer scale, and that distance is measured by multiplying the number of ocular units by a factor of 10. For example, if an object is 10 ocular units long, then its true length is 100 μm (10 ocular units × 10 μm = 100 μm).
6. Repeat this procedure at each magnification (4× and 10×).
7. For each magnification, record this information and label it on the base of the microscope for future reference. The ocular micrometer within the microscope is now calibrated for the duration.

Objective Distance Between Hatch Marks (Microns)

4×: 25 μm
10×: 10 μm
40×: 2.5 μm

Figure 1-4
Centrifuge with a horizontal centrifuge head. In this model, the specimen tubes are loaded into "buckets" *(foreground)*, which in turn are inserted into the rotor arms. (Courtesy Jouan, Inc.)

As the specimen is centrifuged, centrifugal force drives the particles through the liquid to the bottom of the tube. When the centrifuge stops, the specimen cups fall back to the vertical position.

This type of centrifuge has two disadvantages. At excessive speeds (greater than 300 revolutions/min), air friction causes heat buildup. Also, some remixing of the sediment with the supernatant (fluid) may occur when the specimen cups fall back to the vertical position.

The second type of centrifuge head available is the *angled centrifuge head* (Figure 1-5). The specimen tubes are inserted through drilled holes that hold the tubes at a fixed angle, usually about 52 degrees. This type of centrifuge rotates at higher speeds than the horizontal-head centrifuge, without excessive heat buildup.

In addition to a standard on/off switch, most centrifuges have a timer that automatically turns the centrifuge off after a preset time and a tachometer or dial to set the speed of the centrifuge. Some centrifuges do not have a tachometer and always run at maximum speed. A centrifuge also may have a braking device to rapidly stop it. *The centrifuge should never be operated with the lid unlatched.*

Specimens must be centrifuged for a specific time at a specific speed for maximum accuracy. A centrifuge that is run too fast or for too long may rupture cells and destroy

Figure 1-5
Centrifuge with an angled centrifuge head. (Courtesy Becton-Dickinson.)

the morphology of cells in the sediment. A centrifuge that is run too slowly or for less than the proper time may not completely separate the specimen or concentrate the sediment. Information regarding speed and time of centrifugation should be developed for all laboratory procedures and should be followed for maximum accuracy.

Success in use of a centrifuge requires that it be exactly balanced. Similar tubes containing equal weights of sample should be placed in specimen cups opposite each other. Water-filled tubes may be used to balance the centrifuge.

The centrifuge should be cleaned immediately if anything is spilled inside it. Tubes sometimes crack or break during centrifugation. Pieces of broken tubes must be removed when the centrifuge stops. If these are not removed, they could permanently damage the centrifuge.

The operator's manual should list maintenance schedules of the different components of the centrifuge. Some centrifuges require periodic lubrication of the bearings. Others may need the brushes checked or replaced regularly. A regular maintenance schedule prevents costly breakdowns and keeps the centrifuge running at maximum efficiency.

A microhematocrit centrifuge is used to separate blood cells of different densities from the plasma in which the cells are suspended (Figure 1-6). With a small blood sample collected in a microhematocrit tube, the microhematocrit centrifuge rapidly

Figure 1-6
Microhematocrit centrifuge used to determine the packed cell volume. (Courtesy Becton-Dickinson.)

provides the packed cell volume (PCV) and a visual assessment of lipemia, hemolysis, jaundice, and leukocytosis. Plasma from the hematocrit tube may be placed in a refractometer to determine total plasma protein concentration. Using a microscope to examine the microhematocrit tube, microfilariae present can be seen in a spun hematocrit sample near the interface of the plasma and the white blood cell "buffy coat."

◆ Refractometer

A refractometer, or total solids meter, is used to measure fluid-specific gravity or protein concentration. The most common uses of the refractometer are determination of the specific gravity of urine or other fluids and the protein concentration of plasma or other fluids.

A refractometer is a cylindric instrument with a built-in prism and calibration scale (Figure 1-7). *Refraction* is bending of light rays as they pass from one medium (e.g., air) into another medium (e.g., urine) with a different optical density. Refractometers are calibrated to a zero reading (zero refractive index) with distilled water at a temperature between 60° and 100° F.

Although refractometers measure the refractive index of a solution, scale readings in the instrument have been calibrated in terms of specific gravity and protein concentrations (g/dl). The specific gravity or protein concentration of a solution is directly proportional to its concentration of dissolved substances. Because no solution can be more dilute or have a lower concentration of dissolved substances than distilled water, the scale calibration and readings (either specific gravity or protein con-

Figure 1-7
Refractometer or total solids meter. (Courtesy A.O. Reichert Scientific Instruments.)

PROCEDURE 1-3

Refractometer use

1. Inspect and clean the prism cover glass and cover plate.
2. Place a drop of sample fluid on the prism cover glass.
3. Point the refractometer toward bright artificial light or sunlight.
4. Bring the light-dark boundary line into focus by turning the eyepiece.
5. Read and record the result using the appropriate scale (specific gravity, protein).
6. Clean the refractometer following the manufacturer's recommendations.

---

centration) are always greater than zero. The refractometer is read on the scale at the distinct light-dark interface.

Various refractometer models are available. Some are temperature compensated between 60° and 100° F. As long as the temperature remains between these two extremes, even as the refractometer is held in the hands, the temperature fluctuation will not affect the accuracy of the reading.

The advantages of a refractometer over other instruments used for similar purposes are precision, accuracy, durability, simplicity of operation, moderate expense, and the small sample volume required.

The specific gravity of a urine sample can be determined with just a drop of urine. This becomes significant in some renal diseases if only small amounts of urine are available and specific gravity measurement is essential for diagnosis, prognosis, and treatment.

Similarly, the plasma protein concentration can be determined from the small amount of plasma in a spun microhematocrit tube. The tube is broken above the cell-fluid interface after reading the hematocrit, and the plasma is placed on the refractometer prism (Procedure 1-3).

Care and Maintenance

The refractometer should be cleaned after each use. The prism cover glass and cover plate are wiped dry. Some manufacturers suggest cleaning the cover glass and plate with alcohol. The manufacturer's cleaning instructions should be consulted.

The refractometer should be calibrated regularly (weekly or daily, depending on use). Distilled water at room temperature placed on the refractometer should have a zero refractive index and therefore read zero on all scales. If the light-dark boundary deviates from the zero mark by more than one-half division, the refractometer should be adjusted by turning the adjusting screw as directed by the manufacturer's instruction manual. The refractometer should not be used if not calibrated to zero using distilled water.

◆ Chemistry Analyzers

Many veterinarians are purchasing their own chemistry analyzers as they become increasingly dependent on clinical chemistry data to diagnose disease and monitor therapy. Manufacturers of chemistry analyzers have become aware of the veterinary market, and many of them now have veterinary models available accompanied by an increasing number of analytic tests.

Although most chemistry analyzers are accurate, other factors determine their appropriateness for a veterinary practice laboratory. Ease of operation, availability of applicable tests, shelf life of reagents, technician time and skill needed or available, and degree of calibration and quality control needed should be considered before an instrument is purchased. Talking with someone who operates the same instrument in another veterinary facility is one way of evaluating a chemistry analyzer. Most sales representatives have a list of people who have purchased the instrument and can vouch for its quality. Many manufacturers offer lease programs for chemistry analyzers.

Types of Chemistry Analyzers

Photometric colorimetry, also called *direct colorimetry*, is based on a solution's color increasing as it becomes more concentrated. Colorimetric instruments differ from spectrophotometers in that colorimeters use filters to separate light into wavelengths, whereas spectrophotometers use prisms or gratings to separate light into wavelengths. Both types of analyzers are wet chemistry instruments that generate light of specific wavelengths, send the light through a liquid sample, measure the intensity of the emergent light, convert the light intensity into electrical energy, and display the electrical energy digitally or on a meter (Figure 1-8).

Several manufacturers have developed dry chemistry analyzers. Reagents are provided on impregnated, premeasured reagent strips or pads. The sample (serum, plasma, or whole blood) is placed on the reagent pad or strip and inserted into the analyzer. The analyzer reads a bar code similar to a UPC symbol to identify the assay being performed and automatically adjusts the analyzer to the proper light wavelength and temperature. The entire reaction takes place on the reagent pad or strip and usually involves a color change. These analyzers use reflective photometric prin-

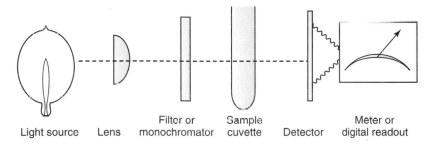

Light source | Lens | Filter or monochromator | Sample cuvette | Detector | Meter or digital readout

Figure 1-8
Components of a spectrophotometer.

ciples to measure the concentrations of solutions being analyzed. The reagent pads or strips are solid and light cannot pass through them. The degree of color change is proportional to the solution's concentration. The analyzer measures the solution's concentration by the intensity of the light reflected from the reagent pad or strip and generates a digital reading or computer printout.

The advantages of using these dry chemistry analyzers versus wet chemistry analyzers are ease of operation, elimination of the necessity to handle and measure liquid reagents (a common source of error), and elimination of test tube or curette costs. One disadvantage may be the initial purchase cost of the analyzer.

Manufacturers of wet chemistry analyzers are continuing to improve the simplicity and accuracy of their analyzers to compete with the increasingly popular dry chemistry analyzers. Dedicated-use analyzers are available for certain tests. These analyzers sample for only one substance, such as blood glucose. They are generally found in larger laboratories, where larger analyzers are used to run panels or batteries of tests. Dedicated analyzers can be used if only a single test is requested or in emergency situations.

Instrument Use and Care

Chemistry analyzers are sensitive instruments that must be carefully maintained. Veterinary technicians should follow the manufacturer's operating instructions. Instruments generally have a warm-up period to allow the light source, photodetector, and incubator, if present, to reach equilibrium before they are used. Ideally, laboratory personnel should turn on the instrument in the morning and leave it on all day. The instrument is therefore ready to use at any time during the day, especially in emergency situations.

Following the manufacturer's maintenance schedule prolongs the life of the chemistry analyzer. A schedule sheet should be established for each instrument in the laboratory, which allows quick and easy review of the maintenance history of any instrument (Figure 1-9). Most manufacturers have a toll-free number to call if problems arise.

Day/year	Tech	Clean printhead (weekly)	Check light source (monthly)	Clean and inspect thermocuvette (monthly)	Check linearity (monthly)	Clean syringe (monthly)	Change purge valve tubing (every 2 mos)	Change O rings (annually)	Other
January									
January									
January									
January									
February									
February									
February									
February									
March									
March									

Figure 1-9

A maintenance schedule can be prepared for each instrument so that maintenance procedures are not overlooked.

◆ Electronic Cell Counters

Chemistry analyzers have become more affordable and available in veterinary laboratories as have electronic cell counters used in veterinary hematology. A number of electronic cell counters used in human medical laboratories have been adapted to veterinary use. This adaptation was necessary because of the variation in blood cell size among different animal species. Some companies have developed dedicated veterinary multispecies hematology systems that count cells and determine the hematocrit, hemogloblin concentration, mean corpuscular hemoglobin concentration (MCHC), a partial white blood cell (WBC), and platelet counts.

Types of Electronic Cell Counters

An impedance counter counts cells by measuring the cells' ability to alter electric resistance as they pass through a small aperture. Two electrodes are placed in an electrically conductive fluid, and a bridge with a small aperture is placed between the two electrodes. Cells to be counted are suspended in the fluid and drawn through the aperture. The concentration of cells and the size of the aperture ensure that most cells pass through the aperture one at a time. Horse, goat, and sheep blood must be diluted more than the blood of other species because of their characteristically high red blood cell (RBC) counts.

When a cell passes through the aperture, it decreases or impedes the electrical flow between the two electrodes. The instrument electronically counts the impedances and reports them as counted cells. The degree of impedance (measured as a voltage pulse) is proportional to the cell volume, so that the counter can distinguish cell types based on the varying cell volumes. Most impedance counters have threshold cell-size settings that allow the instrument to exclude cells or particles below the threshold setting in the cell count. Veterinary practices need a cell counter with an adjustable threshold that can accommodate varying red and white blood cell sizes among different animal species. Impedance counters provide red blood cell, white blood cell, and platelet counts, along with mean corpuscular volume. They use the number of red blood cells per unit volume to calculate the hematocrit.

Darkfield illumination counters measure cell numbers by detecting light diffraction as a cell passes through a light beam. These counters produce a microscopic focal point of light. The cells are uniformly suspended in solution and drawn through the focal point of light one at a time. When the light hits a cell, it is measurably diffracted. This diffraction sets up an impulse that is used to electronically count the cells. Darkfield counters are not discriminating enough to measure mean cell volumes. Some newer electronic cell counters use a laser light beam. They use the same principles as the darkfield counters and can determine mean cell volumes.

Multifunctional instruments combine either impedance or darkfield illumination counters with photometric capability to measure hemoglobin concentration. Additionally, they may be programmed to calculate the mean corpuscular hemoglobin and mean corpuscular hemoglobin concentration.

When white blood cell or platelet counts are performed, a lysing solution is added to the blood sample to destroy red blood cells so that they do not interfere with the counts. When red blood cell counts are performed, white blood cells and platelets also are counted, but their numbers are so few compared with red blood cells that they normally are not a significant source of error. Error resulting from the presence of white blood cells is usually less than 1%. An elevated white blood cell count may elevate the reported red blood cell count using an electronic cell counter.

Advantages, Sources of Error

Electronic cell counters offer a fast, reliable method for the determination of cell counts. They minimize technician error and require decreased technician time to provide results. Several manufacturers offer cell counters with variable threshold settings needed for veterinary hematology. A visit to the commercial exhibits at any major veterinary meeting provides information about and demonstrations of many of the instruments currently available. Depending on the degree of sophistication desired, the initial cost of an electronic cell counter can range from less than a thousand dollars to thousands of dollars.

Electronic cell counters do, however, pose problems. Voltage fluctuations may cause undetectable errors. Pumps, tubing, and valves must be maintained. Diluting fluid and dusty glassware may be contaminated with particles large enough to be erroneously counted as cells. The aperture may become partially or totally obstructed. The threshold setting may be improperly set on a counter with a variable threshold control.

Cold agglutinins may cause a decreased red blood cell count because of red blood cell clumping. Before processing, refrigerated blood samples must be warmed to room temperature. Fragile lymphocytes, as seen with some lymphocytic leukemias, may rupture in the lysing solution used to lyse red blood cells. This rupturing can result in a decreased white blood cell count. The presence of spherocytes (abnormally small, round red blood cells) may alter the mean corpuscular volume, thus reducing the calculated hematocrit. Elevated serum viscosity may interfere with cell counts.

Maintenance

Electronic cell counters, similar to chemistry analyzers, are sophisticated instruments that require careful maintenance. The manufacturer's recommendations for routine maintenance should be followed. Daily maintenance for many electronic cell counters requires flushing the entire system with bleach and fresh diluting solution to keep the aperture open. Background counts are done periodically to make sure the diluting solution is not contaminated or the glassware and tubing are not dirty. The vacuum pump must be checked at regular intervals to ensure that the proper amount of blood and diluting fluid is being drawn into the counter.

QUALITY CONTROL

One of the responsibilities of a veterinary technician in a clinical laboratory is to provide accurate results of analyses. The various steps performed to ensure this accuracy are collectively known as *quality control* or *quality assurance*.

◆ Instrument Quality Control

A well-planned and carefully executed quality-control program entails evaluation of equipment performance, the technician's analytic skills, and variation of results obtained by different technicians performing the same test.

Depending on the chemistry analyzer or electronic cell counter in the laboratory, an individual quality control program uses a number of solutions. Control serum consists of pooled, freeze-dried serum from many patients (usually human) that must be accurately rehydrated before use. "Assayed" control serum has been analyzed repeatedly for each of the many constituents present in serum (e.g., glucose, urea nitrogen, calcium). Data are statistically analyzed, and a range of acceptable values for each constituent is established. The manufacturer of the control serum provides a chart listing the range, or lowest acceptable value to highest acceptable value obtained during the many assays, and the mean, or average value, for each constituent.

Control serum is used for technician and instrument assessment. It is handled exactly as are patient test samples and should be regularly assayed (with each test batch, daily, or weekly) at the same time patient serum samples are assayed. After the assay is completed, the control value should fall within the manufacturer's reported range. If it does not, the assays of the patient and control samples must be repeated.

Individual laboratories may produce their own control serum. Serum samples obtained from at least 20 clinically healthy animals of one species are pooled and analyzed numerous times in the laboratory. Data collected from these tests can be statistically analyzed to establish appropriate ranges and mean values. This procedure is time consuming, especially for smaller laboratories. For this reason, purchasing commercial control sera is much more convenient.

Aliquots of control serum are placed in small tubes, covered tightly, and frozen and used one at a time. At regular intervals (with each test batch, daily, or weekly), one of the aliquots of control serum is assayed at the same time patient serum is assayed. The results of the control serum are recorded on a chart or log for each assay (Figure 1-10). The values for tests performed on control serum should not significantly vary from one time to another.

Some analytic instruments require a blank to prepare them for assays. A blank contains all of the reagents used in the assay except the patient specimen. The instrument is adjusted to read 100% transmittance (or zero absorbence) using the blank. "Blanking" the instrument means instructing it to ignore chemicals or colors contained in the reagents that might interfere with the assay.

A *standard* is a solution containing an exact known amount of a constituent and is used to calibrate some instruments. Most of the newer instruments available no longer require a blank or standard for use, but control samples are required for any quality-control program.

◆ Accuracy, Precision, Reliability

Accuracy, *precision*, and *reliability* are terms frequently used to describe quality control and are the standards for any quality-control program. *Accuracy* is how closely results agree with the true quantitative value of the constituent. *Precision* is the

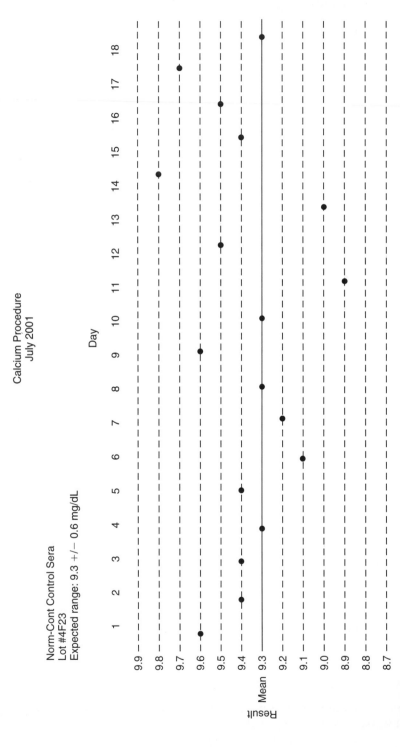

Figure 1-10
Results of periodic quality-control tests on control samples can be charted to detect any deterioration in accuracy.

magnitude of random errors and the reproducibility of measurements. *Reliability* is the ability of a method to be accurate and precise.

◆ Errors

Three types of errors are common to all systems: clerical, random, and systematic. Clerical errors are avoidable and include incorrect labeling, delays in transporting samples, incorrect calculations, transcription errors, and sampling the wrong patient. A well-trained and conscientious staff produces few clerical errors. Some of the most common prob lems related to sample handling are mislabeling and incomplete or incorrect requisition forms. All tubes, slides, and sample containers should be labeled with the owner's last name and the patient's name, species, identification number if available, and date.

Systematic errors cause shifts or trends in results obtained with a specific assay method. They often result in gradual changes, causing the mean value of results to shift in one direction (elevated or decreased). Some factors causing systematic errors include inaccurate standard sera, reagent instability, and method nonspecificity (using a test method unsuitable for the constituent being assayed).

Random errors are caused by variation found in glassware and pipettes, electronic and optic variations of instruments, and variation in temperature controls and timing. These errors occur in all parts of a system and increase the variability of results.

◆ Applied Quality Control

Instrument maintenance is required to prolong the life of the instrument and to prevent expensive "down time." All instruments are accompanied with an owner's manual. If the manual has been misplaced, the manufacturer should be contacted for a replacement. The manual lists the instrument components that must be inspected and attended to regularly. A notebook listing a schedule with the types of maintenance required for each instrument facilitates instrument maintenance. A page is dedicated to each instrument and includes the following (see Figure 1-9):

- Instrument name
- Serial number
- Model number
- Purchase date
- Points to be checked
- Frequency of checks
- Record of test readings
- Changes made to restore accuracy and precision of readings
- Cost and time associated with necessary repairs and restoration
- Name or initials of the person performing the maintenance

Control serum is analyzed to check the accuracy of an assay method. Some manufacturers provide a quality-control service in which "test" samples are sent to many laboratories for assay each month. The results from all the laboratories are collected and compared. From these results the manufacturer can identify laboratories with accuracy problems.

Ideally, control serum should be tested with each batch of tests run. Controls with normal and/or abnormal concentrations of constituents are run because an assay method may not perform the same at all concentrations tested by a particular method. Normal control serum has constituent concentrations that approximate levels normal for that constituent. Abnormal control serum has constituent concentrations that are either higher or lower than normal. These abnormal concentrations represent concentrations seen clinically in disease conditions. If an abnormal concentration of a constituent is found in a patient sample, the results can be trusted if the abnormal control serum concentration was assayed as "in range."

For example, a dog with uncontrolled diabetes mellitus could have serum glucose levels many times higher than the normal 91 mg/dl $+$ 12 mg/dl. By using an abnormal control serum that has an abnormally high glucose concentration, the veterinary technician can feel confident that the elevated patient glucose reading is accurate if the abnormal control serum assays are in range.

Results obtained using control serum are recorded and kept in a permanent record. The veterinary technician should graph results so that changes or trends can be visually detected (see Figure 1-10).

Data may be analyzed in two ways: detection of shifts or trends and determination if results for control samples are within the range established by the manufacturer. If a control serum result does not fall within the range, it should be retested. If it still fails to come into range, the reagents, instrument, and technique must be checked. When control values are successively distributed on one or the other side of the mean, the mean has shifted and a systematic error is involved.

The frequency of control testing depends on the laboratory's goals. To ensure reliability, control samples must be tested when a new assay is set up, a new technician runs the test, a new lot number of reagents is used, or when an instrument is known to perform erratically. Ideally, a control sample is tested with each batch of patient samples. A problem with a particular assay may require an increase in the frequency of control testing.

If attention is paid to detail and as many sources of all three types of error as possible can be eliminated, the laboratory can provide reliable results. Sloppy, inattentive work habits can lead to diagnostic and therapeutic disasters that may result in the death of an animal. Careful attention to detail ensures the veterinarian has all the correct information needed to make a proper diagnosis, prescribe appropriate treatment, and offer an educated prognosis.

⬮ LABORATORY RECORDS

Laboratory records are divided into internal and external record systems. Complete, up-to-date records are necessary for both systems. Numerous computer systems are now available for almost all the records generated in the veterinary clinic or hospital. Patient information, inventory, ordering information, sales records, and laboratory data can be stored on a computer. Clinics using a computer system should be sure to keep backup records in case of computer failure or "infection" with computer viruses.

◆ Internal Records

By using internal records, the laboratory logs assay results and obtains methods. The records consist of a procedures book and quality control data and graphs. The procedures book contains the instructions for all analyses run in the laboratory. Each procedure is described on a separate page. The easiest way to maintain the book is to insert the instruction sheets accompanying each commercial test kit in a three-ring binder, along with pages for any other procedures performed in the laboratory. Each procedure not performed with commercial kits is described on a separate page, including the name of the test, synonyms (if any) for the test, the rationale, reagent list, and step-by-step instructions for a single analysis. Individual pages can be inserted into plastic overlays for protection. The procedures book is reviewed periodically and updated as needed. Those who keep a procedure book on a computer should make sure an up-to-date hard copy backup is available.

Quality-control records are essential because they document the reliability of assay results and identify results that may be inaccurate. In addition to logs, daily quality-control data can be depicted graphically, allowing early identification of subtle performance changes by instruments, reagents, or technicians (see Figure 1-10).

◆ External Records

Laboratory personnel communicate with people throughout the veterinary clinic or hospital and in other laboratories through the use of external records. They consist of request forms that accompany the sample to the laboratory, report forms for assay results, laboratory log books with individual test results, and a book containing pertinent information on samples sent to reference laboratories. In a clinic or hospital with an internal computer network, all personnel can access much of this information as needed.

Information provided on a request form includes the patient's full identification (including identification number, if available) and presenting signs; date and method used to obtain the sample; pertinent history; tests desired; any special notes regarding sample handling; and to whom and by what method results are to be reported (telephone, fax, e-mail, or written report).

The report form should include complete patient identification and presenting signs, test results (including appropriate units), and notation of any extraordinary observations or explanatory comments, if applicable. For additional backup, the laboratory staff should keep a logbook to record test results. If the original laboratory report form is lost in transit, the results are retrievable.

◼ SUPPLIES AND REAGENTS

◆ Prepackaged Supplies and Reagents

When possible, reagents and supplies should be purchased in ready-to-use form. Although the initial purchase price may be higher, ready-to-use reagents or test kits offer several advantages over reagents prepared in the laboratory. Labor costs and investments in supplies and special equipment necessary for bulk-reagent preparation are eliminated. Test kits often have reagents premeasured and packaged individually for each test, so that fewer chances exist for inaccurate measurements, spoilage after opening, and contamination. Test-kit reagents are often packaged to aid proper mixing of reagents and samples. Instructions included with kits are often clear and easy to follow. Finally, many kits and ready-to-use reagents are packaged in small amounts and in a manner that maximizes shelf life, so that even laboratories with a small workload use the reagents before their expiration date.

◆ Purchasing Reagents and Supplies

Purchasing reagents and supplies is easy for most practices. Most veterinary pharmaceutical companies and supply houses have sales representatives who regularly visit practices in their sales territories. Many other companies have catalogs for customers to order pharmaceuticals and supplies. Orders can be mailed, telephoned (usually toll free), e-mailed, or faxed to the companies, and the merchandise is shipped in a short time if items are in stock. Important points to remember when ordering are the following:

- The practice should be identified by name, address, and account number.
- If applicable, the date the order must be received is stated.
- Any handling or shipping specifications should be specified.
- Each item ordered should be identified by description and catalog number, followed by the quantity desired.

The complete order should be written on paper before placing a telephone or e-mail order. The supplier provides an up-to-date catalog. The few minutes spent in preparation save telephone time and help avoid confusion that could otherwise result in an incomplete or incorrect order.

A supplier may be temporarily out of stock or discontinue an item; therefore the practice should maintain active accounts with at least two veterinary supply houses.

◆ Reagent Handling and Storage

Generating consistently reliable test results is impossible with improper, inferior, outdated, or contaminated reagents. Most common problems can be avoided by observation of some general guidelines. Outdated reagents should never be used. Containers should be capped, which avoids evaporation and contamination. All instructions must be carefully read and all reagents stored at the proper temperature. Reagents should not be exposed to prolonged sunlight or artificial light, which may inactivate the reagent. When preparing reagents, veterinary technicians should avoid contamination and incorrect measurements.

◆ Stains

Clinical microscopy is an important part of a veterinary laboratory. Because so much of microscopy depends on proper staining technique, stain quality must be maintained. Stains are commonly used in veterinary laboratories (Table 1-1). Nearly all of the stains listed in Table 1-1 are available in ready-to-use form or in a form that requires little preparation.

The two most common problems related to stain integrity are dye depletion in solutions and excessive precipitate accumulation in the stain solutions. Solutions should be replaced at least once a month, more often if they are heavily used. New stain should not be added to old stain; the stain solution is completely changed. Bottles should be kept tightly capped when not in use to prevent concentration changes resulting from evaporation. The stain must be filtered every few weeks. If a dip staining method is being used, the precipitate settles at the bottom of the stain container and not on the slide. Keeping the containers tightly capped when not in use also prevents contamination, colonization by microbes, and pH changes. When applying a stain, a clean pipette or dropper must be used. A "contaminated" pipette must never be returned to the stain source's container; this action may result in the contamination of an entire stock solution.

◆ Items Required for Specific Tests

Equipment, supplies, and reagents are necessary for various laboratory procedures (Tables 1-2 to 1-7). These tables list them on a test-by-test basis. Details pertaining to methodology and specific supply and reagent use are discussed throughout the remainder of this book. References listed at the end of each chapter, in addition to other textbooks of clinical pathology and laboratory technology, provide additional information.

TABLE 1-1	

Common stains and their use

Stain	Use
Romanowsky stains (Wright's, modified Wright's stains)	General cytology and demonstration of bacteria
Gram	Demonstration of bacteria and Gram reaction
New methylene blue	General cytology, reticulocyte count, demonstration of Heinz bodies
Methylene blue	Demonstration of microfilariae
India ink	Demonstration of *Cryptococcus neoformans*
Lactophenol cotton blue	Demonstration of fungal elements
Sudan III and IV oil-red-O	Demonstration of lipids
Iodine	Demonstration of parasites

TABLE 1-2

Equipment, supplies, and reagents required for hematologic tests

Test	Items Needed for Procedure
WBC count	WBC/platelet Unopette (Becton-Dickinson), hemacytometer with coverslip, microscope, cell counter
Platelet count	WBC/platelet Unopette, hemacytometer with coverslip, microscope cell counter
Reticulocyte count	Test tube (12 × 75 mm), Pasteur pipette, pipette bulb, new methylene blue, glass slide and coverslip, microscope, cell counter
Hemoglobin concentration	Cyanide reagents, spectrophotometer, test tube (12 × 75 mm), pipette (20 ml)
Hematocrit	Microhematocrit reader, microhematocrit centrifuge, microhematocrit tubes, sealing clay
Protein (total solids)	Refractometer, microhematocrit centrifuge, microhematocrit tubes, single-edge razor blade
Plasma fibrinogen	56° C heating block or water bath, microhematocrit tubes, single-edge razor blade, microhematocrit centrifuge, refractometer, test tube
Differential cell count	Glass slide, hematologic stain, phosphate buffer, distilled water, microscope, cell counter
Crossmatch	Centrifuge, saline, test tubes (12 × 75 mm), Parafilm, wooden applicator stick, 37° C heating block, refrigerator, glass slide with coverslip, microscope
Erythrocyte sedimentation rate	Sedimentation stand, Wintrobe tubes; 9¾" Pasteur pipettes, clock
Bone marrow evaluation	Microscope, glass slide with coverslip, stain
Bleeding time	Lancet or scalpel, stopwatch, filter paper, clippers, gauze sponge
Lee-White clotting time	Syringe (5 ml), needle (20 ga), 3 test tubes (12 × 75 mm), 37° C water bath
Fibrin degradation products	Thrombo-Wellco test kit (Wellcome), test tubes (12 × 75 mm)

TABLE 1-3

Equipment, supplies, and reagents required for urinalysis

Test	Items Needed for Procedure
Rapid test strip (dipstick) analyses	Reagent test strips, test tube
Protein concentration	Test tube (12 × 75 mm), 3% sulfosalicylic acid, Pasteur pipette with bulb
Occult blood detection	Reagent test strip, blood tablet test kit
Bile detection	Bile tablet test kit, Pasteur pipette
Urobilinogen detection	Reagent test strip
Sediment examination	Test tube (12 × 75 mm), centrifuge, Pasteur pipette with bulb, glass slide with coverslip, stain
Glucose concentration (reducing method)	Reagent tablet, test tube (12 × 75 mm)

TABLE 1-4

Equipment, supplies, and reagents required for parasitologic tests

Test	Items Needed for Procedure
Fecal flotation	Magnesium sulfate, zinc sulfate, sodium nitrate, test tube (16 × 100 mm), strainer, paper cup, distilled water, centrifuge, glass slide with coverslip, wooden applicator stick, microscope, micrometer, cell counter
Ectoparasite evaluation	Potassium hydroxide, glass slide with coverslip, microscope
Microfilariae detection by modified Knott's technique	Distilled water, 37% formaldehyde, Parafilm, methylene blue, conical tube, 1-ml pipette, graduated cylinder, centrifuge, glass slide with coverslip, microscope, micrometer
Microfilariae detection by microhematocrit method	Microhematocrit tube, microhematocrit centrifuge, microscope
Microfilariae detection by glass slide examination	Glass slide with coverslip, microscope
Microfilariae detection by filtration method	Filtration test kit, glass slide with coverslip, microscope

TABLE 1-5

Equipment, supplies, and reagents required for fecal analysis

Test	Items Needed for Procedure
Parasite detection	See Table 1-4
Occult blood detection	Blood table test kit, distilled water, Pasteur pipette with bulb, glass slide
Fiber content	Applicator stick, Pasteur pipette with bulb, glass slide with coverslip, microscope
Qualitative fat content	Applicator stick, Pasteur pipette with bulb, glass slide with coverslip, Sudan or oil-red-O stain, distilled water, acetone, glacial acetic acid, 70% ethanol, Bunsen burner or alcohol lamp, microscope
Trypsin activity	Radiographic film or gelatin, test tube (16 × 100 mm), pipette (9 ml), 37° C heating block or water bath, distilled water, sodium bicarbonate, refrigerator

TABLE   1-6

Equipment, supplies, and reagents required for serologic and immunologic tests

Test	Items Needed for Procedure
Coombs' test	37° C heating block or water bath, refrigerator, test tubes (12 × 75 mm), species-specific Coombs' reagent (Miles Labs), 0.9% saline, glass slide with coverslip, microscope, centrifuge
Rheumatoid factor detection	Test kit, slide agglutination plate
Canine brucellosis test	Test kit, slide agglutination plate
Feline leukemia virus test	Test kit, Pasteur pipette with bulb
Canine heartworm antigen test	Test kit

TABLE   1-7

Equipment, supplies, and reagents required for bacteriologic and mycologic tests

Test	Items Needed for Procedure
Gram-stained slide examination	Glass slide with coverslip, Gram's stain, distilled water, fixative or Bunsen burner, microscope
Dermatophyte detection	Wood's lamp
Microscopic detection of dermatophytes	Glass slide with coverslip, 15% potassium hydroxide, alcohol lamp or Bunsen burner, microscope
Microscopic detention of systemic fungi	Glass slide with coverslip, 15% potassium hydroxide, lactophenol cotton blue stain, microscope
Aerobic culture	Bunsen burner or alcohol lamp, inoculation loop, agar plates, 37° C incubator
Fungal culture	Sabouraud's agar or commercially prepared media kits

Recommended Reading

Burtis CA, Ashwood ER: *Tietz fundamentals of clinical chemistry*, ed 5, Philadelphia, 2001, WB Saunders.

Feldman BV, Zinkl JG, Jain NC: *Schalm's veterinary hematology,* ed 5, Philadelphia, 2000, Lea & Febiger.

Henry JB: *Clinical diagnosis and management by laboratory methods*, ed 20, Philadelphia, 2001, WB Saunders.

Lee GR, Foerster J, Lukens J: *Wintrobe's clinical hematology*, ed 10, Philadelphia, 1999, Lea & Febiger.

Operator's manual for the DuPont analyst, Wilmington, Del, 1993, DuPont Company.

Operator's manual for the reflotron system, Indianapolis, 1985, Boehringer Mannheim Diagnostics.

Pace B: Health information on the Internet, *J Am Med Assoc* 285(20):2672, 2001.

Hematology

MARY ANNA THRALL
M. GLADE WEISER

Accurate hematologic data are essential for diagnosis of many disorders. Blood for hematologic tests should be taken from a large vein and immediately placed in the anticoagulant potassium ethylenediaminotetraacetate (EDTA). Vacuum tubes containing potassium EDTA are commercially available and should be filled with the specified amount of blood. Blood films should be prepared immediately after collection and kept dry at room temperature. If hematologic tests are not performed within 2 hours of collection, the blood tube should be refrigerated.

Blood samples must be adequately mixed before the performance of any tests; inadequate mixing results in erroneous data. For example, red blood cells (RBCs) in horses start to settle within seconds, and a packed cell volume performed on an unmixed sample may be erroneous. Tubes of blood may be mixed by gentle inversion for several seconds by hand or by placement of the tube on a commercially available tilting rack or rotator.

THE COMPLETE BLOOD COUNT

A complete blood count (CBC) provides a minimum set of values that may be determined reliably and cost effectively in the hospital setting. Various techniques are used to determine hematologic values for the CBC, which may be performed manually or with automated systems designed for use in veterinary hospitals. Attention to detail is a prerequisite for accurate performance of the basic components of the CBC.

The CBC should consist of at least the following basic information:
- Packed cell volume (PCV)
- Plasma protein concentration
- Total white blood cell (WBC) count
- Blood film examination: differential WBC count; erythrocyte morphology; estimation of platelet (PLT) concentration
- Reticulocyte count when the patient is anemic

When hematology instruments designed for the veterinary hospital are used, the following determinations may be added to the CBC:

- Hemoglobin concentration
- Mean corpuscular volume (MCV) and other erythrocytic indices
- WBC differential information
- Platelet count

Performing hemoglobin concentration and erythrocyte counts with manual procedures is no longer considered appropriate. These counts were performed historically to calculate erythrocytic indices detailed in traditional textbooks of hematology. Some of the erythrocytic indices are now regarded as useful when measured on more precise and controlled automated hematology analyzers.

When a commercial laboratory performs the CBC, additional values are reported because automated instruments are used. These additional values, which vary in their interpretive usefulness, may include the erythrocyte concentration, hemoglobin concentration, erythrocytic indices, and erythrocyte size distribution histograms. They are packaged together, partly out of necessity, by virtue of the way automated hematology analyzers function. Because these automated systems have been reduced in size and cost, they may be implemented for use in veterinary hospitals.

◆ Instrumentation

Instrumentation designed for veterinary hospital use is available to facilitate generation of hematologic data for the CBC. Options are cost effective and convenient in situations in which three or more CBCs are performed per day. Benefits of instrumentation include reduced labor investment, more complete information, and improvement of data reliability. The brief discussion presented here is not intended to provide an in-depth understanding of instrument system options. Individual users are responsible for becoming familiar with detailed documentation that accompanies specific instruments.

Instrumentation for the veterinary hospital falls into two general categories: electronic cell analysis systems and the quantitative buffy coat analysis system.

Electronic Cell Counters

Electronic cell counters are based on passage of electric current across two electrodes separated by a glass tube with a small opening or aperture. Electrolyte fluid on either side of the aperture conducts the current. Counting occurs by moving cells through the aperture by use of vacuum or positive pressure. Because cells are relatively poor conductors of electricity compared with the electrolyte fluid, they impede flow of current while within the aperture. These transient changes in current may be counted to determine the blood cell concentration. In addition, the volume or size of the cell is proportional to the change in current, allowing the system to catalogue cell sizes. Size information may be displayed in a distribution histogram of the cell population (Figure 2-1).

Figure 2-1
Representative histogram curve showing the distribution of canine erythrocyte volume. From the data in the curve, the mean corpuscular volume (MCV) can be determined. In this example, the MCV is indicated by the vertical line marked *MCV 65 fl.* The position of a counting threshold relative to the cell population is indicated by the vertical line (*T*).

Leukocytes, erythrocytes, and platelets may be analyzed by these systems.

These instruments are calibrated to count cells in specified size ranges, defined by threshold settings, which prevents erroneous interpretation of small debris and electronic noise as cells and to properly separate cell populations in the same dilution, such as platelets and erythrocytes. Because cell populations vary in size between species, some of the threshold settings are species specific. These settings should be established by the manufacturer and are usually set automatically by system software when the user selects the species for analysis in a software menu. Comprehensive hematology systems designed specifically for veterinary applications are now commonly used in veterinary facilities. These systems incorporate the advantages of individual cell analysis that provide sophisticated information about blood cell populations.

The blood sample must be diluted to count cells. For WBC, a dilution is treated with a lytic agent that destroys cell membranes, leaving only nuclei for counting. Erythrocytes (RBCs) may be analyzed on systems that count the RBCs and provide cell size information using a much greater blood dilution to which no lytic agent is added. Erythrocyte analysis on automated systems provides diagnostic information about cell volume and an alternative method for determining the hematocrit (HT). The mean corpuscular volume (MCV) may be directly measured from analysis of the erythrocyte volume distribution. The hematocrit is then calculated by multiplying the MCV by the erythrocyte concentration. On more sophisticated systems, the volume distribution curve of the erythrocyte population is displayed (see Figure 2-1). A relatively new value, termed the *red cell distribution width (RDW)*, is determined by mathematical analysis of the distribution and functions as an index of erythrocyte volume heterogeneity. Abnormally high values indicate increased volume heterogeneity and an underlying disturbance of the erythron. When used in conjunction with the MCV value, the RDW may alert the veterinarian to diseases of erythrocytes that alter RBC size. The same counting and sizing functions exist for counting platelets on more advanced systems.

Hematology Systems with Differential Capability

The newest electronic hematology systems provide complete analysis of platelet, erythrocyte, and leukocyte (WBC) populations, including WBC differential count information with three or more parts. Most provide graphic displays of cell population size analysis. Differential information is calculated from the WBC population size distribution. Some concern exists about use of the differential information in settings other than the professional laboratory. Veterinary facilities tend to rely solely on this differential information and exclude blood film analysis from the hematology procedures.

The automated differential was not invented to be the definitive source of the differential data for all samples. It was invented to sort samples into two categories. The first category includes samples that have relatively normal WBC data that the instrument generates reliably. The second category is abnormal WBC data that may need clarification by a manual differential count and identification of abnormalities on a blood film. No instrument system, no matter how expensive or complex, can reliably analyze all samples covering the range of pathologic abnormalities. The manufacturer must provide the user guidelines for use of these systems in conjunction with blood film review for patients with abnormal WBC data. The added benefit is that other abnormalities in RBC and platelets also may be observed during blood film review.

Quality-Control Procedures

Unfortunately, instrumentation is not regulated for use in veterinary medicine. As a result, veterinary facilities must rely on manufacturers or suppliers for recommendations on use of quality control. Many manufacturers indicate that their system does not need a quality-control program, which is contradictory to all laboratory recommendations for use of instrumentation devices that repetitively interact with patient samples. Human medical laboratories must follow universally accepted standard laboratory practice of implementing specific quality-control programs. For hematology, this practice typically involves three levels of control material and requirements for analysis multiple times per day. This may be simplified in veterinary applications to one level of control material, planned analysis once per day, and unplanned use of control material to troubleshoot questioned system performance. The rationale for a quality-control program is as follows: Clinicians are frequently faced with test results that do not meet expectations. This inherently raises questions about the accuracy of those results. A regular quality-control program provides an additional day-to-day confidence level that patient test results are reliable. In addition, quality-control data is an essential first step in instrument troubleshooting when a problem does occur.

Evaluation of New System Performance

Because performance specifications and quality-control programs for instrument systems are not regulated for systems placed in veterinary medicine, considerable variation may exist in actual performance standards. Some manufacturers, such as Heska Corporation (Fort Collins, CO), perform extensive evaluation to demonstrate that systems meet stated claims for performance in veterinary applications. Veterinary personnel purchasing new instrumentation may want to perform their own evaluation. However, persons not trained in laboratory science may not know how to perform a valid comparative evaluation. Their natural tendency for designing a comparison is to run a few patient samples on another in-house instrument or through a commercial laboratory and compare results with the new instrument being evaluated.

This approach has some problems that may lead the observer to erroneous conclusions. First, commercial laboratories may obtain different results because the analysis takes place some number of hours after the in-house measurements were done. Second, comparison should be avoided with an instrument that is not quality controlled because its performance is not documented to be within specification. In this situation, the new system may have better performance than the comparison system being used as a reference. Third, normally considerable variation exists in results between instrument types and between laboratories. A guideline for acceptable variation on individual samples for these kinds of comparisons is up to 20% for HCT, WBC, and PLT values within the normal range. Most veterinarians are surprised to learn the expected degree of variation between laboratories and instruments. Without this perspective, they are misled when trying to interpret results from individual samples.

A more simple and reliable way to perform an evaluation is to start with a simple reproducibility test. This consists of repetitive analysis of a single sample 10 to 15 times on the instrument. The sample may be either freshly collected animal blood or control material with known values. The results are then placed in a table to facilitate evaluation of the variation. Calculation of the mean of observations and then identification of the minimum and maximum observed values are helpful. Some guidelines for interpretation of minimum and maximum observations are the following: WBC should reproduce as mean ± 10% or less, HCT should reproduce as mean ± 2.5 units or less, MCV should reproduce as mean ± 2 fl or less, and PLT should reproduce as mean ± 15% or less. If the instrument cannot reproduce results, it cannot be accurate. Accuracy is best assessed with the use of control material with documented known values. Meaningful assessment of accuracy using patient samples is probably beyond the scope of most veterinary hospital facilities.

Quantitative Buffy Coat System

The quantitative buffy coat system (QBC; Becton Dickinson, Franklin Lakes, NJ) uses differential centrifugation and estimation of cellular elements by measurements on an expanded buffy coat layer in a specialized microhematocrit tube. It provides a hematocrit value and estimates of leukocyte concentration and platelet concentration. It extrapolates tube volumes to an estimate of concentration based on fixed cell volumes. Partial differential count information is provided in the form of total granu-locytes and lymphocyte/monocytes categories. One limitation of these leukocyte groupings is that abnormalities such as left shift and lymphopenia may be undetected unless the blood film is examined as defined for the minimum CBC.

◆ Manual Procedures

Packed Cell Volume

The packed cell volume (PCV; also called *hematocrit*) is that percentage of whole blood composed of erythrocytes or RBCs. Whole blood is collected in an anticoagu-lant, such as EDTA or heparin, and placed in a capillary tube (75 mm). Microhemat-ocrit tubes should be filled about three fourths full, with one end plugged with clay sealant, placed in a centrifuge with the plugged end facing outward, and then cen-trifuged in a microhematocrit centrifuge for 2-5 minutes (see Figure 1-6). Of the blood cells, RBCs have the highest specific gravity and gravitate to the bottom of the tube, appearing as a dark red layer. The PCV is then measured with a hematocrit tube reader, many of which have a linear scale, so the amount of blood in the tube need not be exact. The bottom of the RBC layer should be at the zero line and the top of the plasma on the top line. The percentage can then be read as the line level with the top of the RBC layer.

A whitish gray layer just above the RBC layer is termed the *buffy coat* and consists of WBCs and platelets. The plasma is the clear to yellow fluid at the top. Plasma ob-tained by this method can be used to determine the plasma protein concentration by refractometry. Plasma color and transparency may be helpful in the determination of a diagnosis and should be recorded.

White Blood Cell Count

The manual Unopette hemacytometer method (Becton-Dickinson, Rutherford, NJ) of counting WBCs is appropriate for most veterinary hospital laboratories. Unopette WBC test kits contain diluting reservoirs and capillary pipettes for making a 1:100 di-lution of blood in ammonium oxalate or acetic acid, which lyse erythrocytes. Cells are counted using a hemacytometer and cover glass. An instruction sheet accompanies the kit.

Briefly, the appropriate amount of blood is added to the diluent, or lysing solution. After about 10 minutes, the reservoir is shaken to evenly mix the cells and is con-verted to a dropper assembly. The iris diaphragm of the microscope must be closed to a point where the cells are most visible. The hemacytometer and coverslip must be free of dust and grease. The hemacytometer, with coverslip applied, is loaded with the solution and placed on the microscope, and the counting grid is found, by using the 4× objective. Cells are counted in the nine primary squares, using the 10x objective (Figure 2-2).

The number of cells counted is multiplied by dilution and volume factors:

Figure 2-2
Nine primary squares of the hemacytometer are used for a Unopette total WBC count.

(Total cells counted + 10% of those counted) × Dilution factor of 100

Counts are expressed as cells per microliter (μl) of blood. For example, if 80 cells are counted:

80 + 8 = 88 × 100 = 8800/μl

Evaluation of Blood Films

Blood films are prepared by placing a small drop of blood on a clean glass microscope slide. The end of a second slide is placed against the surface of the first slide at a 30-degree angle and drawn back into the drop of blood (Figure 2-3). When the blood has spread along most of the width of the spreader slide, it is then pushed forward with a steady, even, rapid motion. A properly prepared blood film is thin, with even distribution of cells. After they air dry, the films should be stained with Wright's or Wright's-Giemsa stain. A particularly good method of Wright's staining has been described.[1] A quick stain that gives acceptable results is Diff-Quik (Dade Behring, Deerfield, IL).

The blood film is used to perform the differential WBC count, estimate platelet numbers, and evaluate morphology of WBCs, RBCs, and platelets. The blood film should be inspected under low-power magnification (10x) to note cell numbers and to scan the feathered edge (Figure 2-4) for platelet clumps, large abnormal cells, and microfilariae. The observer should then select a portion of the film near the thin end, referred to as the *counting area,* and switch to the oil-immersion objective (100x) to complete the evaluation.

Figure 2-3
Blood film preparation. The spreader slide has been drawn back into the drop of blood and the blood has spread along most of its width. The spreader slide will then be pushed rapidly to the right.

Figure 2-4
Gross and microscopic views of different areas on a blood film. The blood film on the glass slide at the top was made by pushing the blood from the drop (indicated *drop of blood*) at the right to the left (*large arrow*). The three major areas of the blood film (*feathered edge, count area, thick area*) are indicated by the lines connected to the respective microscopic views. The rectangular pattern on the glass slide indicates a recommended movement pattern for examining the slide under high magnification. The feathered edge (*left lower*) should be avoided because of artifacts. Erythrocyte central pallor is artifactually absent. Leukocytes may be broken (*arrow*). In the count area (*middle lower*), erythrocytes are present in a monolayer and have central pallor. Leukocytes are flattened so that intracellular detail is best, which makes this the optimal area for evaluation of erythrocyte abnormalities and identification of leukocytes. In the thick area (*right lower*), evaluation of erythrocyte morphology is impossible because the cells are extensively superimposed. Leukocytes are rounded and appear as dark spots, which makes identification difficult.

RED BLOOD CELLS

◆ Classification of Anemia

The function of RBCs, or erythrocytes, is to transport and protect hemoglobin, the oxygen-carrying pigment. Daily production of erythrocytes equals the daily loss from destruction of aged cells in a healthy animal. If RBC production is decreased or destruction and/or loss is increased, anemia results. *Anemia* is a condition with a reduced number of circulating RBCs, reduced PCV, or a reduced concentration of hemoglobin. Anemia may be classified according to bone marrow response, either regenerative or nonregenerative, or RBC size and hemoglobin concentration (MCV, mean corpuscular hemoglobin concentration [MCHC]).

Classification by Bone Marrow Response

This classification is most clinically applicable because it distinguishes between regenerative and nonregenerative anemias. In regenerative anemia, the bone marrow responds to anemia by increasing erythrocyte production and releasing immature erythrocytes. These immature RBCs; that is, polychromatophilic RBCs or *reticulocytes,* can be observed on the blood film and indicate that the marrow is responsive. The ability of bone marrow to respond indicates that the cause of the anemia is probably either blood loss (hemorrhage) or blood destruction (hemolysis). In nonregenerative anemia, the bone marrow is unable to respond to the anemic state, and reticulocytes are absent on blood films, suggesting bone marrow dysfunction. A bone marrow aspiration biopsy is then indicated (see Bone Marrow Evaluation, pp. 58-60), once common endocrine and metabolic causes of nonregenerative anemia are excluded.

Classification by RBC Size and Hemoglobin Concentration

Anemias may be classified as *normocytic* (RBCs of normal size), *macrocytic* (RBCs larger than normal), or *microcytic* (RBCs smaller than normal), depending on RBC size. Normocytic anemia is characterized by RBCs of normal size and is secondary to a variety of chronic disorders. In domestic animals, the most common cause of macrocytic anemia is the transitory increase in RBC size seen with regenerative anemia (reticulocytosis). In people, macrocytic anemia is frequently associated with vitamin B_{12} and folic acid deficiencies. These conditions are rarely, if ever, seen in domestic animals. Microcytic anemia is almost always the result of iron deficiency. Division of immature erythrocytes stops when a critical concentration of hemoglobin is reached. With inadequate iron for hemoglobin synthesis, extra division may occur, resulting in smaller erythrocytes. Although chronic blood loss is the most common cause of iron deficiency in adult animals, inadequate dietary iron results in iron-deficiency anemia in young nursing animals such as kittens and baby pigs.

Anemias may be hypochromic (reduced hemoglobin concentration) or normochromic (normal hemoglobin concentration). A hyperchromic state is not possible. Newly released polychromatophilic erythrocytes (*reticulocytes*) are hypochromic because the full concentration of hemoglobin is not yet attained. Macrocytic hypochromic anemia suggests regeneration. Iron deficiency also results in hypochromic anemia but is also characterized by microcytosis. Most other types of anemia are normochromic.

Erythrocyte Indices

Determination of erythrocyte indices is helpful in classification of certain anemias.

Mean Corpuscular Volume

The MCV is the mean volume for a group of erythrocytes. For many years, the MCV was calculated by dividing the PCV by the RBC concentration and multiplying by 10. The unit of volume is the femtoliter (fl), which is 10^{-15} liters.

MCV (in femtoliters) = PCV (%) × 10/RBC (millions/μl)

, For example, if a dog has a PCV of 42% and an RBC count of 6.0 million/μl, the MCV is 70 fl. Normal ranges for MCV vary among species (Table 2-1).

The size of the erythrocytes can now be determined electronically by automated systems (see Electronic Cell Counters). The PCV can then be calculated by multiplying the MCV by the erythrocyte concentration, which eliminates the need to determine the PCV by microcentrifugation.

Mean Corpuscular Hemoglobin

Mean corpuscular hemoglobin (MCH) is the mean weight of hemoglobin (Hb) contained in the average RBC. It is calculated by dividing the hemoglobin concentration by the RBC concentration and multiplying by 10.

MCH (in picograms) = Hb (g/dl) × 10/RBC (millions/μl)

Normal MCH values vary with the species (see Table 2-1).

Mean Corpuscular Hemoglobin Concentration

The mean corpuscular hemoglobin concentration (MCHC) is the concentration of hemoglobin in the average erythrocyte (or the ratio of weight of hemoglobin to the volume in which it is contained). The MCHC is calculated by dividing the hemoglobin concentration by the PCV and multiplying by 100.

MCHC (g/dl) = Hb (g/dl) × 100/PCV (%)

For example, if a dog has a hemoglobin concentration of 14 g/dl and a PCV of 42%, the MCHC is 33.3 g/dl. The normal range for MCHC is 30 to 36 g/dl for all mammals, with the exception of some sheep and all members of the family Camellidae (camels), which have MCHC values of 40 to 45 g/dl.

TABLE 2-1

Red blood cell characteristics in normal domestic animals

Species	Diameter	Rouleaux	Central Pallor	Anisocytosis	Basophilic Stippling in Regenerative Response	Reticulocytes (Normal PCV)	Poikilocytes	MCV (fl)	MCHC (g/dl)
Dogs	7.0	+	++++	−	−	±1.0%	−	60-77	32-36
Pigs	6.0	++	±±	±±	−	±1.0%	++++	50-68	30-34
Cats	5.8	++	++	±±	±±	±0.5%	−	39-55	30-36
Horses	5.7	++++	±±	−	−	0% (will not increase in response to anemia)	−	34-58	31-37
Cattle	5.5	−	+	++	+++	0% (will increase in response to anemia)	−	40-60	30-36
Sheep	4.5	±±	+	+	+++	0% (will increase)	−	23-48	31-38
Goats	3.2	−	−	−	++	0% (will increase)	++ (in young)	15-30	35-42

◆ Reticulocyte Count

A reticulocyte is an immature erythrocyte that contains organelles (ribosomes) that are lost as the cell matures (Plate 1). These organelles account for the diffuse blue-gray or polychromatophilic staining of immature cells with Wright's stain. When these immature cells are stained with new methylene blue or brilliant cresyl blue, the organelles clump into visible granules referred to as *reticulum.* This reticulum is present as aggregates or chains of blue granules. WBCs do not stain well with this type of stain.

Cats, unlike other species, have two morphologic forms of reticulocytes. The aggregate form contains large clumps of reticulum, is similar to reticulocytes in other species, and is the same cell that stains polychromatophilic with Wright's stain. The punctate form, unique to cats, contains two to eight small, singular, basophilic granules. These cells do not stain polychromatophilic with Wright's stain. In normal, nonanemic cats, about 0.4% of the RBCs are aggregate reticulocytes, whereas 1.5% to 10% of the RBCs are punctate reticulocytes. For a meaningful reticulocyte count in cats, only the aggregate form of reticulocyte should be counted.

A reticulocyte count is an expression of the percentage of RBCs that are reticulocytes. A reticulocyte count should be performed on the blood of all anemic domestic animals except horses, which do not release reticulocytes from the bone marrow, even in the face of regenerative anemia. Reticulocyte concentration is useful in assessing the bone marrow's response to anemia.

Blood is stained by placement of a few drops of blood and an equal number of drops of new methylene blue or brilliant cresyl blue stain in a small test tube. The mixture is allowed to stand for about 10 minutes. Tubes containing premeasured brilliant cresyl blue are commercially available (Curtin Matheson Scientific, Houston, TX). A drop of the mixture is then used to prepare a conventional air-dried blood film, which can then be examined or counterstained with Wright's stain. The percentage of reticulocytes per 1000 erythrocytes is determined.

Reticulocyte counts should be interpreted according to the degree of anemia, because fewer mature erythrocytes are present in anemic animals, and reticulocytes are released earlier and persist longer than in normal animals. Higher percentages may be seen in hemolytic than in hemorrhagic types of anemia. Although reticulocytes are often reported as a percentage, a more useful method is to multiply the percentage by the erythrocyte count, to give reticulocytes/microliter. Guidelines for reticulocyte interpretation are listed in Table 2-2.

If an erythrocyte count has not been performed, reticulocyte counts may be reported as a percentage. Reticulocyte counts can be corrected for the degree of anemia as follows:

Corrected reticulocyte % = Observed reticulocyte % × Patient's PCV/Normal mean PCV

For example, if a dog has a PCV of 15% and an observed reticulocyte count of 15%, the corrected reticulocyte count equals:

15% × 15%/45% = 5%

TABLE 2-2

Interpretation of absolute reticulocyte counts in dogs, cats, and ruminants

	Normal	Nonregenerative Anemia	Moderate Regeneration	Maximum Regeneration
Dogs, cats	>60,000/μl	<60,000/μl	100,000-200,000/μl	Up to 500,000/μl
Ruminants	0	0	±100,000/μl	±300,000/μl

Typical reticulocyte responses for dogs (given as percentage) are as follows:

Normal	Mild regenerative response	Moderate regenerative response	Marked regenerative response
<1%	1% to 8%	9% to 15%	>15%

◆ Erythrocyte Morphology

Normal erythrocyte morphology (Plate 2) varies among different species of domestic animals (see Table 2-1). Morphology of erythrocytes can be categorized according to cell arrangement on the blood film, size, color, shape, and presence of structures in or on erythrocytes.

Cell Arrangement

Rouleaux formation is a grouping of erythrocytes in stacks (Figure 2-5 and Plate 3). Increased rouleaux formation is seen with increased fibrinogen or globulin concentrations. Marked rouleaux formation is seen in healthy horses.

Agglutination of erythrocytes should be distinguished from rouleaux formation (see Figure 2-5 and Plate 4). Agglutination occurs in immune-mediated disorders, in which antibody coats the erythrocyte, resulting in bridging and clumping of RBCs. It is sometimes observed macroscopically and microscopically.

Size

Anisocytosis is a variation in the size of RBCs (Plates 5 and 6) and may be due to the presence of macrocytes (large cells) or microcytes (small cells) or both.

Macrocytes are RBCs that are larger than normal, with an increased MCV. Macrocytes are usually young, polychromatophilic erythrocytes (reticulocytes) (Plate 6).

Microcytes are RBCs with a diameter less than that of normal erythrocytes, with a decreased MCV. Microcytic cells may be seen with iron deficiency (Plate 7).

Color

Polychromasia or polychromatophilic erythrocytes are RBCs exhibiting a bluish tint when stained with Romanowsky (Wright's-type) stain (Plates 6 and 7). The blue tint

Rouleaux formation   Agglutination

Figure 2-5
Drawing depicting rouleaux formation and agglutination.

is due to organelles remaining within the cytoplasm; therefore these are young cells. This is the same cell that, when stained with new methylene blue, or brilliant cresyl blue, appears as a reticulocyte.

Hypochromia is a decreased staining intensity caused by insufficient hemoglobin within the cell (Plate 7). Iron deficiency is the most common cause, although macrocytic erythrocytes often appear hypochromic because of their large diameter. Hypochromic cells should be distinguished from bowl-shaped or "punched-out" cells, which are insignificant. Animals with true hypochromia almost always have microcytosis, as determined by a decreased MCV. Normochromia is a normal staining intensity.

Shape

Abnormally shaped erythrocytes are called *poikilocytes.* This terminology is not helpful because it does not suggest a specific diagnosis. Shape and color changes (Figure 2-6) are considered important when they are frequently associated with specific disorders.

Spiculated cells are erythrocytes with one or more surface spicules. This general term includes schistocytes, keratocytes, acanthocytes, and echinocytes. Specificity is recommended in descriptions of shape changes because certain types of spiculated cells have been associated with certain diseases.

Schistocytes (Plates 1 and 8), which are RBC fragments, are usually formed as a result of shearing of the red cell by intravascular trauma. Schistocytes may be observed with disseminated intravascular coagulopathy (DIC) when erythrocytes are broken by fibrin strands, with vascular neoplasms (e.g., hemangiosarcoma), and with iron deficiency. Animals with DIC usually have concurrent thrombocytopenia. In dogs with hemangiosarcoma, usually acanthocytes and fragments are present (see Figure 2-6 and Plate 9). In iron-deficiency anemia, the fragmentation is apparently the result of oxidative injury, leading to membrane lesions or increased susceptibility to intravascular trauma. Initially the RBC develops what appears to be a blister or vacuole (Plates 7 and

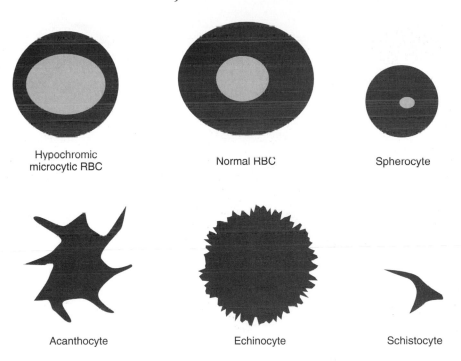

Figure 2-6
Erythrocyte shape and color abnormalities that may be helpful in diagnosis.

10), which is thought to represent an oxidative injury occurring when inner membrane surfaces are cross linked across the cell. Exclusion of hemoglobin may account for the colorless area. These lesions subsequently enlarge and break open to form "apple-stem cells" (Plates 7 and 10) and keratocytes (Plate 10), which are spiculated red cells with two or more pointed projections. The projections from the keratocytes probably then fragment from the cell (Plates 8 and 10). This process is depicted in Figure 2-7.

Acanthocytes or spur cells are irregular, spiculated red cells with a few, unevenly distributed surface projections of variable length and diameter (Plates 6 and 11). They are thought to result from changes in cholesterol concentration at the red cell membrane. They are seen in patients with altered lipid metabolism, such as may occur in cats with hepatic lipidosis and, occasionally, in dogs with liver disease. They are seen quite consistently in dogs with hemangiosarcoma of the liver. The presence of acanthocytes in middle-age to old large-breed dogs with concurrent regenerative anemia is suggestive of hemangiosarcoma.

Echinocytes (burr cells) are spiculated cells with numerous short, evenly spaced, blunt to sharp surface projections of uniform size and shape. Echinocyte formation can be an artifactual, in vitro process associated with pH change from slow drying of blood films; it is then termed *crenation*. Echinocytes have also been associated with renal disease and lymphosarcoma in dogs, after exercise in horses, and with rattlesnake envenomization in dogs (Plate 12).

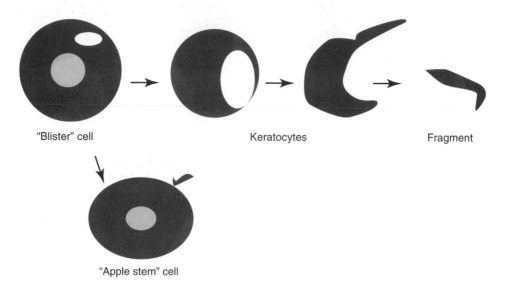

"Blister" cell   Keratocytes   Fragment

"Apple stem" cell

Figure 2-7
Keratocyte formation and fragmentation in RBCs from patients with iron-deficiency anemia.

Spherocytes are darkly staining red cells with reduced or no central pallor (Plates 5 and 13). Spherocytes with a small amount of central pallor are referred to as "imperfect spheres." Spherocytes are not easily detected in species other than dogs. They have a reduced amount of membrane as a result of partial phagocytosis by macrophages, which occurs because of antibody and/or complement on the surface of the RBC. Spherocytes are significant in that they suggest immune-mediated destruction of red blood cells, resulting in hemolytic anemia. They also may be seen after transfusion with mismatched blood. Immune-mediated hemolytic anemia (IMHA) is usually a regenerative anemia, with marked polychromasia and high reticulocyte count. However, in some instances, the anemia is nonregenerative as a result of antibodies against RBC precursors within the bone marrow. In these cases, spherocytes are often difficult to detect because the presence of large polychromatophilic cells facilitates recognition of the small spherocytes. Although spherocytes have a decreased diameter and appear small, their volume is normal, and dogs with IMHA do not have decreased MCV.

Other abnormally shaped erythrocytes, such as leptocytes and bowl-shaped cells, are less important because they are not associated with specific disorders. Other abnormalities, such as stomatocytes, are seen in dogs with rare, inherited disorders (Plate 14).

Leptocytes are thin erythrocytes with increased membrane or decreased volume. Because of this, the cell membrane can fold or become distorted. Leptocytes have a tendency to accumulate in the lower portion of the buffy coat at centrifugation. The most common forms of leptocytes are target cells and folded cells (Figure 2-8 and Plate 11). Target cells are RBCs with a central, rounded area of hemoglobin, sur-

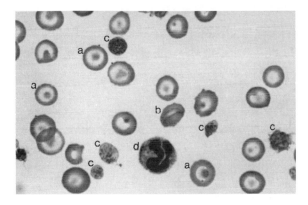

Figure 2-8
Numerous target cells (*a*) and a folded cell (*b*) on a blood film from a dog. *c*, platelets; *d*, neutrophil.

rounded by a clear zone, with a dense ring of hemoglobin around the periphery. Folded cells have a transverse, raised fold extending across the center of the cell. Leptocytes are common in patients with nonregenerative anemia.

Inclusions

Basophilic stippling, the presence of small, dark-blue bodies within the erythrocyte, is observed in Wright's-stained cells containing residual RNA. It is common in immature RBCs of ruminants and occasionally in cats during a response to anemia and is usually characteristic of lead poisoning when seen in dogs (Plate 15).

Howell-Jolly bodies are basophilic nuclear remnants seen in young erythrocytes during the response to anemia (Plate 13). As cells containing nuclear remnants pass through the spleen, phagocytic cells remove the remnants. Consequently, increased numbers may be seen after removal of the spleen or with splenic disorders.

Nucleated erythrocytes represent early release of immature cells during anemia but also may be observed in nonanemic animals (Plate 13). An increase in nucleated RBCs out of proportion to the degree of anemia is sometimes caused by lead poisoning. All red blood cells of nonmammalians, such as birds and reptiles, contain nuclei (Plate 16).

Heinz bodies are round structures representing denatured hemoglobin, caused by certain oxidant drugs or chemicals. The denatured hemoglobin becomes attached to the cell membrane and appears as a pale area with Wright's stain (Plate 17). When stained with new methylene blue (same technique used for reticulocytes), the Heinz bodies appear blue (Plate 18). In dogs, they are 1 to 2 μ in diameter. Unlike other domestic animals, normal cats have Heinz bodies in as many as 5% of their RBCs, and Heinz bodies are often increased in concentration with diseases such as lymphosarcoma, hyperthyroidism, and diabetes mellitus in cats.

◆ Blood Parasites

Parasites may be present in or on erythrocytes. Stain precipitate and drying artifacts are sometimes confused with red cell parasites. Drying artifact usually appears refractile (Plate 19).

Hemobartonella Felis

Hemobartonella felis is a fairly common parasite of feline erythrocytes. The disease is referred to as *hemobartonellosis*, or feline infectious anemia. The organisms appear as small (0.2 to 0.5 μ), coccoid, rod-shaped, or ring-like structures that stain dark purple with Wright's stain (Plate 20). They most frequently appear as short rods on the periphery of RBCs. The parasitemia is cyclic; if hemobartonellosis is suspected, the blood should be examined several times before the infection is ruled out. Once antibiotics are given, the parasite disappears rapidly.

Hemobartonella Canis

Hemobartonellosis is rare in dogs and usually is only observed in splenectomized or immunosuppressed dogs. The organism most commonly appears as a chain of small cocci or rods that stretch across the surface of the erythrocyte (Plate 21). The chains may appear to branch.

Eperythrozoonosis in swine, cattle, and llamas is quite similar to hemobartonellosis; the organisms are closely related. Eperythrozoa appear as small (0.8 to 1.0 μ) cocci, rods, or rings on the RBC surface or free in the plasma. The ring form is most common (Plate 22).

Anaplasma Marginale

This intracellular blood parasite causes anaplasmosis in cattle and wild ruminants. It appears as small, dark-staining cocci at the margin of RBCs (Figure 2-9) and must be differentiated from Howell-Jolly bodies because their sizes are similar. Early in the course of the disease as many as 50% of RBCs may contain parasites. By the time the anemia is severe, usually less than 5% of RBCs are affected.

Cytauxzoon Felis

This is a rare cause of hemolytic anemia in cats. The organism appears as small (1.0 to 2.0 μ), irregular ring forms within erythrocytes, lymphocytes, and macrophages (Figure 2-10).

Babesia Species

Babesiosis of cattle is caused by *Babesia bigemina* and *Babesia bovis.* The disease is also called *Texas fever, redwater fever,* and *cattle tick fever. Babesia* spp. appear as large (3 to 4 μ), pleomorphic, teardrop-shape intracellular organisms, frequently seen

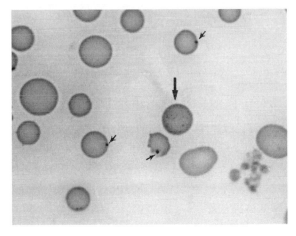

Figure 2-9
Anaplasma marginale (*small arrows*) in blood from a cow. Note the anisocytosis and basophilic stippling (*large arrow*). (1400×)

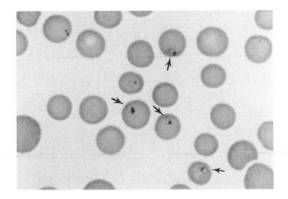

Figure 2-10
Cytauxzoon felis (*arrows*) in blood from an experimentally infected cat. (1400×)

in pairs. Babesiosis in horses (piroplasmosis) is caused by *Babesia equi* and *Babesia caballi,* which are similar to *B. bigemina.* Babesiosis is rare in horses, and the few cases reported in the United States have been seen in the South, especially Florida. Babesiosis in dogs is caused by *Babesia canis* and *Babesia gibsoni.* They are also similar to *B. bigemina,* but *B. gibsoni* is slightly smaller and appears as rings. Only a small percentage of erythrocytes may be affected. The organisms are more commonly observed in RBCs at the feathered edge.

Ehrlichia Species

Ehrlichiosis of dogs (tropical pancytopenia) is caused by *Ehrlichia canis,* an intracellular parasite of monocytes and neutrophils (Plate 23). It is transmitted by the

Figure 2-11
Ehrlichia spp. *(arrows)* in the neutrophils of a horse. (1400×)

brown dog tick. The organism appears as small clusters, called *morulae* (3 to 6 μ), in the cytoplasm (Figure 2-11). The disease may result in neutropenia, thrombocytopenia, and anemia. Chronically affected animals may be severely anemic, with marked leukopenia and thrombocytopenia, but sometimes the only hematologic abnormality is lymphocytosis. The total plasma protein level usually is increased. The organisms are best demonstrated during the acute phase but usually are present in small numbers. Films made from the buffy coat (where monocytes are concentrated) may aid diagnosis. However, in most cases organisms are not seen and the diagnosis is made by serologic testing.

WHITE BLOOD CELLS

Mature and immature neutrophils, lymphocytes, monocytes, eosinophils, and basophils make up the leukocytes (WBCs) found in blood. Each type of cell plays an important role in the body's defense system, and the total concentration of each type is extremely valuable in the diagnosis of various diseases.

◆ Definitions

The following are some definitions of hematologic terms used in this section:
> *-penia:* Decreased number of cells in the blood. For example, *neutropenia* refers to decreased numbers of neutrophils in the blood. *Lymphopenia* describes decreased numbers of lymphocytes in the blood.

Figure 2-12
Various types of counters used for manual cell counts. (Courtesy Becton-Dickinson, Franklin Lobes, NJ.)

-philia or *-cytosis:* Increased number of cells in the blood. For example, *neutrophilia* refers to increased numbers of neutrophils in the blood. *Leukocytosis* refers to increased numbers of leukocytes in the blood.

Left shift: Increased numbers of immature neutrophils in the blood.

Leukemia: Neoplastic cells in the blood or bone marrow. Leukemias are often described as leukemic, subleukemic, or aleukemic, indicating the variation in the tendency for neoplastic cells to be released in the blood.

Leukemoid response: Condition that can be mistaken for leukemia. It is characterized by marked leukocytosis (more than 50,000/μl) and is usually the result of inflammatory disease.

Lymphoproliferative disorders: Conditions in which lymphocytes or plasma cells proliferate abnormally.

Myeloproliferative disorders: A group of bone marrow disorders, usually neoplastic, characterized by proliferation of one, several, or all of the bone marrow cell lines.

◆ Differential White Blood Cell Counts

After examination of the blood film with the 10× objective (see Evaluation of Blood Films), the 100× (oil-immersion) objective is used to count and classify at least 100 nucleated WBCs in the counting area, using a commercially available differential cell counter to keep a running tally of cell types (Figure 2-12). The cells should be counted in the area near, but not on, the feathered edge, where the erythrocytes do not overlap. Broken, "smudged" cells (Plate 24) should be ignored. The quantities of all cell types are then expressed as percentages of the total 100-cell count. The absolute number of each type of cell counted is then obtained by multiplying the percentile fraction by the total WBC count.

Differential WBC counts should always be expressed in absolute numbers to be diagnostically useful. Percentages are not useful for interpretive purposes. For example, a cat has a total leukocyte count of 3000/μl, with 300 (10%) neutrophils and 2700 (90%) lymphocytes. A second cat has a total count of 40,000/μl, with 4000 (10%) neutrophils and 36,000 (90%) lymphocytes. Although the percentages of cells are the same in both cats, the absolute numbers of cells are different. The first cat has neutropenia, with a normal lymphocyte count. The second cat has extreme lymphocytosis, suggesting lymphoid leukemia, with a normal neutrophil count.

Nucleated RBCs (NRBCs) are included in the total WBC count performed on hemacytometers and electronic cell counters. When performing a differential cell count, NRBCs may be counted separately and reported as NRBCs/100 WBCs. The number of NRBCs encountered while counting 100 WBCs is incorporated into the following equation to calculate a corrected leukocyte count[3]:

Corrected WBC count = Observed WBC count × 100/100 + % Nucleated RBCs

An alternative and much more practical method is to include the NRBCs within the 100-cell differential count.[1] For example, an animal has a total WBC count of 10,000/μl, with 5000 (50%) neutrophils, 3000 (30%) lymphocytes, 1000 (10%) monocytes, and 1000 (10%) NRBCs. The corrected WBC count can then be calculated by subtracting the absolute number of NRBCs (1000/μl) from the total WBC count (10,000/μl), giving a corrected total WBC count of 9000/μl (10,000 − 1000 = 9000).

◆ Appearance of Leukocytes in Peripheral Blood

Neutrophil

The nucleus of neutrophils is irregular and elongated; true filaments between nuclear lobes are rare (Plates 2, 8, 13, and 25). The nucleus of equine neutrophils has heavily clumped, coarse chromatin. The cytoplasm stains pale pink, with fine, diffuse granules. Bovine neutrophils have darker-pink cytoplasm. Toxic neutrophils have blue cytoplasm and may contain Döhle bodies, which are small (0.5 to 2 μ), angular, blue-gray granules (Plate 26 and Figure 2-13). Other changes with toxicity include vacuoles in the cytoplasm and increased size. The toxic appearance of neutrophils should be recorded because it signifies rapid replication and may be seen in association with infections.

Band Neutrophil

The nucleus of band neutrophils is horseshoe shaped, with large round ends (Plate 27). Although slight indentations may be present in the nucleus, if the constriction is greater than one third the width of the nucleus, the cell is usually classified as a *seg-*

Plate 1
Numerous reticulocytes in blood from a dog with regenerative anemia. Representative reticulocyte *(arrow)*. *N*, neutrophil. (Brilliant cresyl blue stain.)

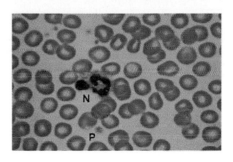

Plate 2
Blood film from a normal dog. Central pallor is evident in the erythrocytes. *N*, neutrophil. *P*, platelet. (Wright's stain.)

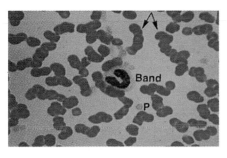

Plate 3
Blood film from a horse. Rouleaux formations are indicated *(arrows)* and a band neutrophil. *P*, platelet. (Wright's stain.)

Plate 4
Low-power magnification of blood film from a dog with erythrocyte agglutination *(arrows)*. (Wright's stain.)

Plate 5
Anisocytosis on a blood film from a dog with immune-mediated hemolytic anemia. The small cells are spherocytes *(short arrow)*. Agglutination is indicated *(long arrow)*. (Wright's stain.)

Plate 6
Large (macrocytic) polychromatophilic erythrocytes *(long arrows)* on a blood film from a dog with regenerative anemia resulting from a bleeding intraabdominal hemangiosarcoma. An acanthocyte is indicated *(short arrow)*. (Wright's stain.)

Plate 7

Microcytic hypochromic erythrocytes on a blood film from a dog with iron-deficiency anemia from blood loss. Blister formation *(short arrow)* and "apple stem" formation *(arrowhead)* are common. A large platelet *(long arrow)* is indicated. (Wright's stain.)

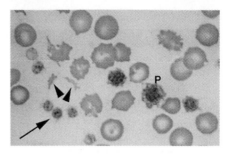

Plate 8

Blood film from a dog with iron-deficiency anemia. Red cell fragments (schistocytes) *(arrowheads)* and normal platelets *(arrow)* are indicated. *P,* giant platelet. (Wright's stain.)

Plate 9

Red cell fragment *(long arrow)* and acanthocytes *(short arrow)* on a blood film from a dog with hemangiosarcoma of the liver and spleen. *P,* platelet; *M,* metarubricyte; *N,* neutrophil. (Wright's stain.)

Plate 10

Blood film from a cat with iron-deficiency anemia resulting from chronic gastrointestinal blood loss. Numerous blister cells *(short arrows)*, a keratocyte *(long arrow)*, and fragments *(arrowheads)* are typical membrane changes. (Wright's stain.)

Plate 11

Acanthocytes *(long arrow)*, target cells *(short arrows)*, and folded cells *(arrowhead)* in a blood film from a dog with hemangiosarcoma. (Wright's stain.)

Plate 12

Many echinocytes *(arrow)* on a blood film from a dog bitten by a rattlesnake. Polychromatophilic erythrocytes *(arrowhead)* do not become echinocytic. (Wright's stain.)

Plate 13
Numerous spherocytes on a blood film from a dog with immune-mediated hemolytic anemia. Several large poly-chromatophilic red cells are present, indicating the anemia is regenerative. *Arrow,* Howell-Jolly body; *M,* meta-rubricytes; *N,* neutrophil; *L,* lympho-cyte. (Wright's stain.)

Plate 14
Stomatocytes *(arrow)* on a blood film from a Schnauzer with inherited stom-atocytosis. *P,* platelet. (Wright's stain.)

Plate 15
Basophilic stippling *(arrow)* on a blood film from a dog with lead poisoning. (Wright's stain.)

Plate 16
Nucleated erythrocytes *(arrow)* on a blood film from a reptile. Reptiles, like birds, have heterophils *(H)* with eo-sinophilic granules, rather than neu-trophils. (Wright's stain.)

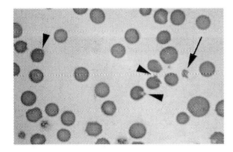

Plate 17
Heinz bodies *(arrowheads)* and frag-ment *(arrow)* on a blood film from a cat with diabetes mellitus. (Wright's stain.)

Plate 18
Many Heinz bodies *(arrow)* on a blood film from the cat mentioned in Plate 17. Heinz bodies are more easily seen with this new methylene blue stain. *Ar-rowhead,* reticulocyte.

Plate 19
Drying artifacts appear as dots *(arrow)* and ring forms *(arrowhead)*. These artifacts can be distinguished from red cell parasites by their refractile, amorphous appearance. (Wright's stain.)

Plate 20
Hemobartonella felis organisms *(arrow)* on the periphery of red cells. Ring forms *(arrowhead)* can be easily visualized because the erythrocyte is lysed. (Wright's stain.)

Plate 21
Hemobartonella canis organisms *(arrow)* appear as chains of cocci across the surface of red blood cells. *Arrowhead,* polychromatophilic erythrocyte. (Wright's stain.)

Plate 22
Eperythrozoon in a blood film from a llama. Numerous organisms *(arrowhead)* are present on the surface of all red cells (high magnification, *inset* in upper right corner) and are free in the plasma, as indicated by their presence between erythrocytes *(arrow)*. (Wright's stain.)

Plate 23
Babesia canis organisms *(arrows)* in erythrocytes on the feathered edge of a blood film from a dog. (Wright's stain.)

Plate 24
Broken nuclei, often termed "smudge cells" *(arrows)*, should be ignored during performance of differential white cell counts. (Wright's stain.)

Plate 25
Blood film from a dog with normal neutrophils *(N)* and monocytes *(M)*. Many of the red blood cells are acanthocytic and fragmented. (Wright's stain.)

Plate 26
Blood film from an ill cat with numerous toxic neutrophils and bands, as evidenced by Döhle bodies *(arrow)*, "foamy" cytoplasm *(arrowhead)*, and basophilic cytoplasm. (Wright's stain.)

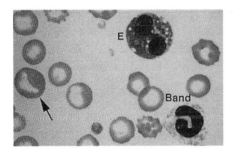

Plate 27
Normal band neutrophil and eosinophil *(E)* from a dog with regenerative anemia, as evidenced by polychromatophilic erythrocytes *(arrow)*. (Wright's stain.)

Plate 28
Metamyelocytes on a blood film from a dog with regenerative anemia, as evidenced by polychromatophilic erythrocytes *(arrow)*. Numerous imperfect spherocytes are also present, suggesting immune-mediated hemolytic anemia. (Wright's stain.)

Plate 29
Normal bovine blood film. Large lymphocyte with nucleolar rings *(arrow)*. (Wright's stain.)

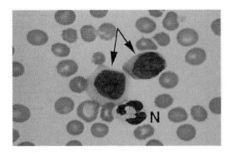

Plate 30
Lymphoblasts *(arrow)* with pale-staining nucleoli within the nuclei. This blood film is from a dog with lymphoblastic leukemia. *N,* neutrophil. (Wright's stain.)

Plate 31
Canine *(C)*, feline *(F)*, equine *(E)*, and bovine *(B)* eosinophils showing varied color and shape of the granules. (Wright's stain.)

Plate 32
Normal basophil *(B)* and platelets *(P)* on a blood film from a dog. Many of the erythrocytes are echinocytes. (Wright's stain.)

Plate 33
Normal feline basophils *(B)*. One basophil *(arrow)* contains darkly staining granules, which are not commonly observed in cats. *E,* eosinophil; *N,* neutrophil. (Wright's stain.)

Plate 34
Large granular lymphocyte *(arrow)* on a blood film from a dog with chronic ehrlichiosis. (Wright's stain.)

Plate 35
Reactive lymphocyte from a cat with hepatic lipidosis. Numerous acanthocytes are present. (Wright's stain.)

Plate 36
Nuclear hyposegmentation in neutrophils *(N)* and eosinophils *(E)* from a dog with Pelger-Huët anomaly. (Wright's stain.)

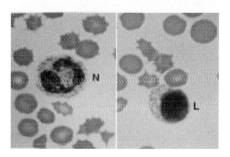

Plate 37
One normal and one vacuolated *(arrow)* lymphocyte from a cat with type A Niemann-Pick disease, an inherited lysosomal storage disorder. (Wright's stain.)

Plate 38
Neutrophil *(N)* and lymphocyte *(L)* that contain granules on a blood film from a cat with GM$_2$ gangliosidosis, a lysosomal storage disease. Numerous erythrocytes are acanthocytic, likely related to the associated liver disease. (Wright's stain.)

Plate 39
Blood film from a cat with mucopolysaccharidosis VI, a lysosomal storage disease. Lymphocytes contain vacuoles and granules *(arrowhead)*. Neutrophils *(arrow)* contain granules (Alder-Reilly bodies). (Wright's stain.)

Plate 40
Blood film from a cat with Chédiak-Higashi syndrome. Fused lysosomes appear as pink granules *(large arrows)* in the cytoplasm of neutrophils. Döhle body *(small arrow)* is indicated. (Wright's stain.)

Plate 41
Large masses or clumps of platelets on a blood film from a horse. (Wright's stain.)

Plate 42
Bone marrow aspirate from a normal dog. Granulocytic cells *(G)* can be differentiated from erythroid cells *(E)* based on nuclear and cytoplasmic characteristics. *L,* lymphocyte. (Wright's stain.)

Plate 43
Bone marrow aspirate from a cat. Primary granules within granulocytic precursors are evident *(arrow)*. All cells are granulocytic except one rubricyte *(E)*. (Wright's stain.)

Plate 44
Bone marrow aspirate from a normal dog. A megakaryocyte *(arrows)* is indicated. (Wright's stain.)

Plate 45
Bone marrow aspirate from a normal dog. A plasma cell *(arrow)* is indicated. Rubricytes *(arrowheads)* have nuclei similar to those of plasma cells but have less cytoplasm. The remaining cells are granulocytic precursors. (Wright's stain.)

Plate 46
Bone marrow aspirate from a cat with erythremic myelosis. Undifferentiated cells have cytoplasmic projections *(arrow)*. Numerous cells are in mitosis *(arrowheads)*. (Wright's stain.)

Plate 47
Blood film from a cat with erythremic myelosis (bone marrow is shown in Plate 46). Two rubriblasts *(arrows)* and a cytoplasmic fragment *(arrowhead)* are indicated. *M*, megakaryocyte. (Wright's stain.)

Plate 48
Bone marrow aspirate from a dog with late-stage lymphoblastic leukemia. Note the almost complete absence of granulocytic and erythroid precursors. Numerous lymphoid cells contain cytoplasmic granules. *N*, neutrophil. (Wright's stain.)

Figure 2-13
Döhle bodies (*arrows*) in toxic neutrophils in blood from a cat with pyothorax.

mented neutrophil. More immature neutrophils (myelocytes, metamyelocytes) are rare in peripheral blood (Plate 28).

Lymphocyte

Small lymphocytes are about 7 to 9 μ in diameter and have a slightly indented nucleus (Plate 13). The chromatin is coarsely clumped, and the cytoplasm is light blue and quite scanty. Chromocenters, areas of condensed chromatin, should not be confused with nucleoli; chromocenters appear as dark clumps within the nucleus. Medium-size to large lymphocytes are 9 to 11 μ in diameter, with more abundant cytoplasm. The cytoplasm may contain pink-purple granules. Normal bovine lymphocytes may contain nucleolar rings and may be large and difficult to distinguish from neoplastic lymphoid cells (Plate 29).

Lymphoblast

Lymphoblasts are immature lymphoid cells that contain a nucleolus within the nucleus (Plate 30). The nucleolus is a light-blue structure, often surrounded by a ring of chromatin. Lymphoblasts may be observed rarely in the blood of healthy animals. Their presence should be recorded because increased numbers suggest a lymphoproliferative disorder.

Monocyte

Monocytes are large cells that contain variably shaped nuclei (Plate 25). The nucleus is occasionally the shape of a kidney bean but is often elongated and lobulated. The nuclear chromatin is more diffuse in monocytes than in neutrophils, in which it is coarsely clumped. The cytoplasm of monocytes is blue-gray and may contain vacuoles and/or small, fine, pink granules. Monocytes may be difficult to distinguish from band neutrophils or metamyelocytes that are toxic. If a left shift is not present, the cells in question are probably monocytes.

Eosinophil

Eosinophils contain a nucleus similar to that of neutrophils, but the chromatin is usually not as coarsely clumped. The shape of the eosinophilic granules varies considerably among species (Plate 31). The granules in canine eosinophils often vary, with small and large granules within the same cell, and stain less intensely than those of other species; they usually are hemoglobin colored (Plates 27 and 31). Feline eosinophils contain granules that are small, rod shaped, and numerous. The rod shape of the granules is more easily observed in broken than in intact eosinophils. Equine eosinophil granules are large and round to oval, staining an intense orange-red. Eosinophil granules in cattle, sheep, and pigs are round and much smaller than those in horses. They are uniform in size and stain an intense pink.

Basophil

The nucleus of basophils is similar to that of monocytes. Basophil granules in dogs are few in number and stain purple to blue-black (Plate 32). Equine and bovine basophil granules are usually more numerous and may completely pack the cytoplasm. Feline basophil granules are round, stain light lavender (Plate 33) and rarely contain dark granules.

Although morphologic abnormalities of leukocytes are sometimes diagnostically useful, quantitative data obtained from the CBC are usually more helpful. A brief description of some acquired and inherited leukocyte morphologic abnormalities follows.

◆ Acquired Morphologic Abnormalities

Nuclear Hyposegmentation

Such hyposegmentation usually simply reflects early release of band neutrophils. Pseudo–Pelger-Huët anomaly has been reported and is either a variant on a normal inflammatory response or may be due to an idiosyncratic drug reaction. In general, in pseudo–Pelger-Huët anomaly, fewer neutrophils are hyposegmented than in the congenital anomaly.

Nuclear Hypersegmentation

Canine and feline neutrophils with five or more lobes are considered hypersegmented. This is usually due to aging of neutrophils, either *in vivo,* as would be seen with endogenous or exogenous glucocorticoids, which prolong the half-life of circulating neutrophils, or *in vitro,* as a result of prolonged storage of blood before making blood films. Hypersegmented neutrophils also are seen in blood films from Poodles with Poodle macrocytosis.

Toxic Change

The most common disease-induced cytoplasmic changes in neutrophils are referred to as *toxic changes* and are associated with conditions such as inflammation, infection, and drug toxicity. These changes are more significant when they occur in dogs; if severe they often suggest bacterial infection. However, toxic changes are seen quite commonly in cats that are not severely ill. Types of toxic change include cytoplasmic basophilia, Döhle bodies, vacuoles, or "foaminess" (Plate 26), and, rarely, intensely stained primary granules (toxic granulation). These "toxic" changes are thought to be due to decreased time of neutrophil maturation within the marrow.

Intracytoplasmic Neutrophil Inclusions in Infectious Diseases

Canine distemper inclusions may appear in RBCs and are pale blue to magenta. Rickettsial inclusions (*Ehrlichia* species) are rarely seen within the cytoplasm of neutrophils (see Figure 2-11), as are the gametocytes of *Hepatozoon canis*.

"Atypical" Lymphocytes

Azurophilic granules in the cytoplasm of lymphocytes (Plate 34) are often associated with chronic antigenic stimulation, especially in canine ehrlichiosis. "Reactive" lymphocytes (Plate 35) have increased basophilia in the cytoplasm, may have more abundant cytoplasm, and sometimes contain a larger, more convoluted nucleus. These changes are usually due to antigenic stimulation secondary to vaccination or infection.

◆ Inherited Morphologic Abnormalities

Pelger-Huët Anomaly

Most of the neutrophils and eosinophils in heterozygotes for Pelger-Huët anomaly have hyposegmented nuclei. Cells have an immature-shaped nucleus (band or myelocyte form) but a coarse, mature chromatin pattern (Plate 36). Neutrophils function normally and affected animals are healthy.

Lysosomal Storage Disorders

In this group of rare inherited diseases, a substance is abnormally stored within cells, usually because of an intracellular enzyme deficiency. Numerous types have been reported in animals. Clinical signs vary, depending on the specific enzyme deficiency. Most types have either skeletal abnormalities or progressive neurologic disease. Because most cells of the body are affected, the stored substance often may be seen in leukocytes, usually monocytes, lymphocytes, or neutrophils. The appearance of the

TABLE 2-3

Lysosomal storage disorders and associated changes

Disorder	Species	Vacuolated Lymphocytes	Granulated Neutrophils
Mucopolysaccharidosis I	Dog, cat	+	±
Mucopolysaccharidosis VI	Dog, cat	+	+++
Mucopolysaccharidosis VII	Dog, cat	+	+++
Niemann-Pick, type A	Cat	+++	−
Niemann-Pick, type C	Cat	+	−
GM$_1$ gangliosidosis	Cat	++	−
GM$_2$ gangliosidosis	Dog, cat, pig	+	+++
Fucosidosis	Dog	+	−
α-Mannosidosis	Cat	++	−
Acid lipase deficiency	Cat	++	−

leukocytes varies, depending on the type of lysosomal storage disease. Lymphocytes may be vacuolated (Plate 37) or contain granules (Plate 38) and/or neutrophils may contain granules (Plates 38 and 39). Examples of these disorders and the accompanying leukocyte abnormality are provided in Table 2-3.

Birman Cat Neutrophil Granulation Anomaly

Neutrophils from affected cats contain fine eosinophilic to magenta granules. This anomaly is inherited as an autosomal recessive trait. Neutrophil function is normal and affected cats are healthy. This granulation must be distinguished from toxic granulation and the granulation seen in neutrophils of cats with mucopolysaccharidosis and GM$_2$ gangliosidosis, two of the lysosomal storage disorders.

Chédiak-Higashi Syndrome

Neutrophils in cats with Chédiak-Higashi syndrome have large, fused 0.5 to 2 μ lysosomes within the cytoplasm and stain lightly pink or eosinophilic (Plate 40). Approximately one in three or four neutrophils contains fused lysosomes. Granules of eosinophils appear slightly plump and large. These cats have a slight tendency to bleed because platelet function is abnormal. Although neutrophil function is also abnormal, affected cats are generally healthy.

PLATELETS

◆ Platelet Count

Platelets (thrombocytes) are a very important component of hemostasis. The best procedure for platelet evaluation is examination of the blood film. When platelet numbers appear decreased, detrmining platelet concentration by a more quantitative procedure is appropriate. This measurement should be performed in a commercial laboratory because the expertise required to manually count platelets is difficult to develop and maintain. Hemacytometer and electronic methods are used to count platelets.

Most domestic animals have increased bleeding if the platelet count drops below 20,000 50,000/μl. Platelet numbers should be evaluated in the counting area of the blood film (see Figure 2-4). The size of the oil-immersion field depends on the type of microscope used. With the use of older microscopes, an average of three to five or more platelets per oil-immersion field is considered adequate. When using newer models, veterinary technicians should see eight to ten platelets per oil-immersion field.

If platelet numbers appear decreased, the 10$\times$ objective should be used to scan the feathered edge for clumps of platelets (Plate 41). Platelet clumping is common in cats. If clumps are observed, platelets are probably adequate in number. The presence of unusually large platelets (Plate 9) may suggest early release of platelets from the bone marrow and should be noted. Platelets, especially in cats, may be larger than erythrocytes. If decreased platelet numbers are suspected on the basis of the blood film examination, a platelet count is indicated.

PLASMA PROTEINS

◆ Plasma Protein Concentration

Plasma protein concentration estimation by refractometry is an important component of the CBC in all species. The plasma used to determine the PCV is used by breaking the hematocrit tube just above the buffy coat–plasma interface. The plasma is allowed to flow onto the refractometer prism (see Figure 1-7). The refractometer is then held to a bright light and the reading is made at the dividing line between the bright and dark field. The protein value (in grams per deciliter) is read directly from a scale inside the refractometer. Lipemia results in a false increase in the total protein reading.

◆ Plasma Fibrinogen Concentration

Fibrinogen is a plasma protein important in coagulation and inflammation. Increased plasma fibrinogen concentrations are common in inflammatory conditions, particularly in cattle. Fibrinogen determination is thus an important component of the CBC in cattle.

Two microhematocrit capillary tubes are filled, as for a PCV, and centrifuged in a hematocrit centrifuge for 5 minutes. The plasma protein concentration is determined by refractometry (see above) with one tube. The other tube is suspended in a 56° C (133° F) water bath for 5 minutes, then centrifuged again to spin down the precipitated fibrinogen. (Heating plasma to 56° C precipitates fibrinogen but not albumin or globulin.) The protein concentration is then measured by refractometry in the fibrinogen-free plasma. The difference between the two plasma protein readings is the fibrinogen concentration, in mg/dl. For example, if the total plasma protein level in the unheated tube is 8.3 g/dl and the plasma protein level in the heated tube is 7.5 g/dl, the fibrinogen concentration is 800 mg/dl (0.8 g/dl). The normal plasma fibrinogen concentration in cattle is 200 to 800 mg/dl.

EVALUATION OF COAGULATION

Coagulation tests are employed to diagnose various bleeding disorders. Hemostasis is normally achieved by complex interrelationships among vessel walls, platelets, and coagulation factors. Coagulation factors are plasma proteins, most of which are synthesized in the liver. Fibrin and aggregates of platelets make up the hemostatic plug, or clot, within the vessel lumen or wall.

The coagulation mechanism is usually divided into two pathways, extrinsic and intrinsic, which terminate in a common pathway leading to fibrin production. The intrinsic pathway of coagulation occurs intravascularly and is essential. The extrinsic, or tissue pathway, enhances coagulation. Various coagulation tests have been developed to evaluate the intrinsic and extrinsic pathways.

◆ Coagulation Tests

Blood samples for coagulation tests should be collected carefully, with minimal tissue damage and minimal venous stasis. Samples should never be collected through indwelling catheters. The preferred anticoagulant for coagulation tests is sodium citrate. Samples for whole blood clotting time and activated coagulation time do not require an anticoagulant. Unless numerous coagulation tests are performed in the veterinary hospital laboratory, blood samples should be sent to nearby commercial laboratories for testing.

The blood should be placed in an ice bath at the time of collection and then centrifuged, and the plasma separated within 30 minutes of collection. The plasma can then be stored in an ice bath and is stable for most tests for 4 hours. If the sample is to be mailed to a commercial laboratory, the plasma should be rapidly frozen in dry ice, then packed in dry ice (about 10 lb) in a polystyrene container.

Coagulation tests that can be performed in a veterinary hospital laboratory are discussed next.

Whole Blood Clotting Time

The whole blood clotting time (Lee-White method) is a test of the intrinsic clotting mechanism. The whole blood clotting time tests are not commonly performed because the activated clotting time is more sensitive. The veterinary technician collects 3 ml of blood in a plastic syringe, noting the time blood first appears in the syringe (using a stopwatch). Then 1 ml of blood is placed in each of three 10- × 75-mm tubes that have been rinsed with saline. The tubes are then placed in a 37° C (98.6° F) water bath or are held in the hand. The first and then the second tubes are tilted at 30-second intervals until coagulation occurs. The third tube is tilted in a similar manner. The time elapsed between the appearance of blood in the syringe and clot formation in the third tube is the clotting time. The normal whole blood clotting time for dogs is 2 to 10 minutes, horses 4 to 15 minutes, and cattle 10 to 15 minutes.

An alternative, more simple method is to collect the blood in a glass syringe and simply tilt the syringe back and forth until the blood clots. Blood normally clots in 2 to 10 minutes if a glass syringe is used.

Activated Clotting Time

The activated clotting time (ACT), another test of the intrinsic clotting mechanism, is the ideal screening test for use in veterinary practices. The ACT procedure uses diatomaceous earth as an activating agent. This shortens the normal clotting time, thus increasing the sensitivity of the whole blood clotting time. Commercially available ACT tubes are prewarmed in a 37° C (98.6° F) water bath. A plastic syringe is used to carefully draw 2 ml of blood, which is then injected into the ACT tube, and a stopwatch is started at the time of injection. The tube is inverted five times to mix and is replaced in the water bath for 1 minute, after which the tube is removed from the bath at 5-second intervals and tilted. The endpoint is the first evidence of clotting. Normal values are about 60 to 90 seconds. Severe thrombocytopenia (fewer than 10,000 platelets/μl) and abnormalities associated with the intrinsic coagulation cascade prolong the activated clotting time.

Bleeding Time

If an animal has a type of bleeding disorder that suggests inadequate platelets, such as petecchiae, epistaxis, or hematuria, but platelet numbers are adequate, the bleeding time should be determined. A clean site devoid of hair (e.g., the nose) is chosen and a deep puncture is made with a lancet or #11 Bard Parker scalpel blade. The time when blood appears is noted. Without touching the skin, the veterinary technician uses a filter paper to remove the blood at 30-second intervals. The endpoint is when blood no longer appears from the puncture site. The normal bleeding time for domestic animals is 1 to 5 minutes. Bleeding time is prolonged with platelet defects (qualitative or quantitative), increased capillary fragility, and von Willebrand's disease.

Large hospitals or commercial laboratories should perform more sophisticated platelet function tests for platelet aggregation or adhesiveness.

Activated Partial Thromboplastin Time

The activated partial thromboplastin time (APTT) is another test of the intrinsic clotting mechanism. If the ACT is prolonged, citrated plasma should be taken to a reference laboratory for an APTT. Citrated plasma is incubated with an activator of Factor XII, platelet substitute (cephaloplastin). After addition of calcium, the time to form fibrin is determined exactly by manual or semiautomated methods using fibrometers. The APTT also may be used in conjunction with known factor-deficient plasmas to identify a specific factor deficiency. Citrated plasma is stable for 4 hours in an ice bath. Each laboratory should establish its own normal range, which should not exceed ±3 seconds from the mean (e.g., mean APTT of 17 seconds, with a normal range of 14 to 20 seconds). A variety of acquired and hereditary disorders, in addition to administration of heparin, can reduce one or more factors necessary for the normal intrinsic coagulation cascade.

One-Stage Prothrombin Time

The one-stage prothrombin time (OSPT) is a test of the extrinsic clotting mechanism. Citrated plasma is added to a thromboplastin-calcium mixture, and the time to form fibrin is exactly determined manually or with a fibrometer. The test is independent of platelet function.

The patient's citrated plasma, along with that of a normal control, should be placed in an ice bath and transported to the laboratory within 2 hours of collection. Each laboratory should establish its own normal values for OSPT. Duplicate determinations should agree within 1 second. The normal range for dogs is 7 to 10 seconds. The test should not be performed in the veterinary hospital laboratory unless it is needed fairly frequently. Commercial reagents with detailed instructions are available (General Diagnostics, Morris Plains, NJ).

A prolonged OSPT may be associated with severe liver disease, disseminated intravascular coagulation, or hereditary or acquired deficiencies of any factors of the extrinsic coagulation cascade. The test is sensitive to vitamin K deficiency or antagonism, such as warfarin toxicity.

BONE MARROW EVALUATION

◆ Collection

A bone marrow aspiration biopsy is indicated in patients with unexplained blood findings that suggest marrow failure or neoplasia when it is not possible to make a diagnosis by careful examination of the peripheral blood. Indications include nonregenerative anemia, leukopenia, thrombocytopenia, possible lymphoproliferative or myeloproliferative disorders, and abnormalities of immunoproteins. Core biopsy is indicated when attempts to obtain an aspirate have been unsuccessful, as is often the case in patients with myelofibrosis, a condition in which the bone marrow becomes filled with fibrous connective tissue.

Bone marrow biopsy needles should be constructed of strong steel and have a short beveled point and a large hub for ease of use (Figure 2-14). Osgood and Rosenthal bone marrow biopsy needles (Becton-Dickinson, Rutherford, NJ) are quite satisfactory (16 to 18 gauge, 1 to 1½ inch). They should be cleaned and autoclaved before each use. Conventional hypodermic needles may be satisfactory in cats with thin bones, but occlusion of the needle often prevents sample collection. Other required equipment includes clippers, soap, and skin disinfectant, a dry 12-ml syringe, local anesthetic, and microscope slides. A small tube containing EDTA is optional.

Technique

The sites most commonly used in dogs and cats are the proximal end of the femur, the humerus, and the iliac crest. The iliac crest usually is used in cattle and horses. A local anesthetic (e.g., 2% lidocaine) injected into the skin, subcutaneous tissue, and periosteum is usually adequate. If the animal struggles, a short-acting general anesthetic may be required. If the femur is used, the animal should be placed in lateral recumbency, and the biopsy site prepared as for surgery. After infiltration with local anesthetic, the trochanteric fossa is located by placing the thumb on the greater trochanter (Figure 2-15). The needle is advanced toward the fossa with its long axis

Figure 2-14
A, Osgood bone marrow biopsy needle. **B,** Rosenthal bone marrow biopsy needle. (From Banks WJ: *Applied veterinary histology,* ed 2, St Louis, 1993, Mosby.)

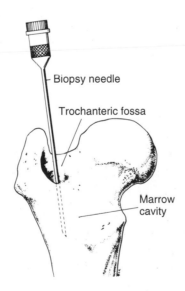

Biopsy needle

Trochanteric fossa

Marrow cavity

Figure 2-15
Placement of a bone marrow biopsy needle in the trochanteric fossa of a dog. (From Banks WJ: *Applied veterinary histology,* ed 2, St Louis, 1993, Mosby.)

parallel to the long axis of the femur. The needle should be directed along the medial aspect of the greater trochanter until it encounters resistance.

When the needle has reached the cortex of the fossa, it should be rotated with short, clockwise movements until it becomes firmly seated in bone. Stabilization of the leg as the needle is advanced is accomplished by the following procedure: the cranial aspect of the thigh and shaft of the femur are grasped and the pelvic limb is elevated to a plane parallel to the table surface. The stylet should remain in the needle, or the lumen may become clogged with bone. The needle is advanced a few more millimeters, the stylet removed, and the syringe attached. Negative pressure is applied only until marrow becomes visible in the syringe barrel. Aspiration of a large volume results in contamination of collected marrow with blood.

The negative pressure is released and the syringe removed. A small drop of marrow is placed on each of several slides. A second slide is dropped gently on the marrow slide. The drop spreads rapidly between the glass surfaces. The slides are then pulled laterally, away from each other, while their surfaces are kept parallel (Figure 2-16). When placing the marrow directly on the slide, the veterinary technician must work quickly because the sample clots within 60 seconds, rendering it useless. An alternative is to quickly place a few drops of collected marrow into an unstoppered commercial EDTA tube, which has had most of the EDTA shaken from it, thus preventing the marrow from clotting. Marrow films can then be made within the ensuing few minutes.

If the iliac crest is used, the needle is placed on the superficial and dorsal portion and directed ventrally and medially. The needle should be firmly seated in bone and advanced several millimeters. Then the veterinary technician proceeds as described above. If a rib is used, the site of biopsy is usually located midway between the vertebra and the costal cartilage. The veterinary technician should avoid damage to the intercostal artery, located caudal to each rib. If the sternum is used, the biopsy needle is positioned so that the long axis is perpendicular to the surface of the sternebrae and the above procedure is followed.

Bone marrow films should be stained as described for blood films.

Figure 2-16
Bone marrow film preparation. A drop of marrow is spread between two glass slides. The slides are about to be pulled laterally, away from each other.

Evaluation of Bone Marrow Films

A systematic approach should be used when evaluating a bone marrow film. The lower-power objective (10×) should be used to scan the entire slide. The veterinary technician should note the number and degree of maturity of megakaryocytes, the degree of overall cellularity, and amount of fat (Figure 2-17). Red cell, or erythroid, and white cell, or myeloid, precursors should be identified, and the ratio of myeloid to erythroid cells, or M:E ratio, estimated. During estimation of this ratio, several fields in different areas of the film should be examined because cells of one type are often seen together. It may be helpful to count 500 nucleated cells and classify them as erythroid or myeloid.

Erythroid and granulocytic precursors usually may be differentiated by their nuclear and cytoplasmic appearance (Plate 42). Nuclei of erythroid precursors tend to be round, with dark, coarse chromatin. These nuclei remain round and become smaller as they mature. The nuclei of granulocytic precursors tend to be less perfectly round, elongating as they mature. The cytoplasm of erythroid precursors is deeply basophilic in more immature forms, becoming polychromatophilic and then pink as the cells mature. The cytoplasm of early granulocytic precursors contains pink primary granules, which disappear as the cell matures.

The completeness and orderliness of maturation in cells in the erythroid and the myeloid series should be noted. Because blast cells divide to ultimately form 16 to 32 mature cells, about 80% of the granulocytic precursors should be the more mature forms, such as metamyelocytes, bands, and neutrophils. About 90% of the erythroid series should be the more mature forms, such as rubricytes and metarubricytes. The

Figure 2-17
Normal canine marrow film containing a megakaryocyte (*arrow*) and erythroid and myeloid precursors. (350×)

erythroid series has complete maturation if significant numbers of polychromatophilic erythrocytes (reticulocytes) are present. Maturation of the myeloid series is complete if mature neutrophils are present. The presence and percentage of other types of cells, such as lymphocytes, plasma cells, and macrophages, should be noted. Erythrophagocytosis, phagocytosis of RBCs by macrophages, and other unusual findings should be recorded.

Marrow Cell Identification

Descriptions of cells found within the marrow follow (Figures 2-18 and 2-19).

Erythrocyte Precursors

RUBRIBLAST.   Rubriblasts have a large, round nucleus, with royal-blue, stippled cytoplasm and a light-blue nucleolus (Figure 2-20).

PRORUBRICYTE.   Prorubricytes are smaller than rubriblasts and have no nucleolus.

RUBRICYTE.   Rubricytes are smaller than prorubricytes. Their nucleus contains dark clumps of chromatin and the cytoplasm becomes hemoglobin colored (see Plate 42 and Figure 2-20).

METARUBRICYTE.   Metarubricytes have a pyknotic nucleus, with cytoplasm colored more like hemoglobin than rubricytes (Plate 42).

POLYCHROMATOPHILIC ERYTHROCYTE.   These are erythroid cells that have had their nucleus extruded. They are larger than mature erythrocytes. When they are stained with new methylene blue or brilliant cresyl blue, precipitated RNA is evident in the cytoplasm (reticulocyte).

Granulocyte Precursors

MYELOBLAST.   The nucleus of myeloblasts is not as round as that of rubriblasts and often is oval. One to two pale-blue nucleoli are present. The cytoplasm is blue-pink as contrasted to the royal-blue cytoplasm of rubriblasts (Plate 43).

PROGRANULOCYTE.   Small, pink granules can be seen in the cytoplasm of progranulocytes. A nucleolus may or may not be present (Plates 42 and 43).

MYELOCYTE.   The nucleus of myelocytes usually is oval and may be eccentric. The cytoplasm stains gray-blue (see Figure 2-19 and Plate 43).

METAMYELOCYTE.   The nucleus of metamyelocytes becomes indented or kidney shaped. Their cytoplasm is less blue than that of myelocytes (see Figures 2-19 and 2-20 and Plate 43).

Figure 2-18
Bone marrow film from a dog with granulocytic hyperplasia. Most of the precursors are myeloid. Plasma cells (*arrows*) appear to be present in increased numbers. Although rubricytic precursors appear to be decreased in number, the decrease is probably relative because this dog is not anemic.

Figure 2-19
Bone marrow film from a dog with granulocytic hyperplasia. *a,* segmented neutrophil; *b,* band neutrophils; *c,* late metamyelocyte; *d,* early metamyelocyte; *e,* myelocyte. (1400×)

Figure 2-20
Normal bone marrow film. *a,* rubriblast; *b,* rubricyte; *c,* band neutrophil; *d,* metamyelocyte; *e,* lymphocyte; *f,* segmented neutrophil. (1400×)

BAND.   Band neutrophils have a horseshoe-shaped nucleus with slightly indented sides (see Figures 2-19 and 2-20 and Plate 43). Myelocytes, metamyelocytes, and bands may be neutrophilic, eosinophilic, or basophilic. Eosinophil precursors contain distinct orange-pink granules, with basophilic cytoplasm. Basophil precursors contain purple or black granules.

Platelet Precursors

MEGAKARYOBLAST.   Megakaryoblast is larger than other blast cells within the bone marrow and contains two reddish nuclei and basophilic, scanty cytoplasm.

PROMEGAKARYOCYTE.   The nuclei of promegakaryocytes partially divide and number 4, 8, 16, or 32. The nuclear lobes remain connected. The cytoplasm does not divide and consists of a rim around the nuclear mass.

MEGAKARYOCYTE.   The cytoplasm of megakaryocytes is abundant and pale blue and contains azurophilic granules. Mature megakaryocytes are large (50 to 150 μ in diameter) (Plate 44).

PLATELET.   Platelets (thrombocytes) are cytoplasmic structures of megakaryocytes. They vary in size and shape and contain azurophilic granules in a pale-blue background. Giant and cigar shapes are not uncommon, especially in cats.

Other Cells Observed in Bone Marrow Films

LYMPHOCYTE.   Small lymphocytes may be seen in bone marrow films, often composing 10% to 15% of the total nucleated cells in cats.

PLASMA CELL.   In a normal animal undergoing antigenic stimulation, plasma cells constitute less than 1% of the nucleated cells of bone marrow. Increased numbers are seen in animals with increased antibody production. Large numbers of immature or abnormal plasma cells in the bone marrow indicate multiple myeloma (a neoplasm of plasma cells). Plasma cells are transformed lymphocytes with abundant basophilic cytoplasm and a round, eccentric nucleus. The nuclear chromatin is usually clumped, resembling the nuclear pattern of rubricytes. They can be distinguished from rubricytes because plasma cells have a more abundant, more basophilic cytoplasm (see Figure 2-18 and Plate 45). Usually a well-defined perinuclear clear zone is associated with the Golgi apparatus. Plasma cells are occasionally filled with round, clear, or pink structures called *Russell bodies.* The cell is then referred to as a *Mott cell.* Russell bodies are thought to be packets of immunoglobulin and are usually associated with intense antibody production.

MONOCYTE AND MACROPHAGE.   These cells may be observed in bone marrow aspirates. Macrophages are best recognized when they contain phagocytized material, such as iron particles, nuclear material, and RBCs.

OSTEOBLAST. These cells are much larger than plasma cells but are somewhat similar. They have abundant basophilic cytoplasm, which is often vacuolated, and eccentric nuclei.

OSTEOCLAST. These are giant, multinucleated cells with abundant granular cytoplasm. Their nuclei are round and do not touch one another, unlike those of megakaryocytes.

◆ Myeloproliferative and Lymphoproliferative Disorders

Leukemia, a neoplastic proliferation of hematopoietic cells within the bone marrow, is classified broadly into *myeloproliferative* and *lymphoproliferative* disorders. Diagnosis is based on finding characteristic blast cells in the blood and/or bone marrow and associated hematologic abnormalities. Specific cell types are identified by their morphologic appearance in Wright's-stained blood and bone marrow films and by their cytochemical staining properties, electron microscopic appearance, and monoclonal antibodies to surface antigens.

Myeloproliferative leukemia includes neoplastic proliferation of erythrocytes, granulocytes, monocytes, and megakaryocytes. Lymphoproliferative leukemia includes neoplastic proliferation of lymphocytes and plasma cells. Multiple cell lines may be neoplastic if the affected stem cell is multipotential. A common example is myelomonocytic leukemia, in which neutrophils and monocytes have been neoplastically transformed.

Myeloproliferative Disorders

Myeloproliferative disorders may involve primitive cells (poorly differentiated leukemia), RBCs (erythremic myelosis), granulocytes (granulocytic leukemia), or megakaryocytes (megakaryocytic leukemia) (Figure 2-21). Typically, normal marrow

Figure 2-21
Giant platelets (*arrows*) in peripheral blood from a cat with megakaryocytic leukemia. (1400×)

cells are displaced by proliferating immature cells. Myeloproliferative disorders occasionally may be difficult to distinguish from marked erythroid regeneration or granulocytic hyperplasia in response to inflammation. A classification scheme similar to that used in humans has been described.[4]

Poorly differentiated leukemia is a proliferation of primitive, undifferentiated cells. These cells are large (12 to 20 μ), with a large, round, eccentric nucleus and basophilic to lavender cytoplasm. The nucleus may contain a nucleolus and the cytoplasm may contain pink granules. Cytoplasmic pseudopod-like structures may project from the cells (Plate 46). If these structures break from cells, they may resemble giant platelets. Undifferentiated cells often have features of erythroid and granulocytic precursors.

Erythremic myelosis is characterized by large numbers of early rubricytic precursors and decreased numbers of mature cells (polychromatophilic red cells). Although erythroid precursors may appear normal, they often have increased cytoplasm (megaloblastoid) as a result of asynchronous nucleus-cytoplasm maturation. Granulopoiesis is usually decreased (Plate 46). Increased numbers of nucleated erythroid precursors, which do not mature to polychromatophilic RBCs, are seen on blood films (Plate 47).

Granulocytic leukemia usually is characterized by an abnormal progression of maturation, such as large numbers of blasts, progranulocytes, and myelocytes with few mature cells. Erythropoiesis usually is decreased.

Lymphoproliferative Disorders

Tumors derived from lymphocytes or plasma cells are classified as *lymphoproliferative neoplasms*. Lymphoproliferative disorders are more common in domestic animals than are myeloproliferative disorders.

Lymphocytic leukemia (Plate 48) differs from malignant lymphoma (lymphosarcoma) primarily in anatomic distribution. Sarcomatous masses are present in lymphosarcoma but not in lymphocytic leukemia. However, about 10% to 25% of dogs and cats with lymphosarcoma develop leukemia. Lymphoproliferative disease arising in the bone marrow (lymphocytic leukemia) has a different biologic behavior, response to therapy, and prognosis. Lymphocytic leukemias are classified as either *chronic lymphocytic leukemia* or *acute lymphocytic leukemia.*

In chronic lymphocytic leukemia, the lymphocytes are small and appear well differentiated. This type of leukemia must be differentiated from physiologic lymphocytosis in excited cats, in which the absolute lymphocyte count may reach 20,000/μl, and from lymphocytosis induced by chronic antigenic stimulation, which is seen in dogs with chronic ehrlichiosis.[5] *Lymphoblastic leukemia* is characterized by large numbers of lymphoblasts in the blood and bone marrow.

Plasma-cell myeloma (multiple myeloma) is a relatively rare lymphoproliferative neoplasm characterized by proliferation of plasma cells or precursors. As implied by the term *multiple myeloma,* plasma cells proliferate at multiple sites in the bone marrow. Although these plasma-cell proliferations may be diagnosed by examination of marrow films, they only infrequently result in plasma cells circulating in the blood. Although markedly increased numbers of plasma cells in the bone marrow (more than 20%) are often a result of neoplasia, this proliferation also may be due to chronic antigenic stimulation.

An important diagnostic and clinical manifestation of plasma-cell myeloma is monoclonal gammopathy, which is detected by serum electrophoresis, a procedure performed in most diagnostic laboratories. Other diagnostic features include Bence Jones protein, which are light chains of immunoglobulins, in the urine and radiographic evidence of osteolysis. Traditionally, two of these four diagnostic features are considered essential to diagnose plasma-cell myeloma. However, dogs with chronic ehrlichiosis may have monoclonal gammopathy and markedly increased numbers of plasma cells in the bone marrow. Fortunately, neoplastic plasma cells usually appear slightly abnormal or immature, with some multinucleated plasma cells present.

HEMOGRAMS IN SELECTED DISEASES

◆ Case 1

A 2-year-old Australian Shepherd was presented for acute onset of hematuria and depression. On physical examination, the dog had pale mucous membranes. The CBC results were as follows:

PCV: 11%
Hb: 4 g/dl
RBCs: 1.57 × 10⁶/μl
MCV: 70 fl
MCHC: 36 g/dl
Total protein: 6.3 g/dl
WBCs: 32,000/μl
Segs: 24,000/μl
Bands: 1000/μl
Lymphs: 6000/μl
Monos: 3000/μl
Nucleated RBCs: 3000/μl
· Platelets: 75,000/μl
Reticulocytes: 314,000/μl (20%)

The blood film demonstrated marked polychromasia and anisocytosis, with many spherocytes (Figure 2-22 and Plate 13). The serum was hemolyzed.

Interpretation

A 20% reticulocyte count (314,000/μl) is evidence of a marked erythroid response. The anemia is regenerative, suggesting blood loss or blood destruction. Many spherocytes are diagnostic for immune-mediated hemolytic anemia. Neutrophilia, with a slight left shift, suggests an inflammatory response, which is typical in immune-mediated hemolytic anemia. Decreased platelets (immune-mediated thrombocytopenia) occur in about one third of affected patients. This case of immune-mediated hemolytic anemia exemplifies the necessity of careful evaluation of blood films; the many spherocytes were diagnostic.

Figure 2-22
Canine blood film from Case 1. What is the diagnosis? (350×)

◆ Case 2

An 8-year-old mixed-breed female dog was presented for evaluation of a mammary tumor, depression, hematuria, and gingival bleeding. The CBC results were as follows:

PCV: 16%
Total protein: 5.0 g/dl
WBCs: 50,000/μl
Segs: 44,000/μl (88%)
Bands: 3000/μl (6%)
Lymphs: 1000/μl (2%)
Monos: 1000/μl (2%)
Nucleated RBCs: 1000/μl (2%)
Platelets: markedly decreased on film, 20,000/μl
Polychromasia: 12%

Numerous schistocytes (RBC fragments) were present, and the neutrophils appeared toxic (basophilic vacuolated cytoplasm, Döhle bodies).

Interpretation

The anemia is regenerative. The presence of schistocytes and decreased platelet numbers suggests disseminated intravascular coagulation (DIC), possibly secondary to the mammary tumor. An ACT, prothrombin time, APPT, and fibrin-degradation product determinations are needed to confirm DIC. The leukogram is evidence of the response to inflammation. The presence of toxic neutrophils suggests a bacterial or endotoxin component to the disease. An appropriate diagnosis is DIC secondary to a mammary tumor.

◆ Case 3

A 4-year-old Thoroughbred horse had been in a trailer accident 5 days previously and sustained severe lacerations and blood loss. The results of a CBC were as follows:
PCV: 18%
Total protein: 5.5 g/dl
WBCs: 15,000/μl
Segs: 13,500/μl
Bands: 500/μl
Lymphs: 500/μl
Monos: 500/μl
Platelets: adequate
    Notes included no polychromasia and an occasional Howell-Jolly body.

Interpretation

Because horses do not release polychromatophilic RBCs (reticulocytes), even in the face of regenerative anemia, the lack of polychromasia is not meaningful. To determine if the anemia is regenerative, the MCV can be calculated (horses release larger cells in regenerative responses), which requires an RBC count. In addition, a bone marrow aspiration could be performed and reticulocytosis evaluated on the bone marrow film. Probably a more practical approach would be to perform the PCV on a weekly basis to determine if it is increasing.

◆ Case 4

A 2-year-old Siamese cat was presented for evaluation of weight loss and anorexia. The CBC results were as follows:
PCV: 10%
Total protein: 8.5 g/dl
WBCs: 25,000/μl
Segs: 4000/μl (16%)
Bands: 1000/μl (4%)
Lymphs: 3000/μl (12%)
Nucleated RBCs: 17,000/μl (68%)
Corrected WBCs: 8000/μl
Reticulocytes: 0%
Platelets: slightly decreased
    The neutrophils had toxic changes: blue, vacuolated cytoplasm, Döhle bodies.

Interpretation

Prorubricytes and rubricytes are very early erythrocyte precursors (Plate 47). Many nucleated RBCs in conjunction with nonregenerative anemia (0% reticulocytes) suggest a myeloproliferative disorder (erythremic myelosis). A bone marrow aspiration and FeLV test are indicated. Note that the nucleated RBC count was included in the 100-cell differential count in this case. The corrected WBC count is obtained by subtracting the absolute number of nucleated RBCs from the observed WBC count. The diagnosis is a type of myeloproliferative disorder, or erythemic myelosis.

◆ Case 5

A 1-year-old male Siamese cat was presented for evaluation of severe depression and anorexia of 3 days' duration. The CBC results were as follows:

PCV: 6%
Hb: 5.1 g/dl
RBCs: 2.27 × 10⁶/μl
MCV: 22 fl
MCHC: 85 g/dl
WBCs: 6000/μl

Many Heinz bodies (80% of red cells affected) were suspected on Wright's-stained film and confirmed with new methylene blue stain (Plates 17 and 18). The blood was brown and hemolyzed.

Interpretation

Heinz bodies are the cause of hemolytic anemia. The hemolysis has resulted in a high hemoglobin value, which has caused an erroneously high MCHC. Further questioning of the client revealed that the cat had been given two acetaminophen (Tylenol) tablets 36 hours previously. Acetaminophen acts as an oxidant of hemoglobin, resulting in Heinz body formation and methemoglobinemia, which resulted in the brown color of the blood. The diagnosis is Heinz body hemolytic anemia subsequent to acetaminophen toxicity.

REFERENCE VALUES

Tables 2-4, 2-5, and 2-6 contain reference ("normal") hematologic values for dogs, cats, horses, cattle, sheep, and pigs.[2]

CROSSMATCHING BLOOD FOR TRANSFUSION

A common treatment for anemia is transfusion of blood. Crossmatching determines if the donor's and recipient's blood is immunologically compatible.

Red cell antigens are structures on the surface of RBCs from one animal that may react with antibodies in the plasma of another animal. These antigen-antibody reactions usually result in clumping or agglutination of RBCs. However, in some species, the antigen-antibody reaction is more likely to result in RBC lysis.

Although erythrocytes of common domestic animals possess antigens, naturally occurring antibodies present in people are relatively rare in animals. However, they

TABLE 2-4

Reference hematologic values for dogs and cats

	Dogs Range (Mean)	Cats Range (Mean)
PCV (%)	37-55 (45)	24-45 (37)
Hemoglobin (g/dl)	12-18 (15)	8-15 (12)
RBC ($\times 10^6/\mu l$)	5.5-8.5 (6.8)	5-10 (7.5)
Total protein (g/dl)	6.0-7.5	6.0-7.5
WBC ($\times 10^3/\mu l$)	6.0-17.0 (11.5)	5.5-19.5 (12.5)
Differential, absolute		
Segs	60%-77%; 3000-11,500 (7000)	35%-75%; 2500-12,500 (7500)
Bands	0%-3%; 0-300 (70)	0%-3%; 0-300 (100)
Lymphs	12%-30%; 1000-4800 (2800)	20%-55%; 1500-7000 (4000)
Monos	3%-10%; 150-1350 (750)	1%-4%; 0-850 (350)
Eosinos	2%-10%; 100-1250 (550)	2%-12%; 0-1500 (650)
Basos	Rare	Rare
Platelets ($\times 10^5/\mu l$)	2.0-9.0	3-7 (4.5)
MCV (fl)	60-77 (70)	39-55 (45)
MCH (pg)	19-23	13-17
MCHC (g/dl)	32.0-36.0 (34.0)	30-36 (33.2)
Bone marrow M:E ratio	0.75-2.5:1 (1.2:1)	0.6-3.9:1 (1.6:1)

From Jain NC: Essentials of veterinary hematology, *Baltimore, 1993, Waverly.*

TABLE 2-5

Reference hematologic values for horses and cattle

	Horses Range (Mean)	Cattle Range (Mean)
PCV (%)	32-52 (42)	24-46 (35)
Hemoglobin (g/dl)	11-19 (15)	8-15 (12)
RBC ($\times 10^6/\mu l$)	6.5-12.5 (9.5)	5-10 (7)
Total protein (g/dl)	6.0-8.0	6.0-8.0
WBC ($\times 10^3/\mu l$)	5.5-12.5 (9.0)	4.0-12.0 (8.0)
Differential, absolute		
Segs	30%-65%; 2700-6700 (4700)	15%-45%; 600-4000 (7000)
Bands	0%-2%; 0-100 (2.0)	0%-2%; 0 120 (20)
Lymphs	25%-70%; 1500-5500 (3500)	45%-75%; 2500-7500 (4500)
Monos	0.5%-7%; 0-800 (400)	2%-7%; 25-840 (400)
Eosinos	0%-11%; 0-925 (375)	2%-20%; 0-2400 (700)
Basos	0%-3%; 0-170 (50)	0%-2%; 0-200 (50)
Platelets ($\times 10^5/\mu l$)	1-6 (3.3)	1-8 (5)
MCV (fl)	34-58 (46)	40-60 (52)
MCH (pg)	15.2-18.6	14.4-18.6
MCHC (g/dl)	31-37 (35)	30-36 (32.7)
Bone marrow M:E ratio	0.94-3.76:1.0 (1.64:1)	0.31-1.85:1.0 (0.71:1)

From Jain NC: Essentials of veterinary hematology, *Baltimore, 1993, Waverly.*

TABLE **2-6**

Reference hematologic values for sheep and pigs

	Sheep Range (Mean)	Pigs Range (Mean)
PCV (%)	24-50 (38)	32-50 (42)
Hemoglobin (g/dl)	8-16 (12)	10-16 (13)
RBC ($\times\ 10^6/\mu l$)	8-16 (12)	5-8 (6.5)
Total protein (g/dl)	6-7.5	6-7
WBC ($\times\ 10^3/\mu l$)	4-12 (8)	11-22 (16)
Differential, absolute		
Segs	10%-50%; 700-6000 (2400)	28%-47%; 3000-10,500
Bands	Rare	0%-2%
Lymphs	40%-75%; 2000-9000 (5000)	39%-62%; 4300-13,700
Monos	0.6%; 0-750 (200)	2%-30%; 220-2200
Eosinos	0.1%; 0-1000 (400)	0.5%-11%; 0-2500
Basos	0%-3%; 0-300 (50)	0%-2%; 0-400
Platelets ($\times\ 10^5/\mu l$)	2.5-7.5 (4.0)	3.25-7.15 (5.2)
MCV (fl)	23-48 (33)	50-68 (63)
MCH (pg)	9-13	16.6-22
MCHC (g/dl)	31-38 (33.5)	30-34 (32)
Bone marrow M:E ratio	0.77-1.68:1 (1.1:1)	$1.77 \pm 0.52{:}1$

From Jain NC: Essentials of veterinary hematology, *Baltimore, 1993, Waverly.*

do occur in cattle, sheep, and pigs. Once a transfusion has been given to an animal, antibodies against the RBC antigen (immune antibodies) are formed. However, because of the lack of naturally occurring antibodies, experts in veterinary medicine generally acknowledge the first transfusion can be given without regard to the blood typing or crossmatching.

Although crossmatching may not be necessary with the first transfusion, subsequent transfusions require crossmatching. Breeding females, especially mares, should always be given properly matched blood to avoid sensitization that results in destruction of the foal's RBCs. Methods used for blood typing vary with the species.

◆ Blood Types

Dogs

At least eight different RBC antigens are present in dogs: DEA 1.1, 1.2, 3, 4, 5, 6, 7, and 8. DEA 1.1 and 1.2 are also referred to as "A" antigens, which are of clinical significance. Because naturally occurring anti-A antibodies do not exist, the first transfusion of A-positive blood into an A-negative recipient does not result in a clinical reaction, but the transfused cells have a shortened life span (7 days). If a previously immunized A-negative dog receives A-positive blood, severe reactions occur in less than 1 hour.

Because no anti-A antibodies occur naturally, crossmatching is of little value unless the animal has been previously sensitized with incompatible blood. A-negative dogs should be kept as blood donors to prevent reactions resulting from the A factor. Blood typing is performed at numerous veterinary teaching hospitals.

Cats

Blood groups of cats include A, B, and AB. Few cats have group AB. The vast majority of cats in the United States have group A, which probably explains the low incidence of transfusion reactions in cats. Type B cats are most likely to be purebred. Transfusing type B cats with type A blood may result in serious transfusion reactions and death. Thus blood for transfusion of purebred cats should be selected by cross-matching.

Cattle

Eleven blood groups have been described in cattle. Anti-J antibodies are the only common natural antibodies in cattle. J-negative donors may be used to minimize transfusion reactions. The lytic crossmatch is required because bovine and ovine erythrocytes have little tendency to agglutinate.

Horses

Sixteen blood antigens have been described in eight systems in horses. Naturally occurring antibodies do not exist, but antibodies may be present as a result of vaccinations containing equine tissue or transplacental immunization. Crossmatching should be done before the first transfusion in a horse, using the lytic and agglutination procedures. Transfusion reactions in horses are commonly fatal.

◆ Crossmatching Procedures

The following procedure can demonstrate hemolysis and agglutination. Blood samples are drawn from the donor and the recipient into individual clot tubes (no anticoagulant used). The clotted samples are centrifuged and the serum transferred to separate, labeled tubes. Using cells from the recipient's and donor's clots, the veterinary technician prepares an approximate 3% red cell suspension (percentage is not critical) in normal saline from each sample. The suspensions are washed three times with normal saline, centrifuging after each washing, until the supernatant is clear and colorless. After the final washing, each tube of washed RBCs is diluted in saline again to about a 3% cell suspension.

Major Crossmatch

Two drops of the recipient's serum and two drops of the donor's red cell suspension are placed in a 12- × 75-mm test tube.

Minor Crossmatch

Two drops of the donor's serum and two drops of the recipient's red cell suspension are placed in a 12-× 75-mm test tube. The tubes are incubated in a 37° C (98.6° F) water bath for 30 minutes. The tubes are centrifuged for 2 minutes at 500 rpm. The supernatant is examined for hemolysis. Slight hemolysis of canine blood is nonspecific. Significant hemolysis in either of the crossmatched tubes indicates incompatibility and the necessity of choosing another donor.

After examination of the supernatant for hemolysis, the tubes are tapped gently to detect grossly visible agglutination. If no agglutination is observed, a small amount of the mixture is transferred to a microscope slide and a coverslip is applied. The veterinary technician then examines it with the 10× objective for agglutination. Agglutination in either tube indicates incompatibility and necessity of choosing a new donor.

References

1. Weiser MG: Hematologic techniques, *Vet Clin North Am* 11:189-208, 1981.
2. Jain NC: *Essentials of veterinary hematology,* Baltimore, 1993, Waverly.
3. Benjamin MM: *Outline of veterinary clinical pathology,* ed 3, Ames, 1978, Iowa State University Press.
4. Jain NC et al: Proposed criteria for classification of acute myeloid leukemias in dogs and cats, *Vet Clin Pathol* 20:63-82, 1991.
5. Weiser MG, et al: Granular lymphocytosis and hyperproteinemia in dogs with chronic ehrlichiosis, *J Am Animal Hosp Assoc* 27:84-88, 1991.

Blood Chemistry

3

JOANN COLVILLE

◉ CHEMICAL ASSAY OF SERUM, PLASMA, OR WHOLE BLOOD

M any veterinary practices own or lease chemistry analyzers to perform routine chemical assays. This focus on in-house laboratory work makes the veterinary technicians' laboratory skills perhaps their biggest asset to the practice.

Evaluation of chemical components of blood has become an important aid in formulation of an accurate diagnosis, prescription of proper therapy, and documentation of the response to treatment. Most chemical assays measure the level of a dissolved substance normally carried in the blood (plasma) or the amount of a substance not normally found in blood, which has been released into the blood from damaged or destroyed cells.

As the person most likely to be in charge of the laboratory, the veterinary technician must become familiar with the types of analytic instruments available (see Chapter 1), the variety of testing procedures used, and the rationale underlying the analyses. The most important contribution the technician can make to the practice laboratory is accurate and reliable test results. For example, in vitro results must reflect, as closely as possible, the actual in vivo levels of blood constituents.

◆ Sample Collection

Most chemical analyses require whole blood, plasma, or serum. The instructions accompany the chemistry analyzers and should be consulted for the type of sample required.

Whole Blood

Whole blood comprises fluid and cells. The fluid component is plasma; the cellular component is made up of red blood cells (RBC), or erythrocytes; white blood cells (WBC), or leukocytes; and platelets, or thrombocytes.

The veterinary technician obtains a whole blood sample by withdrawing the blood into a suitable container with the proper anticoagulant to prevent clotting. As soon as the blood is collected, the blood and anticoagulant are mixed with a gentle rocking motion. Shaking the sample vigorously causes hemolysis, which in turn can affect the results of the assays when chemicals normally found within the erythrocytes are released into the plasma. If the assay is delayed for more than an hour after blood collection, the sample should be refrigerated at 0° C to 4° C. When it is time to perform the test, the sample should be warmed to room temperature (20° C) and gently remixed. Whole blood should not be frozen because blood cells lyse during the freezing and thawing processes.

Plasma

Plasma is the fluid portion of whole blood in which the cells are suspended. It comprises about 90% water and 10% dissolved constituents, such as proteins, carbohydrates, vitamins, hormones, enzymes, lipids, salts, waste materials, antibodies, and other ions and molecules. Procedure 3-1 describes obtaining a plasma sample.

The sample must not be contaminated with any cells from the bottom of the tube after centrifugation. If the sample cannot be centrifuged within 1 hour, it must be refrigerated. If heparinized plasma has been stored overnight after separation or has been frozen, the sample should be centrifuged again to remove any fibrin strands that may have formed. Plasma samples may be refrigerated or frozen. Freezing may affect certain test results; the test instructions should be consulted for all the tests that run before a plasma sample is frozen.

Serum

Serum is plasma from which fibrinogen, a plasma protein, has been removed. During the clotting process, the soluble fibrinogen in plasma is converted to an insoluble fibrin clot matrix. When blood clots, the fluid that is squeezed out around the cellular clot is serum. Obtaining a serum sample is described in Procedure 3-2.

PROCEDURE 3-1

Obtaining a plasma sample

1. Collect a blood sample in a container with the appropriative anticoagulant.
2. Mix the blood-filled container with a gentle rocking motion 12 times.
3. Make sure the container is covered to prevent evaporation during centrifugation.
4. Centrifuge (within an hour of collection) at 2000 to 3000 rpm for 10 minutes.
5. Using a capillary pipette, carefully remove the fluid plasma layer from the bottom layer of cells.
6. Transfer the plasma to a container labeled with the date, time of collection, patient's name, and case or clinic number.
7. Refrigerate or freeze as appropriate.

Centrifuging at speeds greater than 2000 to 3000 rpm or for a prolonged time may result in hemolysis. Freezing may affect some test results; therefore the test instructions should be consulted for all the tests that run before a serum sample is frozen.

Anticoagulants

An anticoagulant is a chemical that, when added to a whole blood sample, prevents or delays clotting (coagulation) of the sample. Some anticoagulants may affect assays, so the test procedure should be consulted for the proper anticoagulant in which to collect the sample. For example, the sodium or potassium salt of an anticoagulant may affect the results of an electrolyte assay by adding sodium or potassium to the sample. The anticoagulant also may remove physically the constituent to be assayed. For example, an oxalate anticoagulant removes calcium from the sample, making it useless for calcium determinations. Other anticoagulants may inhibit certain enzymes and activate others.

HEPARIN. Heparin is the preferred anticoagulant when plasma is required for analysis because it interferes least with chemical assays. Heparin is available as a sodium, potassium, lithium, or ammonium salt. Current belief is that heparin clots by preventing conversion of prothrombin to thrombin during the clotting processes.

To prevent clotting, heparin should be used at 20 units/ml of blood to be collected. The most convenient method for using heparin is to coat the inside walls of a syringe with liquid heparin before the sample is drawn from the patient. Vacuum collection tubes containing the proper amount of heparin are available commercially. These tubes are most convenient when many heparinized samples are needed. The vacuum tubes have a limited shelf life, so they may not be practical for a practice that rarely needs heparinized plasma.

PROCEDURE 3-2

Obtaining a serum sample

1. Collect a whole blood sample in a container that contains no anticoagulant.
2. Allow the blood to clot in its original container at room temperature for 20 to 30 minutes.
3. *Do not* refrigerate the blood until it has clotted.
4. Gently separate the clot from the container by running a wooden applicator stick around the wall of the container between the clot and the wall.
5. Cover the sample and centrifuge at 2000 to 3000 rpm for 10 minutes.
6. Using a capillary pipette, remove the serum from the clot.
7. Transfer the serum to a container labeled with the date, time of collection, patient's name, and clinic or case number.
8. Refrigerate or freeze the sample as appropriate.

Heparin is relatively expensive and may interfere with some chemical assays. For example, it may cause falsely increased inorganic phosphorus levels in blood or may interfere with lactate dehydrogenase activity.

ETHYLENEDIAMINETETRAACETIC ACID.   Ethylenediaminetetraacetic acid (EDTA) is the anticoagulant of choice for hematologic studies because it does not alter cell morphology. It should not be used if plasma samples are to be used for chemical assays. EDTA is available as a sodium or potassium salt and prevents clotting by forming an insoluble complex with calcium, which is necessary for clot formation. To prevent clotting, EDTA is added at 1 to 2 mg/ml of blood to be collected. Vacuum collection tubes containing the proper amount of EDTA are commercially available.

The disadvantages of using EDTA for chemical assays are the following:
- May interfere with color development in some alkaline phosphatase tests
- Binds metallic ions that may be necessary for enzyme activity
- Binds calcium, making it unavailable for assay

OXALATES.   Oxalates are available as sodium, potassium, ammonium, or lithium salts. They prevent clotting by forming insoluble complexes with calcium, which is necessary for clot formation. Potassium oxalate is the most commonly used oxalate salt. To prevent clotting, it is used at 1 to 2 mg per milliliter of blood to be collected. Vacuum collection tubes containing the proper amount of oxalate anticoagulant are available commercially.

Unfortunately oxalates also may bind metallic ions necessary for enzyme activity. Potassium oxalate may inhibit lactate dehydrogenase and alkaline phosphatase activity. Also, because it is a potassium salt it cannot be used with blood samples to be assayed for potassium.

SODIUM FLUORIDE.   Sodium fluoride, best known as a glucose preservative, also has some anticoagulant properties. As an anticoagulant it is used at 6 to 10 mg/ml of blood to be collected. Vacuum collection tubes containing the proper amount of sodium fluoride for anticoagulation are available commercially. Sodium fluoride also may be added to other samples as a glucose preservative even if a different anticoagulant is present. For glucose preservation, sodium fluoride is used at 2.5 mg/ml of blood.

Sample Volume

The amount of blood collected from an animal depends on the quantity of serum or plasma required for the assay and the hydration status of the patient. For example, a well-hydrated animal with a PCV of 50% should yield a blood sample that is 50% cells and 50% fluid. A 10-ml blood sample should yield 5 ml of fluid. In dehydrated animals, hemoconcentration results in a smaller ratio of fluid to cells. A dehydrated animal with a PCV of 70% yields a blood sample that is 70% cells and 30% fluid. This means that only 3 ml of fluid is obtained from a 10-ml blood sample.

As a rule of thumb, enough blood should be collected to yield enough serum, plasma, or whole blood to run all the planned chemical assays three times. This allows for technician error, instrument failure, or the need to dilute a sample without having to collect another sample from the animal.

Factors Influencing Results

Collection of a high-quality sample on which to perform an assay depends on a number of factors. Most adverse influences on sample quality can be avoided with careful consideration of sample collection and handling.

HEMOLYSIS.   When using a syringe for blood collection, the veterinary technician should avoid hemolysis. Hemolysis may result when a blood sample is drawn into a moist syringe, mixed too vigorously after sample collection, forced through a needle when transferring it to a tube, or frozen as a whole blood sample. A syringe must be completely dry before it is used because water in the syringe may cause hemolysis. The needle from a syringe must be removed before blood is transferred to a tube. Forcing blood through a small needle opening may rupture cells. When transferring a blood sample to a tube, the veterinary technician should expel the blood slowly from the syringe without causing bubbles to form.

   Hemolysis, regardless of cause, can greatly alter the makeup of a serum or plasma sample. For example, fluid from ruptured blood cells can dilute the sample, resulting in falsely lower concentrations of constituents than are actually present in the animal. Certain constituents, normally not found in high concentrations in serum or plasma, escape from ruptured blood cells, causing falsely elevated concentrations in the sample. Hemolysis may elevate levels of potassium, organic phosphorus, and certain enzymes in the blood. Hemolysis also interferes with lipase activity and bilirubin determinations. For this reason, plasma or serum is frequently the preferred sample over whole blood, and serum is frequently preferred over plasma.

CHEMICAL CONTAMINATION.   Sterile tubes are not necessary for collection of blood samples for routine chemical assays. However, the tubes must be chemically pure. Detergents must be completely rinsed from reusable tubes so that the detergents do not interfere with test results.

IMPROPER LABELING.   Serious errors may result if a tube containing the sample is not labeled immediately after the sample is collected. The tube should be labeled with the date, time of collection, patient's name, and clinic number. The veterinary technician should double check the sample identification with the request form, if one is used, as the sample is prepared and the test is run.

IMPROPER SAMPLE HANDLING.   Ideally, all chemical measurements should be completed within an hour of sample collection, which is not always feasible. In cases in which it is not feasible to complete measurements within an hour, samples must be properly handled and stored so that levels of their chemical constituents approximate those in the patient's body at the time of collection. Samples must not be allowed to become too warm. Heat may be detrimental to a sample, destroying some chemicals and activating others, such as enzymes. If a serum or plasma sample has been frozen, it must be thoroughly mixed after thawing to avoid concentration gradients. Table 3-1 lists the recommended storage time limits of samples.

TABLE 3-1

Storage recommendations for various constituents in serum or plasma promptly separated from blood cells

Constituent	20° C	0° to 4° C	−20° C	Comments
Alkaline phosphatase	7 days	7 days	1 month	Levels may increase after storage; if frozen, thaw and leave at 4° C until analyzed
Albumin	1 week[1] 4 days[2]	1 month[1] 4 days[2]	2 months[1] 11 days[2]	
ALT (GPT)	1 day	1 week	Unstable	Is not stable during thawing
Amylase	1 month 1 month	7 months 1 month	2 months 1 month	
AST (GOT)	2 days	2 weeks	1 to several months	
Bilirubin	—	1 week	3 months	Protect from light; unstable at room temperature
BUN	8 hours	10 days	Several months	Bacterial contamination should be avoided; store at 4° C or −20° C if longer storage required
Calcium	10 days	10 days	10 days	Cork stopper increases calcium levels
Chloride	Stable	Stable	Stable	

PATIENT INFLUENCES.　If practical, a sample should be obtained from a fasting animal. The blood glucose level can be elevated and the inorganic phosphorus level decreased immediately after a meal. Also, postprandial (after-eating) lipemia results in a turbid or cloudy plasma or serum. Water intake need not be restricted before obtaining a blood sample.

⊘ ENZYMOLOGY

Enzymes are proteins produced inside cells. They induce chemical changes in other substances (called *substrates*) but are not inherently changed. An enzyme may increase the rate of a biochemical reaction by acting as a catalyst to the reaction. Most enzymes are formed and function intracellularly, so they are found in highest concentrations within cells. For this reason, the blood level of most enzymes is low in a healthy animal. The blood level of an enzyme may be elevated if the enzyme has leaked out of damaged cells, or if the cells have increased production of the enzyme and the excess amount has leaked out of the cells into the blood.

TABLE 3-1

Storage recommendations for various constituents in serum or plasma promptly separated from blood cells—cont'd

Constituent	20° C	0° to 4° C	−20° C	Comments
Cholesterol	7 days	—	6 months	
CK	2 hours[3]	6 hours[3]	Unstable[3]	Analyze ASAP as some
	2 days[4]	1 week[4]	1 month[4]	isoenzymes are
				unstable
Creatinine	1 week	1 week	Stable	
Glucose	8 hours	72 hours	Stable	
	(24 hours[5])			
Gamma-GT	2 days	1 week	1 month	
Inorganic phosphorus	—	1 week	3 weeks	
Sorbitol dehydrogenase	Not recommended	2 days[6]	Not recommended	
Total protein	1 week	1 month	Stable	
Uric acid	8 hours[7]	1 week	2 months	

1 — When analyzed using dye-binding methods.
2 — When analyzed using electrophoresis.
3 — "Nonactivated" CK. Does not thaw well.
4 — "Activated" CK.
5 — Sodium fluoride-preserved samples.
6 — Levels drop appreciably. SDH not stable at any storage temperature.
7 — Recommended storage temperature if analyzed on the day of collection.
ALT, *Alanine aminotransferase;* AST, *Aspartate aminotransferase;* BUN, *Blood urea nitrogen;* Gamma-GT, *Gamma glutamyltranspeptidase.*

The substance on which an *enzyme (E)* works is called a *substrate (S)*. Each of many enzymes has a specific substrate. Each enzymatic reaction produces a specific *product (P)* from the interaction of substrate and enzyme. The reaction forms a product but no change in the enzyme.

S + E → P + E

Because blood levels of enzymes are so low, directly measuring enzyme concentrations is difficult. The tests performed to determine enzyme concentrations in blood indirectly measure the enzyme concentration present by directly measuring the enzymatic reaction.

◆ Endpoint versus Kinetic Assays

Enzyme assay methods are classified as *endpoint* or *kinetic*. With endpoint methods, the product formed from enzymatic action interacts with a reagent to produce a color complex. The amount of light absorbed by this color complex is proportional to the amount of color complex present, which indirectly reflects the concentration of the enzyme present in the sample. In other words, the intensity of the color reflects the amount of product produced as a result of the presence of enzyme.

Kinetic methods measure the rate of the enzymatic reaction while it is in progress and usually involve serial measurements of the product concentration per unit of time. The rate of product formation, and hence the rate of the reaction, is proportional to the amount of enzyme present. Enzymes are most active when the substrate concentration is high and the product concentration is zero. If the enzyme concentration in the patient sample exceeds the substrate available in the test reagents, the enzyme activity is no longer proportional to the product formed and the assay is invalid. (The substrate concentration has become a limiting factor to the enzymatic reaction.)

Substrate concentrations must be kept high enough so that they do not invalidate the measurement. Test kits are manufactured so that a large amount of substrate is initially present to avoid this problem. If the amount of enzyme present in the patient sample is doubled, the rate of the reaction is doubled and the amount of product formed is doubled, providing time is constant. If the amount of enzyme present in the patient sample is the same but the time is doubled, the amount of product doubles. Therefore if time and enzyme concentration are kept constant, the rate of the reaction may be determined.

◆ Factors Influencing Enzyme Activity

Enzyme activity may be inhibited by low temperatures and accelerated by high temperatures. Ultraviolet light and the salts of heavy metals, such as copper and mercury, retard enzymes. Enzymes, which are proteins, may be denatured by temperature and pH extremes or by organic solvents. Only a small change in an enzyme's polypeptide chain structure may cause it to lose activity, so samples for enzyme assay must be handled with care.

Each enzyme has an optimum temperature at which it works most efficiently. This temperature is typically listed in the instructions that accompany the test kit or analyzer. Most assays are performed at temperatures between 30° C and 37° C (86° F to 98.6° F). For every 10° C (18° F) above the optimal temperature, the enzymatic reaction doubles. Closely monitoring the incubator or water bath temperature used in enzyme assays is important.

Units of Measurement

Enzyme concentrations are measured as units of activity. These units of measurement may be confusing. For example, enzyme activity is proportional to the enzyme concentration only under certain conditions.

Each investigator who developed an enzymatic analytic method assigned his own unit of measurement to the results, which often reflected the developer's name: Bodansky, Somogyi, and Sigma-Frankel units. Because each of the assays was performed under different conditions (pH, temperature), it became difficult to correlate results reported in one unit to those of another. To avoid this confusion, the International Union

BOX **3-1** ──○

Factors for converting various enzyme units to International Units (IU)

Alkaline Phosphatase
Bodansky Units × 5.37 = IU/L
Shinowara-Jones-Reinhart Units × 5.37 = IU/L
King-Armstrong Units × 7.1 = IU/L
Bessey-Lowry-Brock Units × 16.67 = IU/L
Babson Units × 1.0 = IU/L
Bowers-McComb Units × 1.0 = IU/L

Amylase
Somogyi (saccharogenic) Units × 1.85 = IU/L
Somogyi (37° C; 5 mg starch/15 min/100 ml) × 20.6 = IU/L

Lipase
Roe-Byler Units × 16.7 = IU/L

Transaminases
Reitman-Frankel Units × 0.482 = IU/L
Karmen Units × 0.482 = IU/L
Sigma-Frankel Units × 0.482 = IU/L
Wroblewsky-La Due Units × 0.482 = IU/L

of Biochemistry established a unit of enzyme activity known as the *International Unit* (U or IU). Using this system enzyme concentration is expressed as mU/ml, U/L or U/ml. An International Unit is defined as that amount of enzyme, which, under given assay conditions, will catalyze the conversion of one micromole of substrate per minute. Box 3-1 shows how to convert various units to International Units.

Some laboratories have replaced the IU system with one better related to the Systeme Internationale (SI) set of basic units, which is based on the metric system. In this system the *katal* is the basic unit of enzyme activity, the amount of activity that converts 1 mole of substrate per second.

◆ Terms Used in Enzymology

Enzymes usually are named for the substrate on which they act or the biochemical reaction in which they participate. Most enzyme names end with the *-ase* suffix. For example, *lipase* is an enzyme that catalyzes biochemical reactions that result in the hydrolysis of lipids, or fats, to fatty acids, and lactate dehydrogenase participates in a reaction that involves oxidation, or dehydrogenation, of lactate to pyruvate.

Some enzymes found in different tissues occur as isoenzymes. An *isoenzyme* is one of a group of enzymes with similar catalytic activities but different physical properties. The serum concentration of an enzyme that occurs as isoenzymes is the total of the concentrations of all the isoenzymes present from various tissues. Identification of which isoenzyme is present in the sample also allows identification of the source of that particular isoenzyme. For example, serum alkaline phosphatase is found in many tissues, particularly osteoblasts, those cells involved in the production of bone and hepatocytes, those cells found in liver tissue. If the total serum alkaline phosphatase level is elevated, ascertaining if the increase is from damaged bone cells or damaged liver cells is impossible. However, if the respective levels of the various isoenzymes of alkaline phosphatase are assayed, levels of the isoenzyme from the damaged tissue are elevated, thus identifying the damaged tissue. The alkaline phosphatase assay performed in the practice laboratory is for total serum alkaline phosphatase because individual isoenzyme assay methods have not yet been developed for the practice laboratory.

REFERENCE RANGES

Reference ranges are also known as *normal values*. The reference range for a particular blood constituent is a range of values derived when a laboratory has repeatedly assayed samples from a significant number of clinically normal animals of a given species. Numerous medicine and clinical pathology books list the reference ranges of blood constituents for domestic species. Alternatively, reference ranges may be formulated by local diagnostic laboratories or in individual practice laboratories.

Establishing reference range values for any laboratory is time consuming and expensive. To establish a list of reference values for the laboratory, the veterinary technician would have to assay samples from a significant number of clinically normal animals. Some investigators recommend analysis of at least 20 animals and others more than 100 animals with similar characteristics. Other considerations include the variety of breeds and species most often seen in the veterinary practice; the gender and sexual status, such as intact or neutered, of the tested animals; the environment, including husbandry and nutrition, of these animals; and climate. Climate is a consideration because drastic seasonal changes may affect assay results.

Reference ranges have not been included in the following discussions of blood constituents because of the variations found among different geographic areas. In some areas of the country or in different laboratories, the reference ranges may be wider or narrower than published ranges. The staff members of each practice must decide which reference ranges most accurately reflect the values observed in their patients.

Sample preference varies with each instrument and each assay. One instrument may require whole blood as a sample for an assay. Another instrument may require heparinized plasma or serum. Sample preferences are not included in the following discussions.

Sample handling and special considerations are included in the following discussions as general guidelines. The veterinary technician should always check the test instructions for specific handling instructions or special considerations.

LIVER ASSAYS

The liver is the largest internal organ and is complex in structure, function, and pathology. It has many functions, including metabolism of amino acids, carbohydrates, and lipids; synthesis of albumin, cholesterol, and plasma protein, clotting factors; digestion and absorption of nutrients related to bile formation; secretion of bilirubin, or bile; and elimination, such as detoxification of toxins and catabolism of certain drugs. All of these functions are run by enzymatic reactions.

No single test is superior to any other for detecting hepatic disease. New tests are being developed to allow detection of hepatic disease before the liver is severely damaged.

◆ Enzymes Associated with Hepatocellular Damage

With this type of liver disease, the hepatocytes are damaged and enzymes leak out into the blood, causing a detectable rise in blood levels of enzymes associated with liver cells.

Alanine Aminotransferase

RATIONALE.   Alanine aminotransferase (ALT) was formerly known as *serum glutamic pyruvic transaminase (SGPT)*. In dogs, cats, and primates, the major source of ALT is the hepatocyte. For this reason it is considered a liver-specific enzyme in these species. Horses, ruminants, pigs, and birds do not have enough ALT in the hepatocytes for this enzyme to be considered liver-specific. Other sources of ALT are renal cells, cardiac muscle, skeletal muscle, and the pancreas. If any of these tissues is damaged, the blood level of ALT may rise. ALT is used as a screening test for liver disease because it is not precise enough to identify specific liver diseases. No correlation exists between the blood levels of the enzyme and the severity of hepatic damage.

SAMPLE HANDLING AND SPECIAL CONSIDERATIONS.   Hemolysis and lipemia should be avoided because they can artificially increase the enzyme concentration. Storage of samples at room temperature or in the refrigerator for 24 hours has no effect on results.

SAMPLE STABILITY.   Serum or plasma samples to be assayed for ALT may be stored for 1 day at 20° C and 1 week at 0° C to 4° C. Samples should not be frozen.

Aspartate Aminotransferase

RATIONALE.   Aspartate aminotransferase (AST) was formerly known as *serum glutamic oxaloacetic transaminase (SGOT)*. AST is present in hepatocytes but also is found in significant amounts in many other tissues, including erythrocytes, cardiac muscle, skeletal muscle, the kidneys, and the pancreas. Therefore AST is not considered liver specific. An increased blood level of AST may indicate nonspecific liver damage or may be caused by strenuous exercise or intramuscular injection. The most common causes of increased blood levels of AST are hepatic disease, muscle inflammation or necrosis, and spontaneous or artifactual hemolysis. If the AST level is elevated, the serum or plasma sample should be examined grossly for visible hemolysis. One may check for hemolysis by performing a hematocrit on the patient's whole blood.

SAMPLE HANDLING AND SPECIAL CONSIDERATIONS.   Hemolysis and lipemia result in elevated blood concentrations of AST. AST levels also are elevated if the blood sample was stored before assay. Because the upper acceptable limit of AST concentration in horses is much higher than for other species, test methods developed for species other than horses may not be suitable for use in equine samples.

SAMPLE STABILITY.   Samples for AST analyses can be stored for 2 days at 20° C, for 2 weeks at 0° C to 4° C, and for several months at −20° C.

Sorbitol Dehydrogenase

RATIONALE.   The primary source of sorbitol dehydrogenase (SD) is the hepatocyte. It is present in the hepatocytes of all common domestic species but is especially useful for evaluating liver damage in large animals, such as sheep, goats, swine, horses, and cattle. Large animal hepatocytes do not contain diagnostic levels of ALT, so SD offers a liver-specific diagnostic test. The plasma level of SD rises with hepatocellular damage or necrosis. SD assay can be used in all species to detect hepatocellular damage or necrosis, thus eliminating the need for other tests, such as ALT assay. The disadvantage of SD analysis is that SD is unstable in serum and its activity declines rapidly. Samples should be assayed for SD within 12 hours of collection. SD tests are not readily available to the average veterinary laboratory.

SAMPLE HANDLING AND SPECIAL CONSIDERATIONS.   SD is an unstable enzyme and its activity deteriorates rapidly. Samples should be analyzed within 12 hours after collection. Hemolysis does not appear to affect results.

Glutamate Dehydrogenase

RATIONALE.   Glutamate dehydrogenase (GD) is found in high concentrations in the hepatocytes of cattle, sheep, and goats. An increase in this enzyme is indicative of hepatocyte damage or necrosis in cattle and sheep. GD could be the enzyme of choice for evaluating ruminant liver function, but no standardized test methodology has been developed for use in a veterinary practice laboratory.

◆ Enzymes Associated with Cholestasis

Blood levels of certain enzymes become elevated with cholestasis (bile duct obstruction) or a metabolic defect in liver cells.

Alkaline Phosphatase

RATIONALE.   Alkaline phosphatase (AP) is present as isoenzymes in many tissues, particularly osteoblasts in bone, chondroblasts in cartilage, and cells of the hepatobiliary system in the liver. Because AP occurs as isoenzymes in these various tissues, the source of an isoenzyme or location of the damaged tissue may be determined by special analytic methods in commercial or research laboratories.

In young animals, most AP comes from osteoblasts and chondroblasts because of active bone development. In older animals, most AP comes from the liver as bone development stabilizes. Assay for AP in a practice laboratory determines the total blood AP concentration.

AP concentrations are most often used to detect cholestasis in dogs and cats. Because of wide fluctuations in normal blood AP levels in cattle and sheep, this test is not as useful for detecting cholestasis in these species.

SAMPLE HANDLING AND SPECIAL CONSIDERATIONS.   Sample hemolysis or storage at room temperature for 24 hours has little effect on results. However, samples kept at room temperature for more than 24 hours may show an increased AP value. EDTA or oxalate anticoagulants should not be used.

SAMPLE STABILITY.   Samples for AP analysis can be stored for 8 days at 20° C (a slight rise may be seen after 2 to 3 days), 8 days at 0° C to 4° C, and 8 days at −20° C.

Gamma Glutamyltranspeptidase

RATIONALE.   Gamma glutamyltranspeptidase (GGT) is sometimes referred to as *gamma glutamyltransferase*. GGT is found in many tissues, but its primary source is the liver. Cattle, horses, sheep, and goats have higher blood GGT activity than dogs and cats. Other sources of GGT include the kidneys, pancreas, intestine, and muscle cells. The blood GGT level is elevated with liver disease, especially with obstructive liver disease.

SAMPLE HANDLING AND SPECIAL CONSIDERATIONS.   Hemolysis does not affect test results, but prolonged contact with erythrocytes may affect results.

SAMPLE STABILITY.   Samples for GGT determination can be stored for 2 days at 20° C, 1 week at 0° C to 4° C, and 1 month at −20° C.

◆ Other Tests of Liver Function

Various other tests may be used to evaluate liver function. Only bile acids and bilirubin analysis are discussed here. Other liver function tests are discussed in Chapter 8.

Bile Acids

RATIONALE.   Bile acids are synthesized from cholesterol in liver cells. After synthesis they are secreted into the bile canaliculi and stored in the gall bladder (except in the horse) until they are carried in bile to the duodenum. There the bile acids aid in fat digestion. Bile acids are reabsorbed in the terminal ileum and carried back to the liver by the portal circulation, where they are again secreted back into bile. Only 5% to 10% of the bile acids are lost in feces and need to be replaced by new synthesis.

Normally the serum level of bile acids in peripheral blood is low because the liver effectively removes 75% to 90% of the bile acids being returned to the liver from the ileum via the portal circulation. The serum bile acid level is elevated normally after a meal because the gall bladder has contracted and released increased amounts of bile into the duodenum. For this reason blood drawn for bile acid testing needs to be from a fasting animal. An elevated serum bile acid level may indicate a liver or portal circulation abnormality.

Elevated serum bile acid levels indicate liver diseases such as congenital portosystemic shunts, chronic hepatitis, hepatic cirrhosis, cholestasis, or neoplasms. Bile acid levels are unspecific regarding the type of liver problem that exists and are therefore used as a screening test for liver disease. Bile acid levels may detect liver problems before an animal becomes icteric (see Bilirubin). They also may be used to follow the progress of liver disease during treatment.

SAMPLE HANDLING AND SPECIAL CONSIDERATIONS.   Samples for bile acid assay should be drawn from a fasting animal. Hemolysis and lipemia may falsely decrease measurements.

SAMPLE STABILITY.   Information regarding sample stability is not available.

Bilirubin

RATIONALE.   Bilirubin is a metabolite of the heme portion of hemoglobin. When red blood cells die, the pigment portion of heme, or porphyrin, is metabolized to bilirubin, which is considered a waste material. Bilirubin is carried to the liver bound to the plasma protein albumin. Until it is taken into the liver, bilirubin is insoluble in water and must be bound to water-soluble albumin to stay in solution. After it is taken into the hepatocytes it is conjugated with certain sugars, especially glucuronic acid, or glucuronate, and becomes water soluble. To be eliminated from the body, bilirubin is carried to the intestines by the bile, where it is converted to urobilinogen by bacterial enzymes. Some of the urobilinogen is resorbed back into portal circulation and carried back to the liver. Some of this reabsorbed urobilinogen escapes into peripheral blood and is carried to the kidneys for elimination. The urobilinogen that remains in the intestines is converted to urobilin and is eliminated in feces.

Unconjugated and conjugated bilirubin are found in plasma. Assays can directly measure total bilirubin (conjugated bilirubin plus unconjugated bilirubin) and conjugated bilirubin. Conjugated bilirubin is sometimes referred to as *direct bilirubin* because test methods directly measure the amount of conjugated bilirubin in the sample. Unconjugated bilirubin is sometimes referred to as *indirect bilirubin* because its concentration is indirectly calculated by subtracting the conjugated bilirubin concentration from the total bilirubin concentration of the sample.

Bilirubin is assayed to determine the cause of jaundice, to evaluate liver function, and to check the patency of bile ducts. Blood levels of conjugated (direct) bilirubin are elevated with hepatocellular damage or bile duct injury/obstruction. Blood levels of unconjugated (indirect) bilirubin are elevated with excessive erythrocyte destruction or defects in the transport mechanism that allow bilirubin to enter hepatocytes for conjugation.

SAMPLE HANDLING AND SPECIAL CONSIDERATIONS. Hemolysis produces artificially low values if the diazo assay method is used. The test instructions should be consulted. Lipemic blood samples should not be used. Because bilirubin is sensitive to light, samples should be stored in the dark. Direct exposure to sunlight for an hour may decrease a sample's bilirubin level by up to 50%. Unconjugated bilirubin is more light sensitive than conjugated bilirubin.

SAMPLE STABILITY. Samples for bilirubin determinations are not stable when stored at 20° C. Samples protected from light can be stored for 2 weeks at 0° C to 4° C and up to 3 months at −20° C.

KIDNEY ASSAYS

The kidneys play a major role in maintaining homeostasis in animals. Their primary functions are to conserve water and electrolytes in times of a negative balance and increase water and electrolyte elimination in times of a positive balance; excrete or conserve hydrogen ions to maintain blood pH within normal limits; conserve nutrients, such as glucose and proteins; remove the end products of nitrogen metabolism, such as urea, creatinine and allantoin, so that blood levels of these end products remain low; produce renin (an enzyme involved in controlling blood pressure), erythropoietin (a hormone necessary for erythrocyte production), and prostaglandins (fatty acids used to stimulate contractility of uterine and other smooth muscle, lower blood pressure, regulate acid secretion in the stomach, regulate body temperature and platelet aggregation, and control inflammation); and aid in vitamin D activation.

Urine and blood may be analyzed to evaluate kidney function. Chapter 5 details urinalysis procedures and Chapter 8 specific kidney function tests.

Blood Urea Nitrogen

Some references use the term *serum urea nitrogen* (SUN) instead of *blood urea nitrogen* (BUN).

RATIONALE. Urea, a nitrogenous compound, is a product of amino acid breakdown in the liver. BUN levels are used to evaluate kidney function based on the ability of the kidney to remove nitrogenous waste (urea) from blood. This renal function test is not very sensitive; about 75% of the kidney tissue must be nonfunctional before elevated values are detected. In healthy animals, urea is passively filtered out of plasma by the renal glomeruli. Some urea returns to the blood through the renal tubules but most is excreted in the urine. If the kidney is not functioning properly, sufficient urea is not removed from the plasma, leading to increased BUN levels.

SAMPLE HANDLING AND SPECIAL CONSIDERATIONS. Hemolysis has little effect on results. High-protein diets may cause an elevated BUN level because of increased amino acid breakdown, not because of decreased glomerular filtration. Postprandial (after-eating) lipemia may result in a turbid final solution if a "wet" chemistry assay system, which uses liquid reagents, is used. A "dry" chemistry assay system uses dry reagents.

Contamination of the blood sample with urease-producing bacteria (e.g., *Staphylococcus aureus, Proteus* spp., and *Klebsiella* spp.) may result in decomposition of urea and subsequently decreased BUN levels. To prevent this, analysis should be completed within several hours of collection or the sample should be refrigerated.

SAMPLE STABILITY.   Samples for BUN determination can be stored for 8 hours at 20° C, 10 days at 0° C to 4° C, and several months at −20° C.

Creatinine

RATIONALE.   Creatinine is formed from creatine, which is found in skeletal muscle, as part of muscle metabolism. Creatinine diffuses out of the muscle cell and into most body fluids, including blood. If physical activity remains constant, the amount of creatine metabolized to creatinine remains constant and the blood level of creatinine remains constant. The creatinine in blood is filtered through the glomeruli and eliminated in urine. Creatinine also may be found in sweat, feces, and vomitus and may be decomposed by bacteria.

Blood creatinine levels are used to evaluate renal function, based on the ability of the glomeruli to filter creatinine from blood and eliminate it in urine. Like BUN, creatinine is not an accurate indicator of kidney function because nearly 75% of the kidney tissue must be nonfunctional before blood creatinine levels rise. Creatinine blood levels are not affected by a high-protein diet.

SAMPLE HANDLING AND SPECIAL CONSIDERATIONS.   Hemolysis has little effect on results.

SAMPLE STABILITY.   Samples may be stored for 1 week at 30° C to 37° C and almost indefinitely at −20° C.

PANCREAS ASSAYS

The pancreas is actually two organs, one exocrine and the other endocrine, held together in one stroma. The endocrine part of the pancreas is involved with carbohydrate metabolism through secretion into the blood of insulin, which lowers blood glucose levels, and glucagons, which elevate blood glucose levels. This is discussed later in this section and in Chapter 8.

The exocrine part of the pancreas secretes an enzyme-rich juice that contains enzymes necessary for digestion into the small intestine. The three primary pancreatic enzymes are trypsin, amylase, and lipase.

◆ Trypsin

Rationale

Trypsin is a proteolytic enzyme that aids digestion by catalyzing the reaction that breaks down the proteins of ingested food. Trypsin activity is more readily detectable in feces than in blood. For this reason, most trypsin analyses are done on fecal samples. Trypsin is normally found in feces, and its absence is abnormal.

Two fecal test methods are used in the laboratory: the test tube method and the x-ray film test. The test tube method involves mixing fresh feces with a gelatin solution (Knox gelatin). The test solution does not become a gel if trypsin is present in the sample to break down the protein (gelatin). If trypsin is absent, the solution becomes a gel. The x-ray film test uses the gelatin coating on undeveloped x-ray film to test for the presence of trypsin. A strip of x-ray film is placed in a slurry of feces and bicarbonate solution. If trypsin is present in the fecal sample, the gelatin coating is removed from the film upon rinsing with water. If no trypsin is present, the gelatin coating remains on the film after rinsing. The test tube method is considered more accurate than the x-ray film test in evaluating fecal trypsin proteolytic activity.

Sample Handling and Special Considerations

Only fresh feces should be used. Fecal trypsin activity may be decreased if the patient has recently eaten raw egg whites, soybeans, lima beans, heavy metals, citrate, fluoride, or some organic phosphorus compounds. Calcium, magnesium, cobalt, and manganese in the feces may increase trypsin activity. Proteolytic bacteria in the fecal sample may result in false-positive, or apparently normal, results, especially in older samples.

Sample Stability

Veterinary technicians should not use fecal samples more than 1 day old. Proteolytic bacteria in the feces may cause false-positive results.

◆ Amylase

Rationale

The primary source of amylase is the pancreas. Its function is to break down starches and glycogen in sugars, such as maltose and residual glucose. Increased levels of amylase appear in blood during acute pancreatitis, flare-ups of chronic pancreatitis, or obstruction of the pancreatic ducts.

Two amylase test methods are available: the saccharogenic method and the amyloclastic method. The saccharogenic method measures production of reducing sugars as amylase catalyzes the breakdown of starch. The amyloclastic method measures the disappearance of starch, as it is broken down to reduce sugars through amylase activity.

The rise in blood amylase level is not always directly proportional to the severity of pancreatitis. Determinations of blood amylase and lipase activities are usually requested at the same time to evaluate the pancreas.

Sample Handling and Special Considerations

Calcium-binding anticoagulants, such as EDTA, should not be used because amylase requires the presence of calcium for activity. Hemolysis may result in falsely elevated amylase levels. Lipemia may reduce amylase activity. The saccharogenic method is not recommended for canine samples because maltase in canine samples may artificially elevate assay results. Normal canine and feline amylase values can be up to 10 times higher than those in humans. Therefore samples may have to be diluted if tests designed for human samples are used.

Sample Stability

Samples can be stored for up to 7 days at 20° C and up to 1 month at 0° C to 4° C.

◆ Lipase

Rationale

The primary source of lipase is the pancreas. The function of lipase is to break down the long-chain fatty acids of lipids. Blood levels of lipase increase during episodes of pancreatitis. Test methods for determination of lipase levels usually are based on hydrolysis of an olive oil emulsion into fatty acids using the lipase present in patient serum. The quantity of sodium hydroxide required to neutralize the fatty acids is directly proportional to lipase activity in the sample. Most of these test procedures are time consuming.

Lipase assay may be more sensitive for detecting pancreatitis than amylase assay. The degree of lipase activity, like amylase activity, is not directly proportional to the severity of pancreatitis. Determinations of blood lipase and amylase activities usually are requested at the same time to evaluate the pancreas.

Sample Handling and Special Considerations

Calcium-binding anticoagulants, such as EDTA, should not be used. Hemolysis and lipemia should be avoided.

Sample Stability

Samples for lipase assay may be stored for 1 week at 20° C and 3 weeks at 0° C to 4° C.

◆ Glucose

Rationale

The blood glucose level is used as an indicator of carbohydrate metabolism in the body and may also be used as a measure of endocrine function of the pancreas. The blood glucose level reflects the net balance between glucose production, such as dietary intake and conversion from other carbohydrates, and glucose utilization, which is expended energy and conversion to other products. It also may reflect the balance between blood insulin and glucagon levels.

Glucose utilization depends on the amount of insulin and glucagon produced by the pancreas. As the insulin level increases, so does the rate of glucose utilization, resulting in decreased blood glucose levels. Glucagon acts as a stabilizer to prevent blood glucose levels from becoming too low. As the insulin level decreases (as in diabetes mellitus), so does glucose utilization, resulting in increased blood glucose concentration.

Sample Handling and Special Considerations

Serum and plasma must be separated from the erythrocytes immediately after blood collection. Glucose levels may drop 10% an hour if the sample of plasma is left in contact with erythrocytes at room temperature. Mature erythrocytes use glucose for energy, and, in a blood sample, they may decrease the glucose level enough to give false-normal results if the original sample had an elevated glucose level. If the sample originally had a normal glucose level, erythrocytes may use enough glucose to decrease the level to below normal or to zero. If the plasma cannot be removed immediately, the anticoagulant of choice is sodium fluoride at 6 to 10 mg/ml of blood. Sodium fluoride may be used as a glucose preservative with EDTA at 2.5 mg/ml of blood.

Refrigeration slows glucose utilization by erythrocytes. Hemolysis does not affect results. Eating raises the blood glucose level; therefore samples should be taken from fasted animals if possible.

Sample Stability

Samples for blood glucose determination can be stored for 8 hours at 20° C and 72 hours at 0° C to 4° C. The stability of frozen samples has not been determined. A sample should not be thawed and refrozen more than once.

MISCELLANEOUS CHEMISTRY ASSAYS

◆ Creatine Kinase

Rationale

Creatine kinase (CK) was previously known as creatine phosphokinase (CPK). It is produced primarily in striated muscle cells and, to some extent, in the brain. CK is considered one of the most organ-specific enzymes available for clinical evaluation. When skeletal muscle, including cardiac muscle, is damaged or destroyed, CK leaks out of the cells and produces an elevated blood CK level. Although the brain produces some CK, how much CK from the brain actually enters the peripheral circulation is uncertain. CK is frequently assayed if an animal has an elevated blood AST level but shows no clinical signs of liver disease.

Although the CK assay is an organ-specific assay, it cannot determine which muscle has been damaged or indicate the severity of the muscle damage. Anything that damages the muscle cell membrane can cause an increased blood CK level. This damage may stem from intramuscular injections, persistent recumbency, surgery, vigorous exercise, electric shock, laceration, bruising, and hypothermia. Myositis and other myopathies also cause elevated blood CK levels.

CK levels in samples may be artificially increased by oxidizing agents, such as bleach; EDTA; citrate; fluoride; exposure to sunlight; or delay in assay.

Sample Handling and Special Considerations

Hemolysis does not affect results. CK is unstable, so samples should be assayed as soon as possible after collection. The sample should be kept away from ultraviolet light.

Sample Stability

CK is an unstable enzyme; the sample should be analyzed as soon as possible. Samples must not be frozen.

◆ Cholesterol

Rationale

Cholesterol is produced in almost every cell in the body and is especially abundant in hepatocytes, the adrenal cortex, ovaries, testes, and intestinal epithelium. The liver is the primary site of synthesis in most animals.

Cholesterol assay is sometimes used as a screening test for hypothyroidism. Thyroid hormone controls synthesis and destruction of cholesterol in the body. Insufficient thyroid hormone, or hypothyroidism, results in hypercholesterolemia because the rate of cholesterol destruction is relatively slower than the rate of synthesis. Other diseases associated with hypercholesterolemia include hyperadrenocorticism, diabetes mellitus, and nephrotic syndrome. Dietary causes of hypercholesterolemia are rare but may include high-fat diets or postprandial lipemia.

Cholesterol by itself does not cause the grossly lipemic plasma seen after eating; triglycerides also are usually present. Administration of corticosteroids also may cause an elevated blood cholesterol concentration.

Sample Handling and Special Considerations

The test instructions must be consulted for recommendations on sample handling. Hemolysis may elevate colorimetric test results. Fluoride and oxalate anticoagulants may elevate enzymatic method results.

Sample Stability

Blood samples for cholesterol determinations can be stored for 48 hours at 20° C without separating serum or plasma from the cells. Samples are very stable at 20° C if serum or plasma is removed from the cells and are stable for weeks at −20° C.

PLASMA PROTEIN ASSAYS

Plasma proteins are produced primarily by the liver and the immune system, consisting of reticuloendothelial tissues, lymphoid tissues, and plasma cells. Proteins have many functions in the body:
- Help form the structural matrix of all cells, organs, and tissues
- Maintain osmotic pressure
- Serve as enzymes for biochemical reactions
- Act as buffers in acid-base balance
- Serve as hormones
- Function in blood coagulation
- Defend the body against pathogenic microorganisms
- Serve as transport/carrier molecules for most constituents of plasma

More than 200 plasma proteins exist. Some plasma protein concentrations change markedly during certain diseases and can be used as diagnostic aids. Other protein concentrations change little during disease. The most commonly assayed plasma proteins are albumin, fibrinogen, and globulins.

◆ Total Protein

Rationale

Total *plasma* protein measurements include fibrinogen values, whereas total *serum* protein determinations measure all the protein fractions except fibrinogen, which is removed during the clotting process. The total protein concentration may be affected by altered hepatic synthesis, altered protein distribution, and altered protein breakdown or excretion, dehydration, or overhydration.

Total protein concentrations are especially valuable in determining an animal's state of hydration. A dehydrated animal usually has a relatively elevated total protein concentration, whereas an overhydrated animal usually has a relatively decreased total protein concentration. Total protein concentrations also are useful as initial screening tests for patients with edema, ascites, diarrhea, weight loss, hepatic and renal disease, and blood clotting problems.

Two methods are commonly used for determination of total protein levels: the refractometric method and the biuret method. The refractometric method measures the refractive index of serum or plasma using a refractometer. This method is a good screening test because it is fast, inexpensive, and accurate. The biuret method measures the peptide bonds of the protein in serum or plasma. This method is commonly used in analytic instruments in the laboratory. It is a simple method and yields accurate results.

Sample Handling and Special Considerations

Although moderate sample hemolysis does not affect results, marked hemolysis falsely increases total protein values. Lipemic samples should not be used, especially with a refractometric method. Moderate icterus has no effect on the refractometric method. Heat, ultraviolet light, surfactant detergents, and chemicals can break down proteins, leading to artificially low results.

Sample Stability

Information of sample stability is not available.

◆ Albumin

Rationale

Albumin is one of the most important proteins in plasma or serum. It makes up 35% to 50% of the total plasma protein in most animals, and any significant state of hypoproteinemia is most likely caused by albumin loss. Hepatocytes synthesize albumin, and any diffuse liver disease may result in decreased albumin synthesis. Renal disease, dietary intake, and intestinal protein absorption also may influence the plasma albumin level. Albumin is the major binding and transport protein in the blood and is responsible for maintaining osmotic pressure of plasma.

Sample Handling and Special Considerations

Hemolysis may increase the apparent albumin level if the bromocresol green method is used. The test instructions for the method used should be consulted. The sample must be kept covered to prevent dehydration, which can falsely elevate protein levels.

Sample Stability

Samples for albumin determinations can be stored for 1 week (2 days on the clot has no effect) at 20° C, 1 month at 0° C to 4° C, and indefinitely at −20° C.

◆ Globulins

Rationale

The globulins are a complex group of proteins. Alpha globulins are synthesized in the liver and primarily transport and bind proteins. Two important proteins in this fraction are high-density lipoproteins (HDL) and very low-density lipoproteins (VLDL). Beta globulins include complement (C3, C4), transferrin, and ferritin. They are responsible for iron transport, heme binding, and fibrin formation and lysis. Gamma globulins (immunoglobulins) are synthesized by plasma cells and are responsible for antibody production (immunity). Immunoglobulins identified in animals are IgG, IgD, IgE, IgA, and IgM.

Serum protein assays can be performed with serum protein electrophoresis. The principle of electrophoresis is based on the migration patterns of the different serum protein fractions in an electrically charged field. A specific medium is used to trace the migration. The migration pattern depends on the electrical charge, size of the protein molecule, intensity of the electric field, and medium used. Electrophoretic techniques are not normally employed in a practice laboratory.

Because direct assay methods for globulins are often beyond the capabilities of a practice laboratory, indirect measurements are often used. The total *serum* protein concentration minus the albumin concentration gives an approximation of the total *serum* globulin concentration.

◆ Albumin-to-Globulin Ratio

An alteration in the normal albumin-to-globulin (A:G) ratio is frequently the first indication of a protein abnormality. The ratio is analyzed in conjunction with a protein profile. The A:G ratio can be used to detect increased or decreased albumin and globulin concentrations. Many pathologic conditions alter the A:G ratio.

The A:G ratio is determined by dividing the albumin concentration by the globulin concentration. In dogs, horses, sheep, and goats, the albumin concentration is usually greater than the globulin concentration (A:G ratio is more than 1.00). In cattle, pigs, and cats, the albumin concentration is usually equal to or less than the globulin concentration (A:G ratio is less than 1.00).

◆ Fibrinogen

Rationale

Fibrinogen is synthesized by hepatocytes. It is the precursor of fibrin, the insoluble protein that forms the matrix of blood clots, and is one of the factors necessary for clot formation. If fibrinogen levels are decreased, blood does not form a stable clot or does not clot at all. Fibrinogen makes up 3% to 6% of the total plasma protein content. Because it is removed from plasma by the clotting process, no fibrinogen is found in serum. Acute inflammation or tissue damage may elevate plasma fibrinogen

Hyperphosphatemia is an increased serum or plasma phosphorus concentration. Hypophosphatemia is a decreased serum or plasma phosphorus concentration.

Sample Handling and Special Considerations

Hemolyzed samples should not be used. The organic phosphorus liberated from the ruptured erythrocytes may be hydrolyzed to inorganic phosphorus, which results in a falsely elevated inorganic phosphorus concentration. The serum or plasma should be separated from the blood cells as soon as possible after blood collection and before the sample is stored.

Sample Stability

Samples for phosphorus determinations can be stored for 3 to 4 days at 20° C, 1 week at 0° C to 4° C, and 3 weeks at −20° C.

◆ Sodium

Rationale

Sodium is the major cation of plasma and interstitial, or extracellular, fluid. It plays an important role in water distribution and body fluid osmotic pressure maintenance. In the kidney, sodium is filtered through the glomeruli and resorbed back into the body through the tubules in exchange, as needed, for hydrogen ions. In this manner, sodium plays a vital role in pH regulation of urine and acid-base balance. Sodium concentrations are measured by flame photometry, which is usually not available in practice laboratories, or by dry reagent testing. *Hypernatremia* refers to an elevated blood level of sodium. *Hyponatremia* is a decreased blood level of sodium.

Sample Handling and Special Considerations

The sodium salt of heparin should not be used as an anticoagulant because it can falsely elevate the results. Hemolysis does not significantly alter results, but it may dilute the sample with erythrocyte fluid, causing falsely lower results.

Sample Stability

Information regarding sample stability for sodium analysis is not available.

◆ Potassium

Rationale

Potassium is the major intracellular cation and is important for normal muscular function, respiration, cardiac function, nerve impulse transmission, and carbohydrate metabolism. In acidotic animals, potassium ions leave the intracellular fluid as they are replaced by hydrogen ions, resulting in elevated plasma potassium levels, or hyperkalemia. The plasma potassium level also may be elevated in the presence of cellular damage or necrosis, which causes release of potassium ions into the blood. Decreased plasma potassium levels, or hypokalemia, may be associated with inadequate potassium intake, alkalosis, or fluid loss resulting from vomiting or diarrhea.

Sample Handling and Special Considerations

Plasma is the preferred sample because platelets may release potassium during the clotting process, causing artificially elevated potassium levels. Hemolysis should be avoided because the concentration of potassium within erythrocytes is higher than the concentration in plasma. Hemolysis releases potassium into the plasma, resulting in artificially elevated potassium levels. The sample should not be refrigerated until the plasma has been separated from the cells, because cooler temperatures promote loss of potassium from the cells without evidence of hemolysis. Samples should not be frozen without first separating the blood cells because the resulting hemolysis makes the sample unsuitable for testing.

Sample Stability

Information on sample stability for potassium analysis is not available.

◆ Magnesium

Rationale

Magnesium is the fourth most common cation in the body and the second most common intracellular cation. Magnesium is found in all body tissues. More than 50% of the magnesium in the body is found in bones, closely related to calcium and phosphorus. Magnesium activates enzyme systems and is involved in production and decomposition of acetylcholine. Imbalance of the magnesium:calcium ratio can result in muscular tetany from release of acetylcholine. Cattle and sheep are the only domestic animals that show clinical signs related to magnesium deficiencies.

Hypermagnesemia refers to an elevated blood magnesium level. Hypomagnesemia is a decreased blood magnesium level.

Sample Handling and Special Considerations

Anticoagulants other than heparin may artificially decrease the results. Hemolysis may elevate the results through liberation of magnesium from erythrocytes. Storage of sample without first separating out the blood cells does not appear to affect results. Unlike calcium concentrations, magnesium concentrations are not affected by contact with cork stoppers.

Sample Stability

Information regarding the stability of magnesium after storage at room, refrigerator, and freezer temperatures is not available.

◆ Chloride

Rationale

Chloride is the predominant extracellular anion. It plays an important role in maintenance of water distribution, osmotic pressure, and the normal anion:cation ratio. Chloride is usually included in electrolyte profiles because of its close relationship to sodium and bicarbonate levels. *Hyperchloremia* is an elevated blood chloride level. *Hypochloremia* is a decreased blood chloride level.

Sample Preference

Serum is the sample of choice. Heparinized plasma is preferred over EDTA plasma.

Sample Handling and Special Considerations

Hemolysis may affect test results by diluting the sample with erythrocyte fluid. Prolonged storage without first separating out the blood cells may cause slightly low results.

Sample Stability

Chloride samples are stable at room, refrigerator, and freezer temperatures if the serum or plasma is separated from the blood cells.

◆ Bicarbonate

Rationale

Bicarbonate is the second most common anion of plasma. It is an important part of the bicarbonate/carbonic acid buffer system and aids in transport of carbon dioxide from the tissues to the lungs. These functions help keep the body pH in balance as acids and bases are continually introduced into the body. The kidney regulates bicarbonate levels in the body by excreting excesses after it has resorbed all that is needed. Bicarbonate levels are frequently estimated from blood carbon dioxide levels. The bicarbonate level is about 95% of the total carbon dioxide measured.

Arterial blood is the sample of choice for bicarbonate determinations. If plasma is used, lithium heparinate is the anticoagulant of choice.

Sample Handling and Special Considerations

The sample should be chilled in ice water to prevent glycolysis from altering the acid-base composition. Freezing the sample results in hemolysis. Most test methods require incubation at $37°$ C.

Sample Stability

Bicarbonate analysis should be completed as soon as possible.

Recommended Reading

Burtis CA, Ashwood ER: *Tietz fundamentals of clinical chemistry,* ed 5, Philadelphia, 2001, WB Saunders.

Duncan JR, Prasse KW, Mahaffey EA: *Veterinary laboratory medicine: clinical pathology,* ed 3, Ames, Iowa, 1994, Iowa State University Press.

Henry JB: *Clinical diagnosis and management by laboratory methods,* ed 20, Philadelphia, 2001, WB Saunders.

Kaneko JJ: *Clinical biochemistry of domestic animals,* ed 5, San Diego, 1997, Academic Press.

Meyer DJ, Harvey JW: *Veterinary laboratory medicine interpretation and diagnosis,* ed 2, Philadelphia, 1998, WB Saunders.

Sirois M: *Veterinary clinical laboratory procedures,* St Louis, 1995, Mosby.

Willard MD, Tvedten H, Turnwald GH: *Small animal clinical diagnosis by laboratory methods,* ed 3, Philadelphia, 1999, WB Saunders.

CHAPTER 4

Diagnostic Microbiology

MUHAMMED IKRAM

The veterinarian's ability to diagnose, evaluate, and manage microbial diseases is enhanced through use of laboratory tests. Often the accuracy and value of these tests depend upon the abilities of the veterinary technician responsible for the laboratory. Veterinary technicians employed in veterinary clinics should be competent to perform such microbiologic procedures. A direct Gram's stain of a clinical specimen sometimes permits tentative identification of an organism. More often, culture on an appropriate medium is essential for both tentative and final identification. In addition, subjective judgment is required for interpretation of Gram's stains, examination of colonies on culture media, and interpretation medium changes and results of other biochemical tests.

EQUIPMENT AND SUPPLIES

◆ The Laboratory

Ideally the practice facility should have a separate room for microbiologic procedures. The room should have good lighting and ventilation; a washable floor and limited traffic; at least two benches, one for processing the samples and one for culture work, with smooth surfaces that are easily disinfected; gas and electrical outlets; ample storage space; and easy access to an incubator and a refrigerator.

◆ Materials for Submitting Samples to a Diagnostic Laboratory

The following materials should be available for submitting microbiologic samples to a diagnostic laboratory:
- Sterile cotton-tipped swabs
- Culturette swabs in transport medium
- Plastic specimen bags

- Sterile screw-capped containers (100 to 200 ml)
- Sterile screw-capped tubes or bottles (10 ml)
- Scissors, forceps, scalpel with blades (stored in 70% alcohol and flamed to sterilize)
- "Discard jar" containing disinfectant for contaminated instruments
- Small hacksaw to cut bone specimens
- Wooden tongue depressors for handling fecal specimens
- Bunsen burner (natural gas or propane gas)
- Racks to hold tubes and bottles
- Refrigerator "cold packs" and polystyrene shipping containers

◆ Stains and Culture Supplies

Supplies for staining and culture of bacteriologic samples are discussed in Bacteriology on p. 107.

◉ LABORATORY SAFETY

Most of the microorganisms encountered in the microbiology laboratory are potentially pathogenic. Therefore the safety of every person working in the laboratory depends on strict observance of rules.

- Veterinary technicians must wear a clean, long-sleeved, knee-length, white laboratory coat to prevent contamination of street clothes and dissemination of pathogens to the general public. Laboratory coats should be washed weekly in hot water and strong bleach. If the coat becomes soiled during daily diagnostic procedures, it is removed immediately and placed in the receptacle designated for dirty linens. All laboratory coats should be washed together. At no time should laboratory coats be mixed with other laundry from the veterinary clinic or with laundry from outside the laboratory.
- Eating, drinking, smoking, handling contact lenses, and applying cosmetics are not permitted in the laboratory. Appropriate signage should state this rule. Persons who wear contact lenses in the laboratory also should wear goggles or a face shield.
- Bench tops are cleaned with disinfectant at the beginning and end of the work period.
- Long hair is tied back or tucked inside the laboratory coat.
- No objects (pencil, fingers) should be put in the technician's mouth while working in the laboratory. Labels should be moistened with water, not with the technician's tongue.
- All containers of cultures of suspected or known pathogens should be taped shut before disposal.
- Spilled cultures are treated with disinfectant and allowed contact for 20 minutes before they are cleaned up.
- Wire loops contaminated with inocula are flamed immediately after use.
- Aseptic technique is always observed when transferring or working with infectious agents or specimens.
- Gas, water, and electrical appliances must be turned off in the laboratory before all staff members leave.

- Contaminated materials (plates, test tubes, slides, pipettes, and broken glass) are placed in appropriate containers for disposal, never in the trash receptacle.
- Mouth pipetting is never used in the microbiology laboratory. Automatic or bulb pipetting devices are used instead.
- The veterinary technician must wash hands thoroughly before leaving the laboratory.
- No food is stored in the laboratory; instead it is stored outside the laboratory in designated cabinets or refrigerators.
- All accidents are reported promptly to the laboratory supervisor or to the veterinarian.

BACTERIOLOGY

◆ Collecting Specimens

Proper collection of a specimen is critical to provide valuable diagnostic information. No matter how good the methods used in the laboratory, satisfactory results are impossible to obtain with samples collected improperly.

The specimen selected must contain the organism causing the problem. Normal flora and contaminants may complicate sample collection and subsequent interpretation of results. The following guidelines apply to proper specimen collection:

1. A complete history and sufficient clinical data must be obtained to help select procedures most appropriate to isolate organisms that may be present. Required data include the owner's name, clinic name, address, and phone number. Species, name, age, sex, number of animals affected or dead, duration of the problem, and major signs observed also should be included. The tentative diagnosis, organism suspected, any treatment given, and type of laboratory investigation required should be included in the record.
2. The specimen must be collected aseptically. Specimen contamination is the most common cause of diagnostic failure. The importance of aseptic collection of microbiologic specimens cannot be overemphasized. Samples should be collected as soon as possible after the onset of clinical signs.
3. Multiple specimens must be kept separate to avoid cross contamination. This practice is essential for intestinal specimens because of the flora that is normally present there.
4. The specimen container is labeled, especially if a zoonotic condition is suspected, such as anthrax, rabies, leptospirosis, brucellosis, or equine encephalitis. Tissues in suspected zoonoses should be submitted in a sealed, leakproof, unbreakable container.
5. The reference laboratory should be consulted for advice on specimen collection and the most appropriate selection of specimen or submission procedure, if necessary.
6. Adequate time should be taken. Obtaining results quickly at the expense of accuracy is counterproductive.
7. The specimen should be sent to the diagnostic laboratory by the fastest possible means. If the sample will be arriving during a weekend, the laboratory staff should be informed ahead of time so that arrangements may be made for pickup.
8. The results should be discussed with the veterinarian promptly in a clear, concise manner. Failure to do so reflects adversely on both the veterinarian and the laboratory.

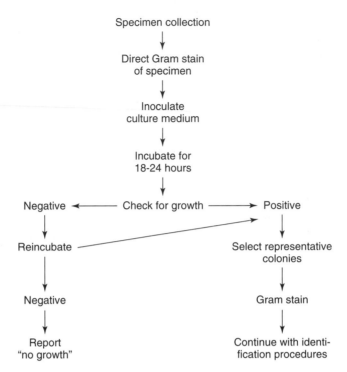

Figure 4-1
Typical sequence of procedures used in processing microbiologic specimens.

Figure 4-1 shows the typical sequences of procedures used in processing micro-biologic specimens.

Abortion Specimens

A range of specimens is particularly important in cases of abortion. Specimens should include a small piece of placenta with one or two cotyledons, fetal stomach contents, amniotic fluid, and a piece of fetal liver, lungs, and spleen. For large animal fetuses aborted before 7 months of gestation, the entire fetus should be sent. The specimens are packed in a leakproof container with several cold packs. If infectious bovine rhinotracheitis is suspected, the technician should submit pieces of lung and liver and a nasal wash.

Sometimes seroconversion coincident with abortion, as in bovine virus diarrhea or brucellosis, may provide more conclusive evidence of the cause than isolation of pathogens. Therefore paired serum samples, one collected at the time of abortion and the other 10 to 14 days later, are required. If leptospirosis is suspected, a midstream urine sample and clotted blood sample should be submitted with placenta and fetal urine.

Leptospirosis Specimens

In diagnosing leptospirosis in cattle, a midstream urine sample is preferred to one collected by catheter. Urination may be stimulated by massaging the cow's vulva.

Another method involves asking the farmer to retain the cows in a nearby corral until the veterinary technician arrives. Then the cows are run into the shed, where a veterinary technician is waiting for urine collection. This procedure induces a few to urinate spontaneously.

The easiest container for collection of a midstream urine sample is an approximately 200-ml plastic container. Then 20 ml is decanted into a screw-capped bottle containing 1.5 ml of 10% formalin. This should be performed within 10 minutes of collection or the *Leptospira* organisms may die and disintegrate. The formalin kills the leptospires but preserves their morphology.

When attempting to diagnose leptospirosis, veterinary technicians should collect paired blood and urine samples from clinically ill animals and from at least 10 animals that have been in contact with them. Suspected brucellosis and leptospirosis samples must be handled with caution.

Milk Specimens

Milk is cultured to identify the organisms that cause mastitis. If milk samples are not collected aseptically, microorganisms from the skin of the udder and from the air may contaminate the specimen, making culture results erroneous. If possible, milk samples should be collected from the cow after mastitis is noticed and before treatment is commenced. Culturing samples within 3 days of the last treatment usually results in a negative culture and meaningless findings. The udder should not be washed before obtaining samples unless it is dirty. The udder may be washed with warm water and disinfectant at the recommended strength. The veterinary technician should dry the udder and teats thoroughly with single-service paper towels.

Using 70% ethyl alcohol or 70% to 90% isopropyl alcohol, veterinary technicians should wipe the two teats farther from them first and then the two nearer teats, taking care to swab the teat sphincter. Sterile bottles or tubes with screw caps should be used for collection. Containers such as plastic bags (e.g., Ziploc bags) are not satisfactory.

The collection tube is held as near to horizontal as possible. The first few squirts of milk from each teat are discarded and then a little milk from each quarter is directed into a separate tube that has been labeled. Samples are taken from the two nearer teats first and then the farther ones so that the arm does not accidentally brush against the disinfected teats before samples are collected. The samples should be collected as quickly as possible with caution not to contaminate the cap of the container. The forefinger should be held against the palm of the hand taking the sample, while the thumb is used to collect the milk. Screening of samples with the California mastitis test before culturing is recommended.

The milk samples are refrigerated, not frozen, as soon after collection as possible until they can be cultured. If mastitis resulting from *Mycoplasma* species is suspected, ampicillin may be added at 1 to 10 mg per milliliter of milk sample to control contaminant bacteria. These milk samples are kept at room temperature so that the *Mycoplasma* species can multiply in the sample. Another milk sample should be taken without adding antibiotics to check for the more common mastitis-causing organisms, such as *Streptococcus agalactiae, Staphylococcus aureus, Streptococcus uberis, Escherichia coli,* and *Nocardia* species.

Urine Specimens

Normal voided urine may contain small numbers of bacteria. Differentiation of these small numbers from significant bacteriuria is important. Urinalysis therefore must be quantitative to yield meaningful results. Contamination with preputial or vulvar flora must be avoided. Ideally the vulva or prepuce should be thoroughly cleaned with detergent, after which at least 5 ml of a midstream sample are collected in a sterile tube. The presence of infection is determined from the number of organisms present. A bacterial count of at least 10,000/μl suggests an active infection. For diagnostic purposes, however, urine samples must be collected aseptically by catheter or cystocentesis. Midstream samples or samples collected by manual compression of the bladder are unacceptable.

Additional specimens should be submitted 72 to 96 hours after the start of antimicrobial therapy to monitor progress. Common pathogens isolated from urine samples include *E. coli, Staphylococcus aureus,* streptococci, and *Proteus* and *Pseudomonas* species.

Fecal Specimens

Feces should be collected in a fecal cup when freshly voided or directly from the rectum using aseptic precautions. In large animals, a disposable rubber glove or sleeve is useful. Once inverted and tied off, the glove may be submitted, containing the specimen. In small animals, a sterile cotton swab may be used to collect samples from the rectum; contamination of the swab with anal skin microflora is avoided. A sample of at least 1 g is needed for bacteriologic examination.

A single negative fecal culture does not rule out involvement of infectious agents, such as intermittent excretion of *Salmonella* species. Serial samples should be submitted. The most common organisms associated with intestinal infection are members of the family Enterobacteriaceae.

Specimens from Abscesses and Wounds

If the abscess has not ruptured, the area is shaved, swabbed liberally with alcohol, and allowed to dry. If the pus is liquid, a good sample may be obtained with a sterile syringe and wide-bore needle. When possible, scrapings are obtained from the wall of the abscess because causative organisms are more likely to be viable there. Several milliliters of material, rather than a swab sample, are collected for culture.

To culture wounds, the surrounding area should be disinfected and superficial debris lifted away. The surface of open wounds frequently contains contaminating bacteria. Gross observation of pus for color, odor, and presence of "sulfur granules" can be helpful, as is a direct smear for Gram's staining. The swab must be taken near the edge of a wound because the center frequently contains only necrotic debris. Abscesses are drained by aspiration as deeply as possible, avoiding the surface of the wound. The most common pathogens involved with abscesses and wounds are *E. coli* and *Staphylococcus, Streptococcus, Proteus, Pseudomonas, Nocardia, Corynebacterium, Fusobacterium,* and *Clostridium* species.

Specimens from the Eye

Organisms from the eye, such as *Moraxella* and *Streptococcus* species, are often fastidious. Culture of corneal scrapings is obtained best with a swab rolled into the conjunctival sac, or lachrymal secretions collected with a sterile swab by application of the specimen directly onto a blood agar plate. If this is not possible, the end of the swab is deposited into about 2 ml of sterile saline and cultured within 2 hours of collection. Other pathogens isolated from the eye include *E. coli* and *Staphylococcus, Pasteurella, Pseudomonas,* and *Chlamydia* species.

Genital Specimens

CERVICOVAGINAL MUCUS ASPIRATE.   Cervical mucus may be collected in a sterile artificial insemination pipette introduced through a speculum. A syringe attached to the pipette by a short length of rubber tubing is used to aspirate the mucus. About 3 ml should be collected and expressed into vials containing Cary-Blair, transport medium, a transport broth used for culture of *Campylobacter fetus* and other genital organisms. If *Taylorella equigenitalis* is suspected, use Amies transport medium containing charcoal.

VULVAR SWAB.   The Culturette swab (Marion Scientific, Kansas City, MO; Baxter, Mississauga, Ontario) should be applied to the vulvar mucosa, particularly around the clitoral fossa. The swab is then cultured for *Ureaplasma diversum* and *Mycoplasma* species. Swabs that cannot be sent to the laboratory on the same day of collection should be stored at 4° C and shipped at 4° C with an ice pack. If the sample is to be held more than 2 days, it should be stored and shipped frozen at −70° C. *Mycoplasma* species are sensitive to drying; therefore *dry swabs should not be submitted.* If mycoplasmal infection is suspected, tissue specimens are the preferred specimen. If swabs are submitted, they should be submitted only in Stuart agar medium (Fisher Scientific, Pittsburgh, PA).

Specimens from the Ear

Ear swabs are most often collected from dogs. Usually both ears should be individually swabbed because comparison of the cultured organisms helps differentiate normal from abnormal flora. Organisms commonly involved in ear infections are *Staphylococcus aureus, Pseudomonas aeruginosa, Malassezia pachydermatis,* and *Proteus* and *Streptococcus* species.

Culture of Anaerobes

Because most anaerobes survive exposure to air for less than 20 minutes, collection of samples for anaerobic culture on swabs is completely useless. Acceptable anaerobic specimens include the following: blocks of tissue (2-inch cube minimum) in a closed sterile container; material placed in Becton-Dickinson's Anaerobic Specimen Collector (bioMerieux, Hazelwood, MO); and pus and exudate collected in a sterile syringe, with the air expelled and the needle plugged with a rubber stopper or bent backward on itself.

Specimens should be cultured as soon as possible after collection. The specimen is inoculated onto a blood agar plate and into thioglycollate broth, which is a liquid medium used to grow anaerobes. The blood agar plates are put into an anaerobe jar, which provides an anaerobic environment during incubation. A self-contained system, such as a Gas Pack (Oxoid, Columbia, MD), may be used. In addition, other commercial anaerobe culture systems are available such as the API Anaerobic System. In cases in which demonstration of specific toxin is required, at least 20 ml of ileal contents or a loop of ileum with contents should be submitted.

Conditions in which isolation of anaerobes may be significant include soft-tissue abscesses, postoperative wounds, peritonitis, septicemia, endocarditis, endometritis, gangrene, pulmonary infection, and foot rot in cattle, sheep, and swine. The isolated anaerobe may be the sole etiologic agent or a partner in a synergistic relationship with another bacterium. For example, liver abscesses seen at slaughter in otherwise healthy feedlot cattle commonly yield the anaerobe *Fusobacterium necrophorum* and the aerobe *Actinomyces pyogenes.*

For conditions involving *Clostridium chauvoei, Clostridium septicum, Clostridium novyi,* and *Clostridium sordellii,* most laboratories use the fluorescent antibody technique in diagnosis. Specimens include affected muscle and a rib containing bone marrow.

◆ Interpreting Results of Bacteriologic Tests

A diagnosis of the cause of a disease is based on clinical signs, gross pathologic observations, the organisms isolated, and the results of other laboratory tests. However, the significance of the isolated organisms depends on whether the samples were collected aseptically. Also important are length of time elapsed between death and collection of specimens and the interval between collection and examination of the specimens. The following should be borne in mind:

- Some organisms, such as the family Enterobacteriaceae, are ubiquitous, and their isolation might merely represent postmortem invasion of tissues, fecal contamination of samples, or soil contamination.
- *Clostridium* species and other anaerobes are rapid postmortem invaders. Bone marrow is often the last tissue to be invaded, so an unopened rib containing bone marrow may be a useful specimen.
- Otherwise healthy animals excrete many organisms, such as *Salmonella* and *Leptospira* species. A distinction must be made between subclinical infection and disease.
- *Mycobacterium paratuberculosis* and *Salmonella* and *Leptospira* species often are excreted intermittently. Therefore collection of serial samples after a negative result is justified.
- The diagnosis of fungal infection must be made cautiously if the fungus is known to survive outside the animal body. Histopathologic examination may determine whether the organism was present as a contaminant or was invading the tissue.

Table 4-1 summarizes bacterial pathogens of veterinary importance, species affected, resultant diseases or lesions, and specimens required for diagnosis.

Text continued on p. 128.

TABLE 4-1

Summary of veterinary bacterial pathogens, animal species affected, resultant disease or lesions, and specimens for diagnosis

Organism	Species Affected	Disease or Lesion	Specimens
***Actinobacillus* Species**			
A. lignieresii	Cattle, sheep	Granulomatous lesions containing pus; most commonly affects tongue (wooden tongue); found in rumen and on tongues of normal animals	Fresh tissue and pus
A. equuli	Foals, occasionally pigs and calves	"Sleepy foal" disease; abortion, navel illnesses	Fresh liver, spleen, bone marrow; abortion material
A. suis	Young pigs, foals	Fatal septicemia in animals <6 weeks; arthritis, pneumonia, or abscesses in older animals	Fresh liver, spleen, bone marrow; lung, pus
A. seminis	Sheep	Epididymitis in rams	Fresh semen, testes epididymis
A. salpingitidis	Chickens	Salpingitis and peritonitis in chickens; also isolated from cloaca of healthy chickens	Fresh affected tissue
A. pleuropneumoniae	Pigs	Fibrinous pleuropneumonia	Suspect tissue
***Actinomyces* Species**			
A. bovis	Horses, cattle	Poll evil and fistulous withers can occur as mixed infection with *Brucella abortus*, mandibular osteomyelitis	Fresh tissue, pus
A. suis	Pigs	Chronic granulomatous and suppurative mastitis in sows	Milk
A. viscosus	Hamsters, dogs	Periodontal disease; chronic granulomatous pleuritis	Fresh tissue, pus
A. pyogenes	Cattle, sheep, pigs	Suppurative mastitis and pneumonia	Milk, pus, tissue

Continued

TABLE 4-1

Summary of veterinary bacterial pathogens, animal species affected, resultant disease or lesions, and specimens for diagnosis—cont'd

Organism	Species Affected	Disease or Lesion	Specimens
***Aeromonas* Species**			
A. hydrophila	Fish, reptiles, mammals, amphibians	Fish: generalized or localized infection, hemorrhagic septicemia; frogs: "red leg;" snakes: infectious stomatitis; mammals: neonatal infection in puppies; ubiquitous organism: may be primary or secondary pathogen	Fresh affected tissue
A. salmonicida	Trout, salmon	Furunculosis in trout and less commonly salmon	Fresh affected tissue or whole fish
***Bacillus* Species**			
B. anthracis	Cattle, sheep, pigs, people	Anthrax, fatal septicemia in sheep, cattle, pigs; acute pharyngitis with hemorrhagic swelling of throat region	Fresh blood smear from ear vein; collect tissues with great caution
B. cereus	People, cats, dogs	Can cause food poisoning	Fresh fecal material
***Bacteroides* Species**			
B. nodosus	Sheep	Foot rot in conjunction with *Fusobacterium necrophorum*	Fresh smear from lesion
B. melaninogenicus	Many species	Associated with other bacteria in such conditions as peritonitis, pericarditis, suppurative arthritis, and pneumonia	Fresh affected tissue
***Bordetella* Species**			
B. bronchiseptica	Pigs, dogs, lab animals	Atrophic rhinitis in pigs; respiratory infection in dogs, associated with distemper virus; snuffles in rabbits and guinea pigs	Fresh nasal swabs or lungs

Borrelia Species

B. anserine	Poultry	Fowl spirochetosis, a fatal disease of chickens, turkeys, geese, and other fowl; acute septicemia, diarrhea, and anemia; transmitted by fowl ticks	Fresh blood, spleen, or liver smears
Other *Borrelia* species	Pigs, cattle	Associated ulcerative granuloma after trauma	Fresh scrapings or biopsy material
		Enzootic/foothill abortion	Fetal blood

Brucella Species

B. abortus	Cattle, pigs, sheep, goats	Abortion; orchitis	Fresh fetal stomach contents, placenta, blood serum, milk, testes
	Horses	Chronic bursitis, fistulous withers, poll evil	Fresh material from lesions
B. melitensis	Goats, sheep, cattle	Abortion	As under *B. abortus*
B. ovis	Sheep	Abortion; epididymitis in rams	Fresh testes
B. suis	Pigs, occasionally cattle	Abortion; orchitis in boars	Fresh uterus, spleen, lymph nodes, semen, testes in boars
	Horses	Bursitis	Fresh material from lesions
B. canis	Dogs	Abortion (Beagles); infertility; epididymitis; orchitis	Fresh blood serum, lymph nodes, bone marrow

Campylobacter Species

C. fetus ss *fetus*	Cattle	Abortion; infertility; fecal-oral route	Fresh vaginal mucus
C. fetus ss *fetus*	Sheep	Epizootics of abortion in sheep; oral infection; resides in intestine of cattle and sheep	Fetal stomach, cotyledons

Continued

TABLE 4-1

Summary of veterinary bacterial pathogens, animal species affected, resultant disease or lesions, and specimens for diagnosis—cont'd

Organism	Species Affected	Disease or Lesion	Specimens
C. fetus ss veneralis	Cattle	Abortion; infertility; venereal infection	Fresh vaginal mucus
C. fetus ss jejuni	Sheep, cattle	Epizootics of abortion; oral infection; healthy carriers, with organisms in intestinal tract	Rectal swabs or feces
C. sputorum ss mucosalis	Piglets	Pigs 2 to 6 weeks after weaning; hemorrhagic proliferative enteropathy; necrotic ileitis and watery diarrhea	Cannot be seen in fresh feces or ileal scrapings; need fixed ileal sections
Chlamydia Species			
C. Psittaci (various strains)	Ewes	Enzootic abortion	Cotyledon, vaginal swab
	Cats	Feline pneumonitis (conjunctivitis, fever, ocular discharge)	Fresh conjunctival scrapings
	Wild and domestic birds, people	Psittacosis/ornithosis—psittacine and other birds	Liver, spleen, kidney, lungs (can ship frozen)
	Cattle	Sporadic bovine encephalomyelitis; serofibrinous peritonitis is typical	Brain, fixed and fresh
	Sheep, calves, pigs (experimental infection in dogs)	Transmissible serositis (polyarthritis)	Synovial fluid or tissue; isolation/stained smears; diagnostic probability in neonates if arthritis is present without navel infection
	Cattle	Epizootic bovine abortion; tick transmitted; not demonstrated experimentally; may need other agents in addition to *Chlamydia* species	Cotyledon, vaginal swab, fetal lung and liver

Clostridium Species

C. *Botulinium* (Types A-G)	Many species	Botulism—types of most importance: A, B, & E—people Cα—wild fowl, pheasants, chickens Cβ—mink, cattle, horses (forage poisoning) D—cattle (South Africa) F—rare in people G—unknown pathogenicity	Fresh serum obtained before death; at necropsy: heart, blood and intestinal contents; suspect feed; presence of toxin must be demonstrated
Cl. chauvoei	Cattle, sheep	Blackleg or blackquarter; gas gangrene	Fresh bone marrow in unopened rib; piece of affected muscle and heart
Cl. septicum	Cattle, sheep, horses, pigs	Malignant edema; gas gangrene/septicemia	As above
	Sheep	Braxy—infection of mucosal and submucosal of abomasum	Fresh and formalinized affected tissue
	Chickens	Necrotic dermatitis—gangrenous necrosis of skin; can be caused by *Cl. novyi* and *Cl. perfringens*, Type A	Fresh affected tissue
Cl. novyi (edematiens) Type A	Cattle, sheep	Gas gangrene of wounds; "big head" of rams, wounds resulting from fighting	Fresh rib with bone marrow; tissue with lesion; liver or whole carcass

Continued

TABLE 4-1

Summary of veterinary bacterial pathogens, animal species affected, resultant disease or lesions, and specimens for diagnosis—cont'd

Organism	Species Affected	Disease or Lesion	Specimens
Type B	Sheep, cattle	"Black disease"—necrotic hepatitis; after fluke damage of liver	As above
Type C (Cl. bubalorum) (Cl. haemolyticum) (Cl. novyi Type D) Cl. perfringens Cl. welchii	Buffalos (Indonesia) Cattle, sheep	Osteomyelitis Bacillary hemoglobinuria or "red water disease," infarcts of liver are characteristic	As above
Type A	People	Food poisoning and gas gangrene; occasional cause of gas gangrene in animals	
Type B	Lambs	Lamb dysentery—severe enterotoxemia of neonates	
Type C	Sheep	"Struck"—acute intoxication	Fresh ileal contents for toxin demonstration; fixed kidney and brain
	Calves, lambs, young pigs	Hemorrhagic enterotoxemia	
Type D	Sheep, occasionally goats, calves	Pulpy kidney disease—enterotoxemia, with focal symmetric encephalomalacia	
Type E	Lambs, calves	Reputed toxemia; not common	
Types A, C	Young chickens	Necrotic enteritis—acute enterotoxemia	Fresh liver and intestine for culture; fixed affected intestine
Cl. tetani	All species	Tetanus	Diagnosis usually based on clinical signs; fresh pus or tissue from invasion site if obvious

Organism	Host	Disease/Condition	Specimen
***Corynebacterium* Species**			
C. bovis	Cattle	Found in mastitis milk samples; pathogenicity uncertain	Milk
C. pseudotuberculosis	Sheep	Caseous lymphadenitis	Fresh and fixed affected lymph nodes
C. renale	Cattle	Cystitis, renal abscess	Fresh urine, kidney, bladder; fixed kidney
C. pilosum	Cattle	Cystitis	Fresh urine, bladder
Rhodococcus equi	Foals	Suppurative bronchopneumonia, multiple abscesses, arthritis	Fresh tissue, joints, abscess wall, lymph nodes
	Pigs	Abscesses in mandibular lymph nodes	Fixed affected tissues
	Cattle	Can be isolated from TB lesions	
Eubacterium suis (anaerobe)	Pigs	Cystitis and pyelonephritis in pigs; occurs in semen	Fresh urine, kidney, bladder, semen; fixed kidney, bladder
C. kutscheri	Mice, rats	Caseopurulent foci in lungs, lymph nodes, liver, kidney, skin	Fresh affected tissue
***Dermatophilus* Species**			
D. congolensis	Cattle, horses, goats, sheep, polar bears	Dermatitis with scab formation and scab; fixed skin biopsy	Swab exudate, fresh plucked hair
***Erysipelotbrix* Species**			
E. rhusiopathiae	Pigs	Diamond skin disease—septicemia, endocarditis, arthritis	Fresh liver, spleen, heart, synovial fluid
	Sheep, cattle, Turkeys, other birds	Polyarthritis / Septicemia	Fixed skin, liver, kidney
***Escherichia* Species**			
Mainly young animals			
E. coli	Cattle, pigs	Calf scours; mastitis; piglet diarrhea; edema disease; hemorrhagic enteritis	Fresh feces, milk, urine, affected tissue
	Chickens	Air sacculitis; coligranuloma	Can be secondary agents and are rapid postmortem invaders

Continued

TABLE 4-1

Summary of veterinary bacterial pathogens, animal species affected, resultant disease or lesions, and specimens for diagnosis—cont'd

Organism	Species Affected	Disease or Lesion	Specimens
***Escherichia* Species—cont'd** Mainly young animals—cont'd *E. coli—*cont'd			
	Dogs	Urinary infections	
	Horses	Acute enterotoxemia in foals	
***Francisella* Species**			
F. tularensis	People, wild animals, domestic animals	Necrotic foci in liver and spleen of wild rabbits and other animals	Fresh liver, spleen; lymph nodes are not involved
***Fusobacterium* Species**			
F. necrophorum	Cattle	Principal agent of foot rot; necrobacillosis of liver in feedlot cattle (associated with *C. pyogenes*); calf diphtheria	Fresh pus or affected tissue; fixed affected tissue
	Sheep	Secondary invader in leg and lip ulceration; infectious bulbar necrosis (heel or foot abscess) in association with *C. pyogenes*	
	Goats	Associated with ulcerative stomatitis	
	Pigs	"Bull nose"—suppurative necrotic infection of nose and face; occurs after trauma	
	Horses	Involved in thrush	
	Fowl	Secondary invader of fowl pox virus lesions	
***Hemophilus* Species**			
H. somnus	Cattle	Infectious thromboembolic meningoencephalitis; pneumonia and polyserositis	Fresh and fixed affected tissue

H. suis and *H. parasuis*	Pigs	Glasser's disease (polyserositis)	
H. gallinarum and *H. paragallinarum* (only need V factor)	Poultry	Fowl (infectious) coryza (nasal discharge and edema of face)	
H. hemoglobinophilus	Dogs	Commensal in prepuce	
Klebsiella Species			
K. pneumoniae	Pigs, cattle	Mastitis	Fresh milk
	Horses	Cervicitis and metritis, septicemia in foals	Fresh liver, spleen, bone marrow
	Dogs	Pneumonia	Fresh lung
Leptospira Species			
L. interrogans	Cattle, sheep, pigs, horses	Cattle: hemoglobinuria and jaundice in calves; abortion, infertility, and agalactia in adults	Fresh kidney taken within 4 hours of death
L. Pomona	Cattle	Pigs: abortion in late pregnancy; kidney lesions in young animals	Urine: 10 ml placed immediately in 1.5 ml of 10% formalin
L. hardjo			
L. grippotyphosa	Cattle, pigs, horses	Horses: fever, jaundice, occasionally abortion and periodic ophthalmia	Fixed kidney, liver
L. icterohemorrhagiae	Cattle, pigs, dogs	Dogs: acute hemorrhagic and icteric disease with *L. icterohemorrhagiae*	
L. canicola	Cattle, pigs, dogs	Uremia or inapparent with *L. canicola*	
L. bratislava	Pigs	Abortion, mummified fetus, stillbirth	Fresh and fixed kidney, uterus, placenta
Listeria Species			
L. monocytogenes	Cows, sheep, occasionally horses, dogs	Abortion; encephalitis	Fresh abortion specimens, brain or liver
	Rabbits, pigs, lambs, raccoons	Liver necrosis	Fixed affected tissues
	Chickens, turkeys, cage birds	Septicemia; necrotic foci in liver and pericardium	

Continued

TABLE 4-1

Summary of veterinary bacterial pathogens, animal species affected, resultant disease or lesions, and specimens for diagnosis—cont'd

Organism	Species Affected	Disease or Lesion	Specimens
***Moraxella* Species**			
M. bovis	Cattle	Infectious keratoconjunctivitis (pink eye)	Fresh swab of eye discharges; place directly on 5% ox blood agar if possible, or place swab in a small amount of sterile saline for rapid transport to laboratory
***Mycobacterium* Species**			
M. bovis	Cattle, pigs, sheep, deer	Bovine-type tuberculosis; granulomas with caseation	Fresh and fixed lesions and affected tissue
M. avium	Pigs, poultry, horses, feral birds and animals	Avian-type tuberculosis; granulomas with caseation	
M. marinum	People, cold-blooded animals	"Swimming pool granuloma" in people	
M. lepraemurium	Rats	Rat leprosy—granulomas	
M. ulcerans	Cats	Skin granulomas that ulcerate	
M. paratuberculosis (*M. johnei*)	Cattle, sheep, goats	Johne's disease	Fresh feces, mesenteric lymph nodes, ileocecal valve or other affected gut; fixed intestine and mesenteric lymph nodes
***Mycoplasma* Species**			
M. mycoides ss *mycoides*	Cattle	Contagious bovine pleuropneumonia	Fresh swabs containing exudates from eye, nostril, trachea, and genitalia should be placed in tubes of *Mycoplasma* broth, chilled to 2° to 3° C and rapidly transported to the laboratory
M. bovis		Mastitis, arthritis, pneumonia	
M. dispar		Pneumonia (calves)	

Mycoplasma Species—cont'd

M. bovigenitalium		Arthritis, vaginitis, seminal vesiculitis	
M. californicum		Mastitis	
M. canadense		Mastitis	
M. bovoculi		Keratoconjunctivitis	
M. agalactiae	Sheep, cattle	Contagious agalactia	Milk
M. conjunctivae		Keratoconjunctivitis	Eyes
M. capricolum		Mastitis, polyarthritis, pneumonia	Exudate, milk
M. ovipneumoniae	Sheep	Pneumonia	Serum, fresh lungs
M. mycoides ss mycoides	Goats	Polyarthritis, septicemia, mastitis, pneumonia	Milk, exudate, fresh lungs
M. mycoides ss capri		Contagious caprine pneumonia	
M. putrefaciens		Mastitis, arthritis	
M. hyorhinis	Pigs	Polyserositis, arthritis (baby pigs)	
M. hyopneumoniae		Enzootic (viral) pneumonia	
M. hyosynoviae		Polyarthritis (12-24 weeks old)	
M. felis	Cats	Conjunctivitis	
M. cynos	Dogs	Pneumonia	
M. felis	Horses	Pleuritis	
M. gallisepticum	Chickens	Chronic respiratory disease	
M. synoviae	Chickens, turkeys	Infectious synovitis	
M. meleagridis	Turkeys	Air sacculitis, bursitis	

Nocardia Species

N. asteroides	Cattle	Acute and chronic mastitis	Fresh milk or affected tissue
	Dogs, cats, other animals	Localized granulomatous lesions with or without lymph node involvement; generalized disease with pneumonia in dogs	Fixed lung or other affected tissue

Continued

TABLE 4-1

Summary of veterinary bacterial pathogens, animal species affected, resultant disease or lesions, and specimens for diagnosis—cont'd

Organism	Species Affected	Disease or Lesion	Specimens
***Pasteurella* Species**			
P. multocida	Many animals	Frequently a secondary invader or opportunist; associated with shipping fever complex in cattle; snuffles ir rabbits; enzootic pneumonia in pigs; primary cause: fowl cholera; hemorrhagic septicemia of cattle; severe mastitis in cattle and sheep	Fresh and fixed lung and spleen or other tissue with lesions
P. hemolytica	Cattle, sheep, pigs, goats, poultry	Associated with pneumonia, shipping fever in cattle; salpingitis of fowl	
P. pneumotropica	Rodents	Pneumonia and abscesses	
P. gallinarum	Chickens	Upper respiratory infection in chickens	
P. anatipestifer	Ducklings	Septicemia in young ducks ("new duck disease")	
P. canis	Cats, dogs	Cellulitis; occasional lymphadenitis	
P. dagmatis	Cats, dogs	Cellulitis; local pain; full swelling	
***Pseudomonas* Species**			
P. aeruginosa	Many animals	Wound infections; bovine mastitis; otitis in dogs and cats; septicemia in chickens	Fresh swabs or affected tissue
P. pseudomallei	People, primates	Melioidosis or pseudoglanders	Fresh pus, nodules, or abscess wall
	Cattle, sheep, horses, dogs, cats, rodents	Septicemia of abscesses in lungs, liver, spleen, lymph nodes, subcutis	Fresh affected tissue
P. mallei	Horses, mules, donkeys	Glanders or farcy (eradicated in North America)	

***Ehrlichia* Species**			
Ehrlichia canis	Dogs	Recurrent tick-borne fever	Blood smear (optimal time 2 weeks postinfection)
Ehrlichia equi	Horses	Fever and edema of legs (California)	Blood smears in febrile period
Ehrlichia risticii	Horses	Potomac horse fever	Blood or buffy coat smear, paired serum samples
Neorickettsia helminthoeca	Dogs	"Salmon poisoning"; carried by metacercariae of intestinal fluke (NW USA)	Fluke eggs in feces, smears of fluid aspirated from mandibular lymph nodes
Colesiota conjunctivae	Sheep	Contagious ophthalmia	Smears from conjunctival scrapings
***Salmonella* Species**			
More than 1000 serotypes			
S. typhimurium	Cattle, sheep, pigs, horses, poultry	Acute septicemia, gastroenteritis	Fresh feces, mesenteric lymph nodes
S. dublin	Cattle		
S. abortus equi	Horses	Abortion	Fetal fluid, fetus, fetal membranes
S. abortus ovis	Cattle	Abortion	
S. bovismorbificans	Cattle	Enteritis	Feces
S. abortusovis	Sheep	Enteritis	Feces
S. choleraesuis	Pigs	Chronic enteritis	Feces
S. typhisuis	Young pigs		Feces
S. gallinarum	Chickens	Pullorum disease	Feces
S. pullorum			
S. arizonae	Chickens, turkeys	Septicema, enteritis	
S. enteritidis			
S. typhimurium	Chickens	Fowl typhoic	
***Serpulina (Treponema)* Species**			
Serpulina (Treponema) hyodysenteriae	Pigs	Swine dysentery (catarrhal hemorrhagic enteritis)	Fresh rectal swabs taken by Culturette swabs; section of spiral colon (3-4 inches) in plastic bag; hold at 0° to 4° C and send to laboratory with ice packs as quickly as possible; DO NOT FREEZE

Continued

TABLE 4-1

Summary of veterinary bacterial pathogens, animal species affected, resultant disease or lesions, and specimens for diagnosis—cont'd

Organism	Species Affected	Disease or Lesion	Specimens
***Staphylococcus* Species**			
S. aureus	Many animals	Suppurative wound infections; abscesses; mastitis	Fresh milk, wound, skin or abscess swabs
S. epidermidis	Many animals	Usually nonpathogenic, but some strains can cause abscesses and skin infections	
S. intermedius	Dogs	Skin infections	
S. hyicus	Pigs	Exudative epidermitis; "greasy pig disease" or impetigo	
***Streptococcus* Species** 18 serogroups:			
S. agalactiae (Group B)	Cattle, sheep, goats	Chronic mastitis	Milk, milk ducts
	Dogs	Neonatal septicemia	Exudate, urine, uterine discharge
	Cats	Kidney and urinary infections	
S. dysgalactiae (Group C)	Cattle	Mastitis (not a common cause)	
	Lambs	Polyarthritis	
S. equi ss equi (Group C)	Horses	Strangles, genital infection	Pus, lymph nodes, uterine or cervical swab
S. equi ss zooepidemicus (Group C)	Horses, cattle, pigs, poultry	Mastitis, abortion, navel infection	Milk, vulvar discharge
S. dysgalactiae ss equisimilis (Group C)	Horses	Abscesses, endometritis	Pus, exudate
Enterococcus fecalis (Group D)	Many species	Endocarditis, mastitis	Feces, milk, urine
S. durans (Group D)		Urinary infection	
S. porcinus (Group E)	Pigs	Jowl abscess, lymphadenitis	Pus, lymph nodes

Organism	Host	Disease	Specimen
***Streptococcus* Species—cont'd**			
S. canis (Group G)		Neonatal septicemia, genital infection	Pus, serum
S. suis (Group R)	Weaner pigs	Meningitis, arthritis, pneumonia	Nasal discharge
S. uberis			
S. pneumoniae	Calves, primates	Pneumonia, meningitis	Nasal discharge, respiratory mucus
***Taylorella* Species**			
T. equigenitalis	Horses	Contagious equine metritis; possible abortion	Fresh cervical or uterine swabs; sheath swabs; place in Amies' transport medium
***Ureaplasma* Species**			
U. diversum	Cattle, turkeys	Vulvovaginitis, pneumonia	
***Vibrio* Species**			
V. metschnikovii	Chickens	Acute gastroenteritis in young chickens	Fresh section of small intestine or whole bird
***Yersinia* Species**			
Y. pseudotuberculosis	Deer, birds, guinea pigs, sheep	Acute septicemic form or chronic with necrotic foci or abscesses through body; diarrhea	Fresh feces, intestine, lung, liver, spleen, lesions
Y. enterocolitica	Deer, birds, sheep, other animals	Enterocolitis	Fixed lung, liver, spleen, intestine, affected tissue

◆ Bacterial Cultures

Culture Supplies

Supplies and equipment needed for culturing and identification of bacteria include the following:

- Small incubator, set at 37° C (98.6° F)
- Small autoclave for preparing culture media and sterilizing instruments and other equipment
- Refrigerator for storing media, reagents, and specimens
- Balance for weighing media in milligrams and grams
- Bunsen burner
- Inoculating needle holders, loops, and 22-gauge nichrome wire
- Waterproof marking pens
- Scalpels, scissors, forceps, and spatulas
- Pasteur pipettes and rubber bulbs
- Pipetting syringe for dispensing liquid media (e.g., Cornwall pipetting syringe)
- Culture media in plates and tubes
- Antimicrobial sensitivity discs (for antibacterials commonly used in the practice)
- Sensitivity disc dispenser (BBL Microbiology Systems, Cockeysville, MD; Oxoid, Columbia, MD; Difco Laboratories, Detroit, MI)
- Distilled water
- Beakers, volumetric cylinders
- Flat-bottom flasks for preparing media from dehydrated powder
- Hot plate with a magnetic stirring facility (Fisher Scientific, Pittsburgh, PA)
- Screw-capped bottles and tubes for storing media
- Racks for bottles and tubes
- Carbon dioxide jar (BBL Microbiology Systems, Cockeysville, MD; Oxoid, Columbia, MD) for isolation of microaerophiles (alternatively, a 1-lb canning jar with a 1-inch piece of candle provides an atmosphere of about 2% carbon dioxide)
- Disinfectant solution for wiping bench surfaces
- Soap, paper towels, and paper towel dispenser
- Plain, sterile, cotton-tipped swabs
- API, Minitek (bioMerieux, Hazelwood, MO), Enterotube II, and urotube (BBL Microbiology Systems, Cockeysville, MD) identification systems
- Organisms for quality control (Difco Laboratories, Detroit, MI) (see following discussion)
- Disposal bin lined with autoclavable bags for disposal of cultures and other contaminated materials

Quality-Control Cultures

Some cultures are required in a laboratory for quality-control purposes. Various procedures and supplies must be monitored for quality and accuracy, including antibacterial susceptibility tests, media, biochemical tests, and certain tests for identification, such as the zone of beta hemolysis around *Staphylococcus aureus* for the CAMP test.

BOX 4-1

Commercial firms supplying microbiologic products

American Scientific Products[2]
1430 Wantegan Rd
McGaw Park, II 60085
(800) 233-4362

Baxter Diagnostic[1,2,3]
Canlab Div
2390 Argentia Rd
Mississauga, Ontario L5N 3P1
Canada
(800) 668-4666

BBL Microbiology Systems[1,6,7,11,13,14]
Div Becton, Dickinson
POB 243
Cockeysville, MD 21030
(800) 638-8663

bioMerieux Vitek, Inc[15]
595 Anglum Road
Hazelwood, MO 63042
(800) 638-4835

Burroughs Wellcome[10]
Wellcome Reagent Div
Order Dept, POB 1887
Greenville, NC 27834
(919) 758-3436 (Ext 2885/6)

Difco Laboratories[1,3,6,18]
POB 1058A
Detroit, MI 48232
(313) 961-0800

Fisher Scientific Company[2,3,6]
Corporate Headquarters
711 Forbes Ave
Pittsburgh, PA 15219
(412) 562-8300

General Scientific Products[a]
8741 Landmark Rd
POB 26509
Richmond, VA 23261
(804) 264-7560

1 - *Dehydrated and prepared culture media in plates and tubes.*
2 - *General laboratory supplies, equipment.*
3 - *Staining kit sets.*
4 - *"Culturette" swabs.*
5 - *Chemicals, laboratory antibiotics, dyes for staining.*
6 - *Antibiotic sensitivity discs.*
7 - *Anaerobic and carbon dioxide systems.*
8 - *Distilled water.*
9 - *Sterile blood.*
10 - *"Streptex" for Lancefield grouping.*
11 - *Minitek identification system.*
12 - *Canine brucellosis diagnostic test.*
13 - *Products obtained through distributors, such as Fisher Scientific or
     American Scientific.*
14 - *Urotube.*
15 - *Enterotube II.*
16 - *Virology supplies.*
17 - *Dermatophyte test medium.*
18 - *Optochin.*

Continued

BOX 4-1

Commercial firms supplying microbiologic products—cont'd

Gibco Products[1,3,8,9]
3175 Staley Rd
Grand Island, NY 14072
(800) 828-6686

Johns Scientific[1,2]
175 Hanson St
Toronto, Ontario
Canada
(800) 268-4410

Marion Scientific[4]
9233 Ward Pkwy
Kansas City, MO 64114
(800) 821-7772

NCS Diagnostic[16]
130 Matheson Blvd
Mississauga, Ontario L4Z 1Y6
Canada
(800) 268-2857

Oxoid USA[1,6,7]
9017 Red Branch Rd
Columbia, MD 21045
(410) 997-2216

Pitman-Moore[13,17]
421 E. Hawley St
Mundelein, IL 60060
(708) 949-3300

Sigma Chemical Co[5]
POB 14508
St. Louis, MO 63178
(800) 325-3010

A selection of control organisms can be obtained on discs from Difco Laboratories (Box 4-1). Media not containing fermentable sugars, such as trypticase soy agar (BBL Microbiology Systems, Cockeysville, MD) and maintenance medium (Difco Laboratories, Detroit, MI), are suitable for maintaining fewer fastidious organisms, such as *Staphylococcus aureus* and Enterobacteriaceae. The bacteria can be stab inoculated into a tube of medium and subcultured about every 2 months.

Streptococcus, Pasteurella, and *Actinobacillus* species die quickly on culture plates. Streptococci may be kept in a tube of cooked meat broth and subcultured about every 4 weeks. *Pasteurella* and *Actinobacillus* species remain viable if mixed with about 0.5 ml of sterile whole blood in a small tube and stored in a deep freeze at −10° C or lower. Otherwise these two genera should be subcultured on blood agar about every 3 days. Control cultures may be kept at room temperature in screw-capped tubes but preferably in a refrigerator at 4° C, which reduces the metabolic rate of the organisms.

Culture Media

Culture medium (plural, media) is any material, solid or liquid, that can support the growth of microorganisms. For bacteriology, culture media may be purchased as dehydrated powder or as prepared agar plates or ready-to-use media for biochemical tests. Most of the commonly used media now may be obtained already prepared from supply houses.

This form is probably most convenient for a small laboratory because preparation time is saved, the manufacturers attend to quality control, and small quantities can be obtained.

BASIC NUTRIENT MEDIA. Nutrient media typically contain peptone, salt, dextrose, water, meat extract, and a solidifying agent, such as agar or gelatin. *Peptone* is partially hydrolyzed protein that may be metabolized readily by bacteria to provide amino acids and other simple nitrogenous compounds. It is the principal nutrient of the medium and is needed for growth. Peptone has some buffering action and contains a considerable amount of inorganic salts. Salt is added to adjust the osmotic pressure of the medium so that it is isotonic for the bacterial cell. Dextrose is a source of carbon and energy for bacteria. Water is added to provide food material in solution form that can be used by bacteria. Usually, distilled water is used to ensure the uniformity of different batches of media. Meat extract provides water-soluble carbohydrates, nitrogen, and vitamins.

Solidifying agents include agar and gelatin. Agar is a dried extract of sea algae known as *agarphytes*. It is a long-chain nonnutrient polysaccharide not attacked by bacteria and is available as a fine, almost colorless powder. For solid medium, 1.5% agar is added; for semi-solid medium, 0.1% to 0.5% agar is added, depending on the degree of solidity required. Agar is a liquid at temperatures greater than 42° C and a solid at temperatures less than 42° C, which is an important consideration during media preparation. Gelatin is a protein obtained from animal tissues and solidifies when present in medium at 12% to 30% concentration. It has two disadvantages:

1. It melts at 28° to 31° C and therefore does not remain solid at 37° C (the usual temperature of bacterial incubation).
2. Bacteria attack the gelatin and liquefy it.

ENRICHED MEDIA. Enriched media are formulated to meet the requirements of the most fastidious pathogens. They are basic nutrient media with extra nutrients added, such as blood, serum, or egg. Examples include blood agar and chocolate agar.

SELECTIVE MEDIA. Selective media contain antibacterial substances, such as bile salts or antibacterials that inhibit or kill all but a few types of bacteria. They facilitate isolation of a particular genus from a mixed inoculum. Examples of selective media are brilliant green agar and MacConkey agar.

DIFFERENTIAL MEDIA. Differential media allow bacteria to be differentiated into groups by biochemical reactions on the medium. Simmons' citrate is a differential medium.

ENRICHMENT MEDIA. Enrichment media are liquid media that favor growth of a particular group of organisms. They contain nutrients that either encourage growth of the desired organisms or contain inhibitory substances that suppress competitors. Examples include tetrathionate broth and selenite broth.

SYNTHETIC MEDIA. Synthetic media are prepared exclusively from pure chemical substances, and their exact chemical composition is known. They are used mainly in experimental work, but a few used for biochemical tests might be included in this category. An example is Koser citrate broth (Difco Laboratories, Detroit, MI).

Preparation of Culture Media

The major firms supplying prepared and dehydrated media are BBL, Difco, Gibco, and Oxoid (see Box 4-1). When the veterinary technician is preparing media from dehydrated powder or granules, the manufacturer's instructions should be followed implicitly. The following directions are not meant to be comprehensive but emphasize important points for beginners preparing media that cannot be obtained commercially:

- Clean glassware is used, rinsed free of detergents and other chemicals. The glassware need not be sterile unless sterilized medium is being decanted into it.
- The appropriate amount of dehydrated medium is weighed and placed in a flask and distilled water is added.
- Distilled water, free from chlorine and heavy-metal ions that may inhibit bacterial growth, should always be used. Containers of distilled water may be obtained commercially.
- The medium is prepared in a container about twice the final volume of the medium, which allows adequate mixing and allows for frothing of the medium during heating.
- Media that do not contain agar usually may be dissolved with gentle agitation. Dehydrated media containing agar, however, are best dissolved by bringing the mixture to a boil, with continuous stirring using a glass rod or a hot plate that incorporates a magnetic stirrer system. Caking at the bottom of the flask may occur if stirring is not adequate.
- Once dissolved, dehydrated media usually are sterilized in an autoclave or pressure cooker at 121° C (15-lb pressure) for 15 minutes. However, some media contain ingredients that cannot tolerate this high temperature, and the manufacturer's instructions indicate the medium should be sterilized at 118° C or 115° C for a slightly longer time. Some selective media, such as brilliant green agar, may be sterilized by boiling for about a minute. *Agar media should be cooled, preferably in a water bath, to 50° to 56° C before the plates are filled.* Agar solidifies at 42° C. One liter of liquid agar medium usually makes 70 to 100 agar plates.
- Some additives to media may not tolerate boiling or autoclaving and therefore must be added after the media have been autoclaved and cooled. These additives must, of course, be sterile. Blood and serum are collected aseptically, whereas certain dyes and sugars are sterilized by passing them through a membrane filter of 0.2-μ pore size to remove bacteria.
- Commercial dehydrated media often contain buffering agents that keep the pH within a desired range (usually pH 6.8 to 7.2). However, as part of quality-control procedures, or if a medium is being prepared from basic ingredients, the pH of cooled media should be checked with an electronic pH meter, but pH paper strips also may be used. The pH is adjusted by adding drops of 1N or 0.1N NaOH or HCl.
- After the poured plates are set, they are allowed to dry at room temperature, or at 37° C for a few hours, to ensure that no surface moisture exists when used. The plates then may be placed in sealed plastic bags and stored in a refrigerator.

BLOOD AGAR. This enriched medium supports the growth of most bacterial pathogens. Trypticase soy agar, blood agar base, Columbia agar, or Eugon agar may be used. The last two base media have extra nutritive value. Bacterial colony size is often larger than when trypticase soy agar is used as the blood agar base.

The blood agar base, such as trypticase soy agar or Columbia agar, is prepared in the usual manner, sterilized, and cooled to 50° to 56° C. Sterile blood is added at 5% to 7%. Sheep blood usually is used because ovine blood accurately reflects hemolytic reactions and is available commercially. The blood may be collected aseptically from a healthy animal using a human donor set; otherwise 10% sodium citrate solution is used at a 1:10 ratio as an anticoagulant.

If the blood has been stored in the refrigerator, the blood should be warmed to room temperature or to 37° C in the incubator before it is added to the agar base. This step avoids thermal shock to the red blood cells. The blood and agar base are mixed before the plates are poured. If bubbles form on the surface of the poured plates, a low Bunsen flame is passed quickly across the surface of the plates before the agar sets. Blood agar should be bright red. A brownish-red color may indicate one or more of the following problems:

- The blood is too old and the red blood cells are hemolyzing.
- The blood was added to the agar base when the medium was too hot.
- Inadequate mixing of the blood with the agar base has prevented oxygenation of the red blood cells.
- Thermal shock has caused hemolysis because refrigerated blood was not warmed before adding it to the molten agar.

If the blood agar plates are contaminated, the veterinary technician should examine them to decide whether the contaminant bacterial colonies are throughout the medium or just on the surface. If colonies are evident throughout, the blood is probably contaminated and should be discarded. If the colonies are only on the surface of the medium, the plates were probably accidentally contaminated after pouring.

Blood agar acts as an enrichment medium and a differential medium because four distinct types of hemolysis can be detected on blood agar. The four types of hemolysis are as follows:

- Alpha (α) hemolysis, partial hemolysis that creates a narrow band of greenish or slimy discoloration around the bacterial colony
- Beta (β) hemolysis, complete hemolysis that creates a clear zone around the bacterial colony
- Gamma (γ) hemolysis, hemolysis that produces no change in the appearance of the medium and no hemolysis around colonies
- Delta (δ) hemolysis, also called *double-zone hemolysis,* a zone of hemolysis surrounded by a narrow zone of hemolysis around a bacterial colony

MACCONKEY AGAR. MacConkey agar is a selective and differential medium. It contains crystal violet, which suppresses growth of Gram-positive bacteria, and bile salts that are selective for Enterobacteriaceae, and a few other bile salt–tolerant Gram-negative bacteria. Growth or no growth on MacConkey agar may be used as a test for primary identification of Gram-negative genera.

The indicators in MacConkey agar are lactose and neutral red. Lactose-fermenting organisms, such as *E. coli* and *Enterobacter* and *Klebsiella* species produce acid from lactose and grow as pinkish-red colonies on this medium. Bacteria that cannot ferment lactose attack the peptone in MacConkey agar, producing an alkaline reaction and colorless colonies. Clinical specimens for routine isolation usually are cultured separately on both blood and MacConkey agars.

Examination of both blood and MacConkey agar cultures, inoculated with the same clinical specimen, can yield considerable information. For example, no growth on the MacConkey agar plate but good growth on the blood agar plate suggests that the isolated pathogen is probably Gram positive.

CHOCOLATE AGAR.   If *Hemophilus* infection is suspected, specimens also should be inoculated on a chocolate agar plate in addition to blood and MacConkey agar plates. In this very nutritive medium, hemolyzed red blood cells have released the "V" and "X" growth factors required by *Hemophilus* species. Hemolytic activity cannot be observed on chocolate agar. Growth of all *Hemophilus* species is enhanced by increased CO_2 tension; some require 10% CO_2 for growth.

BRAIN-HEART INFUSION BROTH.   Brain-heart infusion broth is a useful, general-purpose broth used to increase the number of organisms (preenrichment) before they are plated on solid medium. For example, isolation of *Listeria* species from brain specimens may be difficult, especially those from cattle, without preenrichment. Pieces of the patient's medulla and brainstem are finely cut up or homogenized, and a 10% to 20% suspension is made in the infusion broth. This is refrigerated at 4° C for up to 12 weeks. Subcultures are made on blood agar and MacConkey agar after 1, 3, 6, and 12 weeks of incubation.

Isolating *Listeria* from abortion cases or from animals with the visceral forms of listeriosis typically is not difficult. Specimens from these can be plated directly onto solid medium. Streptococci appear to be especially susceptible to desiccation. When a swab sample is the only specimen available, the likelihood of isolating streptococci may be enhanced by preenrichment. The swab is placed in about 10 ml of infusion broth and incubated at 37° C for 24 hours. A loopful of broth then may be plated out on solid medium.

If testing the sterility of dried milk powder, bone meal, or other substances that may have been subjected to heat treatment in processing, the veterinary technician should first place the sample in nutrient broth for 24 hours at 37° C and then plate it out on agar medium. In an attempt to isolate salmonellae from these samples, about 1 ml of broth is placed into 10 ml of tetrathionate broth for another 24 hours' incubation at 37° C before plating on selective medium.

For culture of blood samples, about 1 ml of the patient's blood sample is added to nutrient broth or a special blood culture medium, which can be obtained commercially. Because a patient's blood contains many substances inhibitory to bacteria, adding the blood sample directly to broth dilutes the effect of these natural inhibitors.

MANNITOL SALT AGAR.   Mannitol salt agar is not routinely used but is a highly selective medium for staphylococci and could be used to isolate *Staphylococcus aureus* from contaminated specimens. The medium has a high salt content (7.5%) and contains mannitol and the pH indicator phenol red. Staphylococci are salt tolerant. *S. aureus,* but usually not *Staphylococcus epidermidis,* ferments mannitol. The resulting acid turns *S. aureus* colonies and the surrounding medium yellow.

PURPLE BASE AGAR WITH MALTOSE.   Purple base agar with maltose is used for presumptive identification of staphylococci. *Staphylococcus aureus* ferments maltose and changes the medium's color from purple to yellow. *Staphylococcus intermedius* produces a slight color change and *Staphylococcus hyicus* produces no color change (i.e., it does not ferment maltose).

HEKTOEN ENTERIC AGAR.   Hektoen enteric agar has a high carbohydrate and peptone content to counteract the inhibitory effects of the bile salts and indicators also in the medium. It only slightly inhibits growth of *Salmonella* and *Shigella* yet still inhibits accompanying microorganisms.

Lactose-positive colonies are differentiated from lactose-negative colonies by the indicators bromthymol blue and acid fuchsin. Added carbohydrate, such as sucrose or salicin, which is fermented more easily than lactose, also further differentiates organisms. The combination of thiosulfate with ferric ammonium citrate causes hydrogen sulfide-producing colonies to become black.

The following summarizes the typical appearance of the more important bacterial organisms on Hektoen enteric agar and the appearance of their colonies.
- *Shigella* and *Providencia* species ⟶ Green, moist, raised colonies
- *Salmonella* and *Proteus* species ⟶ Blue-green, with or without a black center
- Coliforms (rapid lactose fermenters) ⟶ Salmon-pink to orange, surrounded by a zone of bile precipitate

BISMUTH SULFITE AGAR.   In this selective medium, freshly precipitated bismuth sulfite acts with brilliant green to suppress growth of coliforms while permitting growth of salmonellae. Sulfur compounds provide a substrate for hydrogen sulfide production. The metallic salts in the medium stain the colony and surrounding medium black or brown in the presence of hydrogen sulfide.

Atypical colonies may appear if the medium is heavily inoculated with organic matter. This situation may be prevented by suspension of the sample in sterile saline and use of the supernatant for inoculation.

The freshly prepared medium has a strong inhibitory action and is suitable for heavily contaminated samples. Storing the poured plates at 4° C for 3 days causes the medium to change color to green, making it less selective with small numbers of salmonellae being recovered.

The following summarizes the typical appearance of the more important bacterial organisms on bismuth sulfite agar and the appearance of their colonies:
- *Salmonella typhi* ⟶ Black "rabbit-eye" colonies, with surrounding black zone and metallic sheen after 18 hours; uniformly black after 48 hours' incubation
- Other *Salmonella* species ⟶ Variable colony appearance after 18 hours (black, green, or clear and mucoid); uniformly black colonies seen after 48 hours, often with widespread staining of the medium and a pronounced metallic sheen

- Other organisms (coliforms, *Serratia, Proteus* species) → Usually inhibited but occasionally dull green or brown colonies with no metallic sheen or staining of surrounding medium

UREA TUBES.   Urea slants are streaked with inoculum and incubated overnight at 37° C. Urea medium is a peach color. If the bacteria hydrolyze the urea in the medium, ammonia production turns the medium to a pink color. A negative result produces no color change.

SULFIDE-INDOLE-MOTILITY TUBES.   The tube of sulfide-indole-motility medium is inoculated with a straight stab to a depth of about 1 inch. Care is taken to withdraw the wire out along the same line as on entry (see Figure 4-6). Hydrogen sulfide production is indicated by blackening of the medium. Indole production requires addition of 5 drops of Kovac's reagent (BBL, Microbiology Systems, Cockeysville, MD) to the top of the medium. If tryptophan has been broken down to indole by the bacteria in the tube, a red ring immediately forms on top of the medium.

INDOLE SPOT TEST.   This new test detects indole production. A drop of paradimethylaminocinnamaldehyde (DMCA) is placed on a piece of filter paper. A drop of the test culture is then applied with an applicator stick or loop. A green or blue-green color indicates indole production.

SIMMONS' CITRATE TUBES.   Simmons' citrate medium differentiates bacteria according to their use of citrate. Only the slant surface is inoculated. If bacteria use the citrate in the medium, a deep blue color develops. The unchanged medium is green.

TETRATHIONATE BROTH.   Tetrathionate broth is an enrichment broth for isolation of *Salmonella* species. It is prepared according to the manufacturer's instructions. The suspension is mixed thoroughly and heated to sterilize it. The cooled medium is aseptically dispensed in 10-ml quantities into sterile tubes or bottles. An iodide solution must be added to the tetrathionate broth base, at 0.2 ml iodide/10 ml broth base, immediately before use. The iodide solution is made from 6 g of iodine and 5 g of potassium iodide ground together in a mortar. The water is added gradually until a solution is obtained. The solution must be stored in a container whose lid does not contain rubber because the solution attacks rubber.

SELENITE BROTH.   This enrichment broth for *Salmonella* species isolation is prepared by mixing 23 g of selenite in 1 L of distilled water and boiling to sterilize. Excessive heating should be avoided. The solution should not be sterilized in an autoclave. The sterile solution is dispensed into sterile tubes to a depth of at least 5 cm.

TRIPLE SUGAR-IRON AGAR.   This composite medium is used for presumptive identification of salmonellae and for initial differentiation of enteric bacteria (Figure 4-2). The essential ingredients of the medium are 1% lactose; 1% sucrose (or saccharose); 0.1% glucose (dextrose); an indicator system for hydrogen sulfide production;

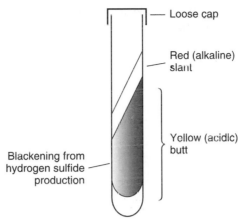

Figure 4-2
Reaction caused by most *Salmonella* species in a triple sugar-iron agar slant.

and pH indicator, phenol red, which colors the uninoculated medium red. All Entero-bacteriaceae ferment glucose, and the small amount (0.1%) is attacked preferentially and rapidly. At an early stage of incubation, both slant and butt turn yellow as a result of acid production. However, after the glucose is metabolized under aerobic condi-tions, and provided the organism cannot ferment lactose or sucrose, the slope reverts to the red (alkaline) condition. The butt, under anaerobic conditions, remains yellow (acidic). To allow this reaction, the triple sugar-iron agar always must be used in tubes with loose caps or plugged with sterile cotton.

If the organism can ferment lactose and/or sucrose in addition to the glucose, the lactose and sucrose are then attacked with resulting acid production, and the medium turns yellow (acidic) throughout. Lactose and sucrose are present in 1% quantities to maintain acidic conditions in the slant, which remains yellow. With organisms that produce hydrogen sulfide, blackening of the medium is partly superimposed on the other reactions. The triple sugar-iron slants should be read after about 16 hours' in-cubation at 37° C. After longer incubation, the blackening tends to reach the bottom of the tube and obscures the yellow butt.

The following summarizes the reactions of *Salmonella* species in triple sugar-iron agar:
- Alkaline (red) slant and alkaline (red) butt: none of the sugars attacked
- Alkaline (red) slant and acidic (yellow) butt: glucose fermentation only
- Acidic (yellow) slant and acidic (yellow) butt: glucose attacked in addition to lactose and/or sucrose
- Blackening along stab line and through medium: hydrogen sulfide production

The triple sugar-iron slant is stab-inoculated with a single colony from the selec-tive medium, using a straight inoculating wire. The wire is pushed down to the bot-tom of the agar and, on withdrawing the wire, the agar slant is streaked. The inocu-lating wire still contains enough bacteria to inoculate a tube of lysine decarboxylase broth. During the search for salmonellae, at least two suspicious colonies should be individually tested in triple sugar-iron agar per brilliant green plate. The triple sugar-iron tubes should be incubated, with loose caps, at 37° C for 16 to 24 hours.

LYSINE DECARBOXYLASE BROTH.   This medium examines the ability of an organism to decarboxylate the amino acid, lysine, to the alkaline end product, cadaverine. The uninoculated medium is usually yellowish purple. Initially, the enterobacteria preferentially ferment the small amount of glucose (0.1%) in the medium. Acid is produced and the indicator, bromocresol purple, turns the medium yellow. However, on further incubation, bacteria that can decarboxylate lysine produce cadaverine, and this alkaline byproduct turns the medium purple (lysine positive). With organisms unable to attack lysine, the medium remains yellow (lysine negative).

LYSINE IRON AGAR.   Lysine iron agar is a sensitive medium for detection of both *Salmonella* and *Arizona* species. The medium is tubed, sterilized, and slanted so that a short slant and deep butt are formed. It is inoculated with a straight needle by stabbing to the base of the butt and streaking the slant. The caps of the tubes must be replaced loosely so that aerobic conditions prevail on the slant. It is incubated at 37° C overnight.

Cultures that rapidly produce lysine decarboxylase cause an alkaline reaction throughout the medium, which turns purple. Organisms that do not decarboxylase lysine produce an alkaline slant and acidic butt and the medium turns yellow. Cultures that produce hydrogen sulfide cause an intense blackening in the medium. Because of determination of the lysine, *Proteus* and *Providencia* cultures produce a red slant over an acidic butt.

METHYL RED.   Glucose phosphate peptone medium tests the ability of an organism to produce large quantities of acidic end-products (methyl red positive) or to produce acetylmethylcarbinol (Voges-Proskauer positive). The test medium is inoculated and incubated at 37° C for 24 to 48 hours. About five drops of the methyl red reagent are mixed in the test medium and the test is read immediately. A positive methyl red test is bright red and a negative is yellow. If the methyl red test is negative, the Voges-Proskauer test may be performed in the same tube. About 1 ml of 40% KOH and 3 ml of a 5% solution of alpha-naphthol in absolute ethanol are added to the tube, and the contents are mixed and allowed to stand for 15 to 30 minutes. A pink color, becoming crimson, indicates production of acetylmethycarbinol (Voges-Proskauer positive). Most enterobacteria are methyl red positive or Voges-Proskauer positive, but not positive to both tests.

Inoculation of Culture Media

ASEPTIC TECHNIQUE.   When a veterinary technician is inoculating media and handling the specimen, care must be taken to prevent contamination. Aseptic (sterile) technique must be used at all times. When obtaining samples from a cadaver or excised organs, the technician must sear the surface of the organ or tissue with a flamed spatula before it is cut open for sample collection. Culture plates are kept closed unless the veterinary technician is inoculating or removing colony specimens

Figure 4-3
Flaming the neck of a culture tube before transfer of a sample.

Figure 4-4
Culture tube cap is held between the last two fingers during transfer of a sample.

for testing. When transferring samples from or to a tube, the technician must flame the tube neck before and after transfer of material and avoid putting down the cap (Figure 4-3). Instead, the cap is held between the last two fingers (Figure 4-4). When flaming an inoculation loop or wire, the technician puts the near portion of the wire in the flame first and then works toward the contaminated end. Placing the contaminated end into the flame first could result in splattering of bacteria, causing aerosol contamination. When the specimen collected is a liquid, a small quantity of well-mixed samples is inoculated at the edge of the plate with a sterile swab or bacteriologic loop. Some labs use presterilized glass rods for streaking samples because Bunsen burners are not always available and glass rods are autoclavable. If the specimen has been initially collected on a swab, this is streaked directly onto the plate.

Streaking Culture Plates

Several methods of streaking an agar plate exist, but the so-called "quadrant" streak method is probably the best (Figure 4-5). In Figure 4-5, area A is the primary streak or "well" of the plate. The bacteriologic loop may or may not be flamed and cooled before making streaks B, C, and D. This depends on the estimated number of bacteria present in the specimen. Employment of two loops, one of which is flamed and cooling while the other is being used, is a practical technique.

Each streaked area is overlapped only once or twice to avoid depositing excessive numbers of bacteria in an area. Otherwise, the resultant colonies are not discrete and isolated. Isolated colonies typically grow in area D of the plate (see Figure 4-5).

Using the entire plate is important, keeping the streak lines close together to include as many streaks as possible and taking care not to overlap the other streak lines. If several types of colonies grow on the plate, each colony is subcultured onto separate plates and the procedure repeated until a pure culture is obtained.

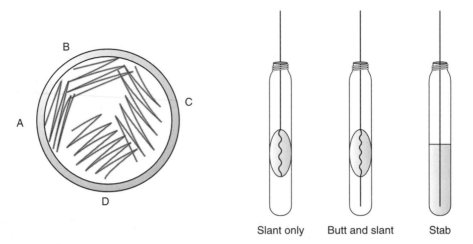

Slant only   Butt and slant   Stab

Figure 4-5
Quadrant method of streaking a culture plate.

Figure 4-6
Inoculation of culture tubes with an inoculating wire.

A convenient system of reporting growth on culture plates is as follows:
- Slight growth (in areas of initial streaking only) → +1
- Low moderate → +2
- High moderate → +3
- Heavy (growth in all areas of streaking) → +4

For opportunistic pathogens, growth should be 3+ or 4+, and organisms should be seen in direct smears at 2+ or higher levels before pathogenic significance is attached to their presence.

Inoculation of Slants

If agar slants are used, only the surface of the slant may be inoculated, or the butt and the surface may be inoculated. To inoculate only the surface of the slant, a straight flamed wire is used to obtain a colony of bacteria from the primary isolation plate. The surface of the slant is streaked in an "S" shape (Figure 4-6).

To inoculate both the butt and slant, the butt of the slant is stabbed with the tip of the inoculating wire and then carefully withdrawn up the same insertion path. The surface of the slant is then streaked in an S shape (see Figure 4-6).

Enough bacteria should be on the wire to inoculate the surface even after stabbing the butt. The tube's cap should be replaced loosely.

Incubation of Cultures

For pathogens that can invade the internal organs of an animal, the optimum growth temperature is usually near 37° C. For some fish pathogens, skin pathogens (such as dermatophytes), and environmental organisms, the optimum growth temperature is lower. Care should be taken to maintain the incubator temperature at 37° C, which is

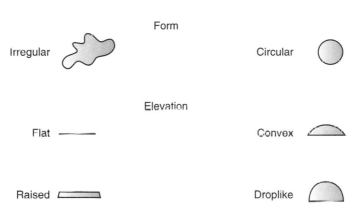

Figure 4-7
Bacterial colonies may be characterized by their form and elevation.

the optimum temperature, because bacterial growth cannot occur above this temperature.

Incubation time depends on the generation time of individual bacterial species and the type of medium on which they are growing. For routine cultures, plates should be incubated for 48 hours, with plates examined after 18 to 24 hours of incubation. Organisms such as *Nocardia* species may take 72 hours before colonies are visible. The culture plates should be inverted during incubation so that moisture does not collect on the surface of the agar, which may cause clumping of colonies.

Some pathogens require carbon dioxide for growth in the culture atmosphere. A candle jar may be used for this purpose. The plates are placed in a large jar, a lit candle is put on top of the plates, and the jar is sealed. The candle flame soon dies, leaving a decreased amount of oxygen and increased carbon dioxide in the jar's atmosphere. (This does not create an anaerobic condition.) The plates are incubated for 18 to 24 hours and then checked for growth. If no growth occurs, the plates are reincubated in the candle jar for another 18 to 24 hours and rechecked for growth. Larger laboratories may have incubators that automatically monitor temperature, CO_2 and O_2 levels, and humidity.

Colony Characteristics

An experienced technician can recognize several bacteria based on gross observation of the colonies. Various colony characteristics, including the following, may help identify the bacterium involved (Figure 4-7):

- Size (in millimeters or described as *pinpoint, medium,* or *large*)
- Color
- Density (opaque, transparent)
- Elevation (raised, flat, convex, droplike)
- Form (circular, irregular)
- Consistency (buttery, brittle, sticky)
- Odor (pungent, sweet, etc.)
- Any hemolysis (alpha, beta, gamma)

◆ Bacterial Staining

Two commonly used stains are Gram's stain and acid-fast stain. Stained smears may be directly examined for bacteria, especially presence, numbers, and type. Information obtained from a direct smear may help in determining the suitability of the specimen for identification, the predominant organism in a mixed specimen, the appropriate medium for culture, and the appropriate antibacterials for sensitivity testing. Staining kits for Gram's and Ziehl-Neelsen (acid-fast) stains are available commercially (see Box 4-1).

Staining Supplies

Supplies needed for staining include the following:
- Microscope with built-in light source and low-power, high-dry, and oil-immersion objectives
- Glass microscope slides (3 inches × 1 inch)
- Coverslips (22 mm × 22 mm)
- Bacterial loopholders and loops
- Gram's stain kit
- Difco TB stain kit (acid-fast staining)
- Staining rack or two glass rods, joined at the ends by rubber tubing
- Dropper or squeeze bottles for stain solutions

Preparation of Staining Solutions

GRAM'S STAIN.   Gram's staining is performed with crystal violet, Gram's iodine, decolorizer, and dilute carbol fuchsin.

Crystal Violet

Crystal violet	2.0 g
Ethanol 95% (vol/vol)	20.0 ml
Ammonium oxalate	0.8 g
Distilled water	80.0 ml

The crystal violet powder is dissolved in the ethanol, and then the ammonium oxalate is dissolved in the distilled water. To aid dissolving, both mixtures are agitated in a bath of hot water. The two solutions are mixed.

Gram's Iodine (Mordant)

Iodine crystals	1.0 g
Potassium iodide	2.0 g
Distilled water	200.0 ml

The iodine and potassium iodide are ground together in a mortar. Distilled water is added slowly. If necessary, it is agitated in a bath of hot water to aid dissolving.

Decolorizer

Ethanol 95% (vol/vol)

Dilute Carbol Fuchsin (Counterstain)

Concentrated carbol fuschin   10.0 ml
Distilled water   90.0 ml

ZIEHL-NEELSEN OR ACID-FAST STAIN. Acid-fast staining uses carbol fuchsin, acid alcohol, and methylene blue or brilliant green.

Concentrated Carbol Fuchsin

Basic fuchsin   1.0 g
Ethanol 95% (vol/vol)   10.0 ml
Ammonium oxalate   5.0 g
Distilled water   100.0 ml

The basic fuchsin is dissolved in the ethanol, then the phenol dissolved in the water is added and allowed to stand for a few days before being filtered into a container.

Acid-Alcohol (Decolorizer)

Concentrated hydrochloric acid   8.0 ml
Ethanol 95% (vol/vol)   97.0 ml

The acid is added to the alcohol.

Methylene Blue (Counterstain)

Methylene blue   8.0 g
Ethanol 95% (vol/vol)   300.0 ml
Distilled water   1300.0 ml
Potassium hydroxide   0.13 g

With Loeffler's methylene blue, the potassium hydroxide is excluded.

Brilliant Green (Alkaline, Alternative Counterstain)

Brilliant green   1.0 g
Sodium hydroxide 0.01%   100.0 ml

MODIFIED ZIEHL-NEELSEN STAIN. Modified Ziehl-Neelsen stain uses carbol fuchsin, acetic acid, and methylene blue.

Dilute Carbol Fuchsin

Dilute carbol fuchsin uses the same formula as Gram's stain.

Acetic Acid (Decolorizer)

Concentrated acetic acid   1.0 ml
Distilled water   200.0 ml

Methylene Blue

Methylene blue uses the same formula as Ziehl-Neelsen stain.

KINYOUN STAIN.   This stain contains basic fuchsin, phenol, and ethanol.

Basic fuschin	4.0 g
Phenol	8.0 ml
Ethanol 95%	20.0 ml
Distilled water	100.0 ml

The basic fuchsin is dissolved in ethanol and the water added slowly while stirring. Then the phenol is added.

FLUORESCENT ACID-FAST STAIN.   This stain uses auramine 0, phenol, acid-alcohol, and potassium permanganate.

Auramine 0	0.1 g
Phenol	3.0 ml
Ethanol 95%	10.0 ml
Distilled water	87.0 ml

The technician should dissolve 0.1 g of auramine 0 in 10 ml of 95% ethyl alcohol. Then 3 ml of liquefied phenol is mixed in 87 ml of distilled water. The first and second solutions are combined.

Acid-Alcohol (Decolorizer)

Hydrochloric acid 0.5 g	
(6 ml of 1M HCl)	
Ethyl alcohol 70%	100.0 ml

The technician adds 0.5 g of hydrochloric acid to 100 ml of 70% ethyl alcohol and mixes solution.

Potassium Permanganate (Counterstain)

Potassium permanganate	0.5 g
Distilled water	100.0 ml

The technician adds 0.5 g of potassium permanganate to 100 ml of distilled water and mixes well.

DMSO ACID-FAST STAIN.   This stain uses basic fuchsin, ethyl alcohol, phenol, glycerol, DMSO, and malachite green.

Primary Stain

Basic fuchsin (certified pure crystals)	4.0 g
Ethyl alcohol 95%	25.0 ml
Phenol 3%	100.0 ml

The basic fuchsin is dissolved in ethyl alcohol, and then the phenol is added. This is mixed well, and then the following is added:

Glycerol	25.0 ml
DMSO, reagent grade	25.0 ml
Distilled water	160.0 ml

This stain is allowed to stand for at least 30 minutes, and then is passed through coarse filter paper.

Combination Decolorizer and Counterstain

Malachite green (96% dye content)	200.0 ml
(Stock solution: 6 g/100 ml distilled water)	
Glacial acetic acid 99.5%	30.0 ml
Glycerol	50.0 ml

Giemsa Stain

Giemsa stain is made from Giemsa powder, glycerol, and methanol.

Concentrated acetic acid	1.0 ml
Distilled water	200.0 ml
Giemsa powder	1.0 g
Glycerol	66.0 ml
Absolute methanol	66.0 ml

Giemsa powder is allowed to dissolve in the glycerol at 55° to 60° C for about 2 hours. Methanol is added and mixed thoroughly. One part of this stock solution is mixed with 40 to 50 parts of neutral distilled water buffered to pH 6.8.

Filtering Staining Solutions

After a staining solution is prepared, it should be filtered into a clean container before use. Commercially prepared staining solutions may require filtering if a precipitate forms.

Quality Control

Each time a clinical specimen is stained, a sample from the control cultures should also be stained. This verifies the quality of the staining procedures and materials.

Gram's Staining Procedure

Gram's staining is used to categorize bacteria as Gram positive or Gram negative, based on their cell wall structure.

PROCEDURE. The sample should be applied thinly on the slide. Swab specimens may be rolled lightly onto the slide. Touching the sterile wire to one colony on the plate is usually sufficient to obtain enough bacteria for application to the slide. The colonies should be young (24-hour culture) because older colonies may not yield proper results, and the stained bacteria often become excessively decolorized.

Bacterial samples from plates are gently mixed in a drop of water or saline on the slide. If the sample is obtained from inoculated broth, two to three loopsful are spread onto the slide. A sample also may be smeared directly onto a slide, such as from tissue or an abscess. Regardless of how the specimen is transferred onto the slide (swab, pipette, wire), care must be taken not to destroy the organisms.

The sample droplet on the slide should be encircled using a wax pencil to help find the area after staining. After the material has dried on the slide, it is passed through a flame two or three times, specimen side up. The technician should be careful to not overheat the slide. The temperature may be tested on the back of the hand. The slide should feel warm but not hot. Heat fixing prevents the sample from washing off, helps preserve cell morphology, and kills the bacteria and renders them permeable to stain.

The Gram's staining procedure is as follows:

- The slide is placed on a staining rack over a sink.
- Crystal violet solution is poured onto the smear and allowed to sit 30 seconds.
- The slide is rinsed gently with water (tap water is acceptable).
- Iodine solution is poured onto the smear and allowed to stand for 30 seconds.
- The slide is rinsed gently with water.
- The smear is washed with decolorizer until no more purple color washes off (usually 10 seconds or less). The technician should not exceed the necessary amount of decolorizer.
- The slide is rinsed with water and replaced on the rack.
- Basic fuchsin or safronin is poured onto the smear and allowed to stand for 30 seconds.
- The smear is rinsed with water.
- The smear is air-dried or blotted between sheets of paper towel.
- The smear is examined microscopically with the 100× oil-immersion lens.

INTERPRETATION OF GRAM'S STAINS. Bacteria that retain the crystal violet-iodine complex and stain purple are termed *Gram positive.* Those that lose the crystal violet or purple color and stain red by safronin or basic fuchsin are classified as *Gram negative.*

The morphology of the bacteria on the smear also is important to note. The bacteria may be bacilli, cocci, coccobacilli or spiral, and arranged randomly or in pairs, chains, or clusters.

Sometimes an organism may stain both Gram positive and negative, which is called a *Gram-variable reaction.* This may occur as a result of excessive decolorization, an overly thick smear, excessive heat fixation, old cultures, or poor quality of stain.

Determining the Gram's stain reaction is an important step in the identification process. Performing the procedure properly and interpreting the results correctly requires practice. To ensure proper staining quality, known (control) Gram-positive and Gram-negative organisms should be stained at least once a week and with each new batch of stain. These control organisms may be kept growing in the laboratory (see Quality Control).

POTASSIUM HYDROXIDE (KOH) TEST. If a Gram-variable reaction occurs, a quick way to check the Gram reaction is with the potassium hydroxide (KOH) test. The procedure is as follows:

1. A loopful (or two, if necessary) of 3% KOH solution is placed on a slide.
2. A generous quantity of surface growth is removed from the culture and transferred to the drop of KOH.
3. The specimen is stirred into the KOH drop with a loop, and then slowly and gently the loop is lifted. After a maximum of 2 minutes of stirring (usually 30 seconds), Gram-negative organisms develop a mucoid appearance and produce a sticky

strand when the drop is lifted with the loop. If the organisms are Gram positive, the mixture stays homogeneous and does not form a strand on lifting.
4. The reaction is recorded as Gram negative (sticky strand and mucoid mass formed) or Gram positive (no sticky strand or mucoid mass formed).

Acid-Fast Stain

This stain is used to detect mycobacteria *(Mycobacterium bovis, Mycobacterium avium, Mycobacterium paratuberculosis)* and *Nocardia* species. Of the various types of acid-fast stains, some are better for mycobacteria and some for *Nocardia* species.

ZIEHL-NEELSEN ACID-FAST STAIN. This method uses carbol fuchsin stain, acid-alcohol decolorizer, and methylene blue counterstain. A thin smear is prepared. The slide is air-dried and heat fixed by passing the slide, specimen side up, through a flame. This process fixes the specimen to the slide and helps preserve bacterial cell morphology. Ziehl-Neelsen staining is performed by the following:
1. Carbol fuchsin stain is used to flood the slide. The slide is then heated over the flame until the stain steams.
2. The technician removes it from the heat and allows it to set for 5 minutes.
3. The slide is rinsed with water (tap water is acceptable).
4. Acid-alcohol is used to decolorize the slide for 1 to 2 minutes until the red color is gone.
5. The slide is rinsed with water.
6. Methylene blue is used to counterstain the slide for 30 seconds.
7. The slide is rinsed with water and dried over gentle heat.
   Acid-fast bacilli (mycobacteria) are stained red, whereas non–acid-fast microorganisms stain blue.

MODIFIED ZIEHL-NEELSEN STAIN WITH BRILLIANT GREEN. To perform this type of staining, the slide is:
1. Flooded with carbol fuchsin for 3 minutes, heated, and then rinsed with water
2. Decolorized with acid-alcohol for exactly 3 minutes
3. Rinsed with water
4. Counterstained with brilliant green (alkaline) for 3 minutes
   With alkaline brilliant green counterstain, overstaining the smear is almost impossible.

MODIFIED ZIEHL-NEELSEN STAIN WITH METHYLENE BLUE. This useful procedure stains bacteria that are partially acid-fast. These organisms resist decolorization by 0.5% acetic acid but not by acid-alcohol. *Brucella* species, *Nocardia asteroides,* and *Chlamydia* species may be stained with this modified Ziehl-Neelsen stain. The slide is:
1. Flooded with dilute carbol fuchsin for 10 minutes
2. Decolorized with 0.5% acetic acid for 20 to 30 seconds
3. Rinsed with water
4. Counterstained with methylene blue for 2 minutes
5. Rinsed and dried

Brucella and *Chlamydia* species stain bright red and are observed as clumps in smears made from fetal stomach contents and cotyledons from abortion cases. *Nocardia asteroides,* in pus or deposits from mastitic milk, are usually in the filamentous phase and some filaments stain red.

KINYOUN ACID-FAST STAIN.   This stain is useful when *Nocardia* species infection is suspected. The procedure is as follows:
1. A fixed smear is flooded with the stain and allowed to set for 3 minutes. No heating is required.
2. After staining, the Ziehl-Neelsen acid-fast stain procedure is followed.

A brilliant green counterstain is sometimes used instead of methylene blue. *Nocardia* species are partially acid-fast and are partially stained red. If counterstained with brilliant green, *Nocardia* species stain red, whereas other organisms stain green.

FLUORESCENT ACID-FAST STAIN.   This is a fluorescent stain for acid-fast bacilli. After a smear is stained with fluorescent dyes, such as auramine 0 and rhodamine, fluorescent microscopy reveals acid-fast bacilli glowing a yellow-orange color against a dark brown color. This method is commonly used for staining *Mycobacterium* species of mammalian origin. The smear is:
1. Heat fixed
2. Stained for 15 minutes at room temperature
3. Rinsed with tap water
4. Decolorized for 2 minutes with acid-alcohol
5. Rinsed with tap water
6. Counterstained with potassium permanganate for 3 minutes
7. Rinsed with tap water
8. Air dried
9. Examined with a fluorescent microscope for fluorescent bacilli

DMSO-ACID-FAST STAIN.   This is a popular method for staining *Mycobacterium* species of avian origin. The smear is:
1. Prepared and heat fixed
2. Stained with carbol fuchsin-DMSO solution for exactly 2 minutes
3. Rinsed with water
4. Counterstained and decolorized in glacial acetic acid malachite green solution for 2 minutes. If an even background of green/blue-green is not obtained, the slide should be returned to the solution for an additional 1 or 2 minutes.
5. Rinsed in tap water
6. Air-dried and examined with the oil-immersion lens

Giemsa Stain

Giemsa stain is used to detect spirochetes and rickettsiae and to demonstrate the capsule of *Bacillus anthracis* and the morphology of *Dermatophilus congolensis.* The smear is:
1. Fixed in absolute methanol for 3 to 5 minutes and air dried

2. Dipped in diluted stain for 20 to 30 minutes. The staining time may be extended as indicated by results. For *Borrelia anserina,* the smear is gently heated while it is covered with Giemsa stain and stained for 4 to 5 minutes
3. Rinsed with water
4. Air-dried and examine for purplish blue-stained bacteria

Specific Diagnostic Procedures That Employ Stained Smears

A summary of the main diagnostic uses of stained smears is given in Table 4-2, but a few useful procedures are discussed here in greater detail.

ABSCESSES, SUPPURATIVE EXUDATES, AND DISCHARGES. Making a Gram-stained smear from this type of material is usually helpful, even if the intention is to attempt to isolate the causative organism. When possible, scrapings should be obtained from the wall of the abscess because organisms are often absent or not viable in the center of these lesions. Wet preparations also are advised because fungi such as *Blastomyces* or *Cryptococcus* species may be involved (see Mycology). The most common pyogenic organisms are summarized in Table 4-2.

STREPTOTHRICOSIS. *Dermatophilus congolensis* causes an infection of the superficial layers of the skin and is characterized by serous scabs, often along the back. Although most animals and human beings seem to be susceptible, the condition is seen mainly in horses, sheep, and cattle.

Specimens should consist of hair plucked from the lesions, which characteristically detach with a considerable amount of scab at the end. To make stained smears from the scab material, a scalpel is used to shave a few bits of scab into a drop of distilled water on a slide. The flakes of scab are allowed to soften for a few minutes in the water, then a smear is made using another slide in a scissor action. Caution must be exercised not to break up the pieces of scab too much or the characteristic filaments of *Dermatophilus* species may be broken up into less diagnostic Gram-positive cocci (zoospores).

The crystal violet stain is left on the smear for only 2 seconds. The organism is intensely Gram positive and if stained too deeply, the characteristic filaments composed of individual zoospores arranged in lines, two or more zoospores across, may be difficult to see. A definitive diagnosis of streptothricosis usually may be made solely from stained smears.

NOCARDIOSIS AND ACTINOMYCOSIS IN DOGS. Infections caused by *Nocardia asteroides* and *Actinomyces viscosus* are fairly common in dogs. The conditions may be clinically indistinguishable, and thoracic and subcutaneous forms are seen in both. Differentiation of these diseases is important because the antibacterial susceptibility of the organism differs. *A. viscosus* is usually sensitive to penicillin, but *N. asteroides* is not.

Smears made from thoracic fluid or serosanguinous pus from subcutaneous abscesses may be stained by the Gram or modified Ziehl-Neelsen method. If granules are

Text continued on p. 154.

TABLE 4-2

Diagnostic uses of stained smears

Disease and Species Affected	Specimen	Causative organism	Appearance in Stained Smears
Gram's Stain			
Abscesses or suppurative conditions	Pus or exudates		
Many animal species		Staphylococcus aureus	Gram-positive cocci, often in clumps
Sheep, cattle		Actinomyces (Corynebacterium pyogenes)	Pleomorphic
Sheep, goats		Corynebacterium pseudotuberculosis	Gram-positive
			All forms, from rods to cocci
Many animal species, group C in horses		Streptococci	Gram-positive cocci, can be in chains
Dogs, cats (bite wounds)		Pasteurella multocida	Gram-negative rods
Many animal species		Pseudomonas aeruginosa	Gram-negative rods
Cattle, sheep, pigs (foot abscesses)		Fusobacterium necrophorum	Slender, long, Gram-positive rods, often with pointed ends
Actinobacillosis (wooden tongue) and actinomycosis (lumpy jaw)	Granules from pus	Actinobacillus lignieresi	Gram-negative rods
Cattle		Actinomyces bovis	Gram-positive, filamentous and branching
Clostridial enterotoxemia Pulpy kidney in lambs	Scraping from small intestine of a recently dead animal	Clostridium perfringens, Type D	Large numbers of Gram-positive, short, thick rods (presumptive evidence only)
Colibacillosis Calves, pigs, lambs <1 week of age	Scraping from small intestine of a recently dead animal	Enteropathogenic strains of E. coli	Numerous Gram-negative rods (presumptive evidence only)
Nocardiosis and actinomycosis Dogs	Pus and granules	Nocardia asteroides, Actinomyces viscosus	Both Gram-positive, filamentous and branching; Nocardia species are modified Ziehl-Neelsen positive

Strangles Horses	Pus	*Streptococcus equi ss equi*	Gram-positive cocci, can be in chains
Dermatophilosis (Streptothricosis) Many species susceptible; seen mainly in sheep, cattle, horses	Scabs	*Dermatophilus congolensis*	Large Gram-positive cocci (zoospores) arranged two or more across in branching filaments
Urinary tract infections Dogs, cats	Very fresh and carefully collected urine	*E. coli, Proteus* and *Enterobacter* species, *Staphylococcus aureus,* fecal streptococci, *Pseudomonas aeruginosa*	Bacteriuria indicated by ≥1 organism(s) per oil-immersion field
Dilute Carbol Fuchsin (Simple) Stain *Campylobacter* infections Infertility in cattle	Vaginal mucus	*Campylobacter fetus ss veneralis*	Comma-shaped rods that can be in short chains resembling seagulls
Abortion in sheep, cattle	Fetal stomach, cotyledons	*Campylobacter fetus ss fetus*	
Foot rot in sheep	Material from lesion	*Fusobacterium (Bacteroides) nodosus*	Rods with knobbed ends (must be present for a diagnosis of foot rot)
	Material from lesion	*Fusobacterium necrophorum*	Long slender rods, often with pointed ends
Swine dysentery	Feces or scrapings from colon	*Serpulina (Treponema) hyodysenteriae*	Numerous long (7 μ) but fine spiral organisms
Various necrotic lesions	Material from lesions	*Fusobacterium necrophorum*	Long slender rods, often with pointed ends
Modified Ziehl-Neelsen Stain Brucellosis Cattle	Vulvar discharge, cotyledons, fetal stomach contents	*Brucella abortus*	Small, red coccobacilli in clumps

Continued

TABLE 4-2

Diagnostic uses of stained smears—cont'd

Disease and Species Affected	Specimen	Causative organism	Appearance in Stained Smears
Modified Ziehl-Neelsen Stain—cont'd			
Brucellosis—cont'd			
Sheep	Cotyledons, fetal stomach contents	*Brucella ovis*	Small, red coccobacilli in clumps
Dogs	Vulvar discharge	*Brucella canis*	Small, red coccobacilli in clumps
Sows	Fetal stomach contents, vulvar discharge	*Brucella suis,* occasionally *Brucella abortus*	Small, red coccobacilli in clumps
Chlamydial diseases			
Cats	Conjunctival scrapings in feline pneumonitis	*Chlamydia psittaci*	Small coccobacilli in clumps; stain red
Sheep, cattle	Fetal cotyledons from bovine and ovine abortions		Similar to *Brucella* species but usually smaller and do not grow on conventional media
Sheep, pigs, calves	Joint fluid in polyarthritis		
Nocardiosis			
Dogs	Pus and granules	*Nocardia asteroides*	Long, branching filaments, many staining red
Bovine mastitis	Sediment from centrifuged milk		
Ziehl-Neelsen (Acid-Fast) Stain			
Acid-fast granulomas			
Cats	Scrapings from lesions	Unknown *Mycobacterium* spp	Large numbers of red, acid-fast rods

Disease / Host	Organism	Specimen	Characteristics
Johne's disease or paratuberculosis			
Cattle, sheep, goats	*Mycobacterium paratuberculosis*	Feces, ileocecal valve smear, mesenteric lymph nodes	Fairly short, red, acid-fast bacteria in clumps; must be in clumps to be diagnostic for Johne's disease
Tuberculosis			
Avian	*Mycobacterium avium* ss *avium*	Suspect lesions	Large numbers of acid-fast organisms; stain red and are often beaded
Swine	*Mycobacterium avium* ss *avium* or *Mycobacterium bovis*	Suspect lesion, often in cervical lymph nodes	Fewer organisms present
Giemsa Stain			
Anthrax			
Cattle, sheep	*Bacillus anthracis*	Blood smear from ear vein	Purplish, square-ended rods, often in chains; surrounded by a capsule
Spirochetosis			
Fowl	*Borrelia anserine*	Whole blood taken during febrile stage (3–5 days after infection); collect from several birds	Helical organisms, 6–30 μ long, 0.2–0.3 μ wide, with 5–8 spirals

present in the pus, they are crushed on the slide using a scalpel. Both *A. viscosus* and *N. asteroides* appear as long, Gram-positive, branching filaments in smears stained by the Gram method. However, *N. asteroides* is partially acid-fast and some of the filaments of *N. asteroides* stain red in smears stained by the modified Ziehl-Neelsen method.

ACTINOMYCOSIS AND ACTINOBACILLOSIS IN CATTLE.   Infections caused by *Actinomyces bovis* in cattle may affect bone and soft tissue, whereas those caused by *Actinobacillus lignieresi* affect soft tissue only. Both conditions often occur as suppurating abscesses in the jaw region. Granules characteristically occur in pus from abscesses caused by both organisms.

Several granules are washed free from pus in distilled water and crushed gently onto a slide. The crushed material is spread to make a thin smear and stain using the Gram method. *Actinomyces bovis* appears as long, branching, Gram-positive filaments, whereas *A. lignieresi* is a moderate-sized, Gram-negative rod.

ACID-FAST GRANULOMAS IN CATS.   This condition in cats is manifested as small granulomatous skin lesions, often on the feet, which tend to ulcerate. They are caused by an unidentified *Mycobacterium* species. A smear may be prepared from scrapings of the lesions or from a biopsy. Smears stained by the Ziehl-Neelsen method show numerous slender, often beaded, red-staining (acid-fast) rods. However, Kinyoun modification of the Ziehl-Neelsen stain is recommended because no heating is required. If the smear is stained with the fluorescent acid-fast stain, small fluorescent bacilli are seen on microscopy. A DMSO acid-fast stain is useful for *Mycobacterium* species of avian origin.

MASTITIS.   Mastitis may be caused by bacterial or mycotic organisms. Several laboratory tests are available to diagnose mastitis, including the California mastitis test, somatic cell count, and milk culture (see Chapter 12). A quick check to detect bacteria can be done by preparing a thin smear of mastitic milk. The smear is heat fixed and stained with Gram's stain or methylene blue. The most common microorganisms involved with mastitis are *Staphylococcus aureus, Streptococcus agalactiae, Streptococcus uberis, E. coli, Corynebacterium* species, and *Pseudomonas aeruginosa.*

CLOSTRIDIAL ENTEROTOXEMIA.   The main clinical signs of clostridial enterotoxemia are diarrhea and often death in circumstances precipitating an intestinal disturbance. Lamb dysentery caused by *Clostridium perfringens* type B does not occur in North America. Type-C enterotoxemia affects neonatal lambs, pigs, and calves. Type-D enterotoxemia, usually seen in feeder lambs, is commonly referred to as "pulpy kidney disease."

The clinical diagnosis can be supported by demonstration of clostridia (large, Gram-positive rods) in stained smears from the small intestinal mucosa of a recently dead lamb. Clostridial organisms are not present in large numbers in the small intestine of healthy animals. Postmortem invasion of the small intestine by clostridia, however, may be rapid.

Fresh ileal contents may be submitted to a laboratory for confirmation. Demonstration and identification of the toxin are necessary for definitive diagnosis.

COLIBACILLOSIS. This disease mainly affects calves, pigs, and lambs younger than 1 week of age. Enteropathogenic *E. coli* strains invade the small intestine, where they adhere to mucosal epithelial cells. Gram-stained smears from the small intestinal mucosa disclose large numbers of Gram-negative rods that are not present in healthy animals. This observation is only significant if the examination is made on a sick animal immediately after death, as postmortem invasion of the small intestine by *E. coli* is rapid. An indirect fluorescent antibody test is available for identification of *E. coli* K-99 antigen (see Chapter 9).

URINARY TRACT INFECTIONS. Urinary tract infections most commonly are seen in dogs and cats. They can be caused by *E. coli, Staphylococcus aureus,* fecal streptococci, *Pseudomonas aeruginosa,* or *Proteus* or *Enterobacter* species. A rapid check for bacteria may be done by Gram's staining a smear of a drop of fresh midstream urine. The presence of at least one bacterium per oil-immersion field in fresh, aseptically collected urine strongly suggests a urinary infection. This diagnosis should be confirmed by bacterial cultures.

◆ Primary Identification of Bacteria

With experience, the veterinary technician can learn to identify pathogenic bacteria using a systematic approach (Figure 4-8).

The specimens are first streaked onto a primary medium, such as blood agar and MacConkey agar. The plates are incubated for 18 to 24 hours and then examined for growth. If an incubated plate has colonies, the veterinary technician must decide if the bacteria should be identified.

Most Gram-positive and Gram-negative organisms grow on blood agar. Gram-positive organisms usually do not grow on MacConkey agar, but this agar supports growth of most Gram-negative organisms. Selection of the colony from the routine blood agar plate is preferable rather than from MacConkey agar. The danger in subculturing from a selective medium such as MacConkey agar is that inhibited organisms may be present as microcolonies on the plate. One of these could inadvertently be the colony of interest. With comparatively few tests, an organism may be identified to the genus level with a fair degree of certainty (Tables 4-3 and 4-4).

Gram's Stain

With a stained smear prepared from a pure culture or a single colony, organisms that have retained the crystal violet-iodine complex and that stain blue-purple must be regarded as Gram positive. If there is a Gram-variable or a doubtful reaction, the KOH test should be performed.

Size, Shape, Arrangement

The size of bacteria varies considerably. The bacteria most frequently studied in the laboratory range from 0.5 to 1 μ in width and 2 to 5 μ in length. Coccoid forms range

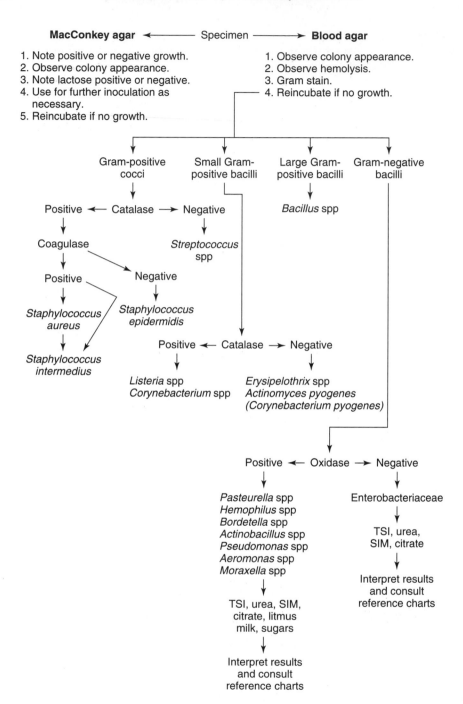

Figure 4-8
Flow chart of procedures used to identify bacteria.

TABLE 4-3

Primary identification of Gram-positive bacteria

Characteristics	Identification												
Shape	C	C	C	C	B	B	B	B	B	B	B	B	B
Acid-fast	−	−	−	−	−	−	−	−	−	+	−	−	−
Spores	−	−	−	−	−	−	−	−	−	−	−	+	+
Motility	−	−	−	+	+	−	−	−	−	−	−	V	V
Growth in air	+	+	+	+	+	+	+	−	+	+	+	+	−
Catalase	+	+	−	−	+	+	+	−	−	V	+	+	−
Oxidase	−	−	−	−	−	−	−	−	−	−	−	V	−
Glucose (acid)	V	+	+	+	+	+	−	+	+	+	+	V	V
O-F test													
Oxidation	+	−	−	−	−	−	−	−	−	+	+	+	−
Fermentation	−	+	+	+	+	+	+	+	+	N	−	+	+
Micrococcus spp	x												
Staphylococcus spp		x											
Streptococcus spp			x	x[1]									
Listeria spp					x								
Corynebacterium spp						x	x[2]	x[3]	x[4]				
Erysipelothrix spp									x				
Lactobacillus spp									x				
Actinomyces spp								x	x[5]				
Mycobacterium spp										x			
Nocardia spp										x[6]	x		
Bacillus spp						x[7]	x[7]	x[7]			x[7]	x	
Clostridium spp									x[7]				x

1 - *Some group-D streptococci.*
2 - Rhodococcus (Coryn.) equi.
3 - Eubacterium (Coryn.) suis.
4 - Actinomyces (Coryn.) pyogenes.
5 - A. viscosus.
6 - N. asteroids *(partially acid fast).*
7 - *Asporogenous variants.*
C, Coccus; B, Bacillus; V, Variable among species; +, >80% of strains positive; −, >80% of strains negative; N, Not tested; O, Oxidation; F, Fermentation.

from 0.75 to 1.2 μ in diameter. Rod forms have a width of 0.1 to 2 μ and a length of 2 to 5 μ. Spirochetes are 3 to 5 μ long.

Bacteria may be organized into four groups according to their shape (Figure 4-9):
1. Coccus: spherical cells, such as *Staphylococcus aureus,* which causes mastitis in animals
2. Bacillus: Shaped like rods or cylinders, such as *Bacillus anthracis,* which causes anthrax in animals and human beings
3. Spiral: Usually occur singly and can be subdivided into loose spirals, such as *Borrelia anserina,* which causes avian borreliosis; tight spirals, such as *Leptospira*

TABLE 4-4

Primary identification of Gram-negative bacteria

Characteristics	Neisseria spp	Branhamella spp	Acinetobacter spp	Enterobacteriaceae	Actinobacillus spp	Pasteurella spp	Aeromonas spp	Pseudomonas spp	Chromobacterium spp	Flavobacterium spp	Alcaligenes fecalis	Bordetella bronchiseptica	Moraxella bovis	Brucella spp	Campylobacter spp	Hemophilus spp	Bacteroides spp
Identification																	
Shape	C	C	B	B	B	B	B	B	B	B	B	B	B	B	B	B	B
Motility	–	–	V	V	–	–	+	+	+	–	+	+	–	–	+	–	–
Growth in air	+	+	+	+	+	+	+	+	+	+	+	+	+	(+)	(+)	(+)	–
Growth on MacConkey agar	–	–	V	+	V	–	+	+	+	–	+	+	–	–	–	–	–
Catalase	+	+	+	+	V	+	+	+	+	V	+	+	V	+	V	V	V
Oxidase	+	+	–	–	+	+	+	+	+	–	+	+	+	+	+	+	–
Glucose (acid)	V	–	+	+	+	+	+	+	+	+	–	–	–	–	–	V	V
O-F test																	
Oxidation	+	–	+	–	–	–	–	+	–	+	–	–	–	–	–	N	–
Fermentation	x	+	+	+	+	+	+	–	+	+	–	–	–	+	–	N	+

Organism-specific markers: Actinobacillus spp (x¹), Pasteurella spp (x²), Aeromonas spp (x³), Brucella spp (x⁴); Moraxella bovis (x), Campylobacter spp (x), Hemophilus spp (x), Bacteroides spp (x).

1 - P. hemolytica.
2 - P. anatipestifer.
3 - A. salmonicida.
4 - B. ovis and B. neotomae.

(), 5-10% CO_2 required by some strains; C, Coccus; B, Bacillus; +, >80% of strains positive; –, >80% of strains negative; V, Variable among species; N, Not tested; O, Oxidation; F, Fermentation.

pomona, which causes red water disease in cattle; and comma-shaped spirals, such as *Campylobacter fetus* subspecies *fetus,* a cause of abortion in cattle

4. Pleomorphic: Shape ranging from cocci to rods

Bacteria are found in a variety of arrangements. Some grow as single cells, whereas others remain attached after dividing and form chains or clusters. Many exhibit patterns of arrangement that are important for their identification (Figure 4-10):

1. Single: Some bacteria occur singly, such as spirilla (singular: spirillum) and most bacilli (singular bacillus).
2. Pairs: Some bacteria occur in pairs, such as *Streptococcus pneumoniae* (diplococcus).
3. Clusters or bunches: Some bacteria occur in clusters, bunches, or groups. For example, *Staphylococcus aureus* forms grapelike clusters.
4. Chains: Some organisms grow in short or long chains, such as *Streptococcus* species.
5. Palisades: Some organisms can be arranged in a palisade or Chinese letter pattern, such as *Corynebacterium* species.

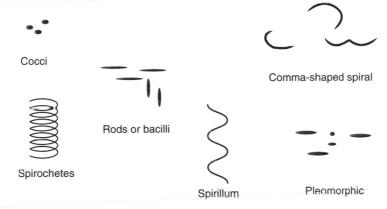

Figure 4-9
Bacterial cell morphology.

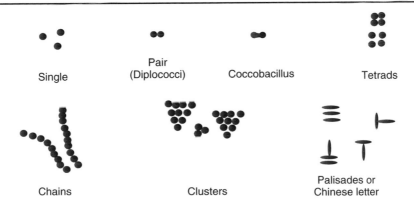

Figure 4-10
Bacterial cell arrangement.

| Central | Subterminal | Terminal | Terminal |

Figure 4-11
Bacterial endospores.

With pleomorphic organisms, such as *Corynebacterium* species, judging whether the organism is a coccus or a bacillus may be difficult. If the Gram-stained smear was made from a pure culture and any of the cells present are definitely rod-shaped, the organism must be regarded as a bacillus for purposes of identification.

Spores

When cultured, a few genera of bacteria form intracellular refractile bodies called *endospores* or, more commonly, *spores.* Organisms in the genera *Bacillus* and *Clostridium* are spore formers. Spores vary in size, shape, and location in the cell and may be classified as follows (Figure 4-11):
* Central: Present in the center of the cell, such as *Bacillus anthracis*
* Subterminal: Present near the end of the cell, such as *Clostridium chauvoei*
* Terminal: Present at the end or pole of the cell, such as *Clostridium tetani*
    Performing a special spore stain is usually not necessary because the endospores can be visualized as nonstaining bodies with Gram's stain.

Other Staining Procedures

Performing a Ziehl-Neelsen, Kinyoun acid-fast, or fluorescent acid-fast stain is not necessary unless *Mycobacterium* species involvement is suspected. The modified Ziehl-Neelsen stain is useful if searching for *Brucella* species or to differentiate between *Nocardia asteroides* (modified Ziehl-Neelsen positive) and *Actinomyces viscosus* (modified Ziehl-Neelsen negative). Both appear as Gram-positive bacilli in a smear from colonies on agar.

Motility

Two methods are commonly used to test motility. In one, young broth culture may be examined microscopically. A moderately heavy suspension is made in a few milliliters of nutrient broth incubated for 2 to 3 hours at room temperature. A loopful of this culture is placed on a microscope slide under a coverslip and examined with the high-dry objective. If the bacteria are obviously motile, with individual cells moving backward or forward among other cells, the answer has been obtained. Brownian movement should not be mistaken for true motility. Brownian movement is the shifting of cells or particles, with little movement relative to each other.

If the organisms are nonmotile on microscopic examination, motility media should be used. Two tubes of a motility medium, such as sulfide-indole-motility (SIM) medium (BBL Microbiology Systems, Cockeysville, MD), are stab inoculated. One tube is incubated at 37° C and the other at room temperature for 24 to 48 hours. Some organisms, such as *Providencia rettgeri,* tend to be motile at ambient temperature but not at 37° C. If growth is restricted to the stab inoculation line, the organism is nonmotile. Diffuse growth throughout the medium means the bacterium is motile. To interpret the results, the tubes are held against a good light and the inoculated tubes compared with an uninoculated one. The SIM medium is unsuitable for motility testing of organisms that produce hydrogen sulfide in this medium because the blackening that results may make the motility test difficult to read.

Catalase Test

The catalase test is performed on Gram-positive cocci and small Gram-positive bacilli. It tests for the enzyme catalase, which acts on hydrogen peroxide to produce water and oxygen. A small amount of a colony from a blood agar plate is placed on a microscope slide and a drop of catalase reagent (3% hydrogen peroxide) is added. If the colony is catalase positive, gas bubbles are produced. No bubble production indicates a negative result.

No blood agar should be transferred with the colony because blood agar can produce a slightly positive reaction. A positive reaction also may occur if a mixed colony is sampled; that is, one with both catalase-positive and catalase-negative organisms growing together. The plate must be streaked carefully to obtain isolated colonies. Staphylococci can be used as catalase-positive controls and streptococci as catalase-negative controls.

Coagulase Test

The coagulase test is performed on catalase-positive, Gram-positive cocci. *Staphylococcus aureus* produces coagulase, an enzyme that coagulates plasma. The test is used to differentiate between coagulase-positive *Staphylococcus aureus, Staphylococcus intermedius,* and coagulase-negative *Staphylococcus,* such as *Staphylococcus epidermidis* or *Staphylococcus saprophyticus.*

TUBE COAGULASE TEST. Lyophilized plasma (purchased from a medical supply house) is diluted according to the manufacturer's directions. About 0.5 ml is placed in a test tube and inoculated with a loopful of the organism from a noninhibitory medium, such as blood agar, which is incubated at 37° C and read hourly for 4 hours. A negative reaction is indicated by no clot formation, whereas a positive reaction is indicated by clots. If the test result remains negative, the sample is incubated again for 24 hours and then read.

SLIDE COAGULASE TEST. The slide coagulase test is a rapid screening test that detects surface-bound coagulase or clumping factor. More than 95% of coagulase-producing staphylococci possess clumping factor.

A loopful of staphylococci from a colony is first emulsified in a drop of water or saline solution to yield a thick suspension. A drop of fresh rabbit or human plasma is then added and stirred with a sterile loop. A positive reaction is indicated by clumping within 5 to 20 seconds.

The Staphyloslide (BBL Microbiology Systems, Cockeysville, MD) agglutination test and Staphaurex (Wellcome) are also commercially available. Staphyloslide detects a cell wall polypeptide-clumping factor. Staphaurex is based on latex agglutination to detect protein A, independent of clumping factor. Staphylococci that yield a negative slide result should be tested with the tube test to confirm the results.

Oxidase Activity

This test depends on the presence of cytochrome C oxidase in bacteria. A drop of 1% tetramethyl-p-phenylenediamine is added to a piece of filter paper in a Petri dish. The filter paper must be damp but not saturated. A short streak of the sample is made on the filter paper using a glass rod or the end of a Pasteur pipette that has been bent into a hook. The sample should be applied with a gentle rubbing action. A nichrome bacteriologic loop should not be used because any traces of iron may give a false-positive result.

In a positive test, the reagent is reduced to a deep purple color within 60 seconds. If the color-change reaction takes longer than this, the test should be regarded as negative. Oxidase reagent tends to be unstable and becomes discolored with time. It should be discarded if it becomes dark purple. *Pseudomonas aeruginosa* can be used as an oxidase-positive control and *E. coli* as an oxidase-negative control.

Acid Production from Glucose

A tube of 1% glucose in peptone broth, containing a pH indicator, is inoculated and incubated for 24 to 48 hours at 37° C. For fastidious organisms, such as *Streptococcus* species, about five drops of sterile serum should be added to the peptone water medium or growth may not occur.

Hyaluronidase Test

Hyaluronidase is an enzyme that has the ability to digest the mucoid capsule of certain bacteria. Blood agar plates are inoculated with *Pasteurella multocida* across the plate. *S. aureus* and *Staphylococcus intermidius* are inoculated at a right angle to *P. multocida* without touching the *Pasteurella* streak. The same procedure is repeated with *Staphylococcus hyicus* on a second blood plate. It is incubated at 37° C for 24 hours. Positive results occur if the mucoid nature of *P. multocida* is lost (dry and flattened) in the vicinity of the hyaluronidase producing Staphylococci species. In case of a negative result, *Pasteurella* species have wet and mucoid colonies.

Optochin Test

The optochin (ethyldrocuprein [EHC]) test is used to differentiate *Streptococcus pneumoniae,* which is sensitive to the optochin chemical. Other alpha-hemolytic streptococci are resistant. A blood agar plate is inoculated heavily (in four directions) with the test organism, and an optochin filter disc is placed into the center of the plate. Gentle pressure is applied to the surface of the disc so that it adheres to the agar plate. The plate is incubated for 18 to 24 hours. *S. pneumoniae* is inhibited by the optochin chemical and shows a zone of inhibition. Other alpha-hemolytic streptococci have growth up to the disc.

Oxidation-Fermentation Test

This test is designed to assess whether carbohydrates are destroyed by oxidation or fermentation. Conventional commercial tubes of media are suitable only for testing such organisms as enterobacteria and *Pseudomonas* or *Aeromonas* species. Other organisms may not grow in the medium. However, the basal medium may be enriched with 2% scrum or 0.1% yeast extract.

Before use, two tubes of oxidation-fermentation medium, with loosened caps, should be heated in a beaker of boiling water to drive off dissolved oxygen. After steaming for a few minutes, the tubes are cooled rapidly under cold running water. Both tubes of media are stab inoculated with the test organism, using a straight wire. Immediately a layer of paraffin oil should be added to a depth of about 1 cm on the top of one of the tubes. It is incubated at 37° C for up to 14 days, although 24 to 48 hours is usually sufficient. The pH indicator in the medium is usually bromthymol blue, which gives the uninoculated medium a green color, turning yellow when acid is produced by the organism's attack on the glucose in the medium. Table 4-5 summarizes the results of the oxidation-fermentation test.

Oxidative organisms, such as *Pseudomonas* species, attack only the glucose, with resultant acid production at the surface of tubes not sealed by paraffin oil.

◆ Identification of Bacteria in Specimens

Enterobacteriaceae

After death, organisms in this family rapidly invade tissues surrounding the intestines. If the animal has been dead for a day or so, the presence of enterobacteria in tissues outside of the bowels must be interpreted with caution. However, enterobacteria

---

TABLE **4-5**

Interpretation of the oxidation-fermentation test

| | Bacterium | | |
| | --- | --- | --- |
Preparation	Enterobacteria *Aeromonas* spp	*Pseudomonas* spp	*Alcaligenes fecalis*
Tube without oil	Yellow	Yellow	Green
Tube with oil	Yellow	Green	Green
Reaction	Fermentation	Oxidation	No reaction

isolated from a recently dead animal, from aseptically obtained mastitic milk samples, and from carefully collected feline or canine urine samples may be regarded as significant.

Septicemia resulting from *E. coli* is rare in animals more than a week of age. The carrier state of *Salmonella* infections is common, and the organisms can be excreted by apparently healthy animals. Figure 4-12 contains a flow chart for presumptive identification of Enterobacteriaceae.

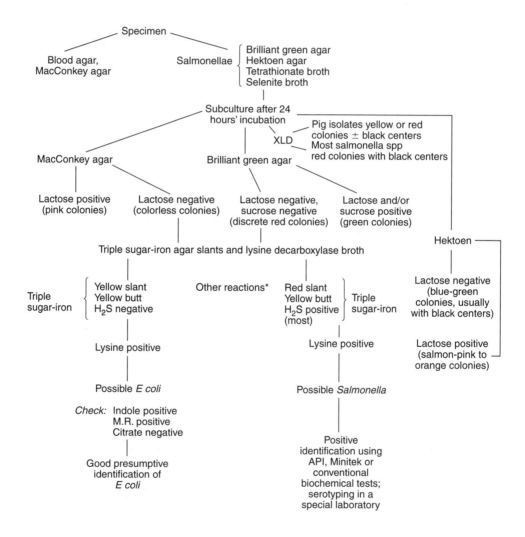

* Identify by biochemical tests if considered significant.

Figure 4-12
Flow chart for identification of Enterobacteriaceae.

CULTURE CHARACTERISTICS. The colonies of the various enteric bacteria on blood agar are not sufficiently distinctive to aid in their identification. Exceptions exist. Colonies of *Proteus vulgaris* and *Proteus mirabilis* swarm over a blood agar plate. The bile salts in MacConkey agar restrict this swarming although it can occur after 72 hours' incubation or if moisture is on the surface of the MacConkey agar. *Klebsiella* and *Enterobacter* species and a few strains of *E. coli* produce mucoid colonies, particularly pronounced after 48 hours' incubation. Table 4-6 shows a short list of reactions for quick differentiation of these three bacteria.

Some strains of *E. coli* may be hemolytic, but this is now thought not to correlate with pathogenicity. *Serratia marcescens* produces an orange-red pigment if incubated at ambient temperatures, but few strains produce pigment at 37° C.

ISOLATION OF SALMONELLAE FROM FECAL AND TISSUE SAMPLES. For isolation of salmonellae, specimens should be inoculated into an enrichment broth, such as tetrathionate and/or selenite and onto selective media, such as brilliant green, Hektoen, and MacConkey agars. A subculture is made on selective media after 24 and 48 hours' incubation of the enrichment broth at 37° C. If the specimens came from pigs or poultry, the more fastidious salmonellae, such as *S. choleraesuis, S. typhisuis, S. pullorum,* and *S. gallinarum* must be considered. These salmonellae often are inhibited by brilliant green agar and do not grow in tetrathionate broth. However, selenite broth and Hektoen, bismuth sulfite, and MacConkey agars usually grow them.

IDENTIFICATION OF SALMONELLA COLONIES. Plates are examined for typical *Salmonella* colonies. On MacConkey agar, they are lactose nonfermenters and appear colorless. On bismuth sulfite agar, they appear as black colonies surrounded by dark halos and/or colonies with a distinct metallic sheen.

On Hektoen Enteric agar, salmonellae are lactose nonfermenters and form blue-green colonies, usually producing hydrogen sulfide (black or dark colonies with black centers). *Salmonella arizonae* may appear as a lactose fermenter (yellow colonies) and may or may not produce hydrogen sulfide. On brilliant green agar, salmonellae form pink colonies surrounded by bright red medium and on xylose/lysine/desoxycholate (XLD) colonies they are red with black centers.

Suspect colonies are inoculated into a few drops of urea medium. Only urease-negative colonies are used to inoculate triple sugar-iron agar, lysine-iron slants, decar-

---

TABLE 4-6

Reactions for presumptive identification of *Klebsiella* and *Enterobacter* species and *E. coli*

Bacterium	Observation			
	Indole	**Methyl Red**	**Citrate**	**Motility**
E. coli	+	+	−	+
Klebsiella spp	−	±	+	−
Enterobacter spp	−	−	+	+

TABLE 4-7

Reactions of Enterobacteriaceae in lysine iron agar

Genus and Species	Slant	Butt	Gas	Hydrogen Sulfide
Escherichia spp	K	K or N	– or +	–
Shigella spp	K	A	–	–
Salmonella	K	K or N	–	+ (–)
typhi	K	K	–	+ or –
paratyphi-A	K	A	+ or –	– or +
Arizona spp	K	K or N	–	+ (–)
Citrobacter spp	K	A	– or +	+ or –
Edwardsiella spp	K	K	– or +	+
Klebsiella spp	K or N	K or N	+ or –	–
Enterobacter				
cloacae	K or N	A	+ or –	–
aerogenes	K	K or N	+ (–)	–
hafniae	K	K or N	– or +	–
Serratia spp	K or N	K or N	–	–
Proteus				
vulgaris	R	A	–	– (+)
mirabilis	R	A	–	– (+)
morganella	K or R	A	–	–
Providencia spp	R	A	–	–

An alkaline or neutral reaction in the butt of this medium indicates decarboxylation.
K, Alkaline; N, Neutral; A, Acidic; R, Red (oxidative deamination).
From Edwards E: Identification of enterbacteriaceae, *Dubuque, Ia, 1989, Burgess Publishing.*

boxylate lysine broth, and malonate broth to determine if the isolates produce typical biochemical reactions for salmonellae. A blood agar plate also is inoculated so that the suspect salmonellae are available for poly "o" testing if results of biochemical tests warrant it. Table 4-7 shows typical reactions of Enterobacteriaceae in lysine-iron agar.

The chances of isolating salmonellae are increased if two tubes of enrichment broth are inoculated per specimen. A tube of tetrathionate broth and a tube of selenite broth should be used. Fecal and tissue samples should be added in 5% to 10% quantities to the enrichment broth. Excessive amounts of inocula inhibit rather than aid the selectivity of enrichment broths.

Selenite broth may be purchased as a prepared tubed medium. Tetrathionate is obtained as a dehydrated tetrathionate broth base.

Table 4-8 summarizes differentiation of Gram-negative bacteria. Not all *Salmonella* strains produce hydrogen sulfide in triple sugar-iron agar. *Salmonella choleraesuis* does not form hydrogen sulfide, but the variant *S. choleraesuis* var. *kunzendorf* does. *Salmonella typhisuis,* which causes disease only in young pigs, is exceptional in that it is lysine negative. Enterobacteriaceae may be identified using API or Enterotube and Minitek biochemical systems (bioMerieux, Hazelwood, MO).

TABLE 4-8

Reactions of Gram-negative bacteria on triple sugar-iron slants and in lysine decarboxylase broth

	Organisms Expected and Lysine Reaction		
Reactions on TSI Slant	Lysine Positive	Lysine Negative	Lysine Variable
Acidic slant Acidic butt No H_2S No gas (reaction may be weak)	*Serratia* spp *Aeromonas hydrophila* ss *proteolytica*	*Aeromonas hydrophila* ss *anaerogenes* *Erwinia* spp *Actinobacillus* spp *Shigella sonnei* *Pseudomonas pseudomallei*	*Pasteurella* spp *E. coli* "inactive" *Pseudomonas* spp (some)
Acidic slant Acidic butt No H_2S Gas in butt (strong reaction)	*E. coli* *Enterobacter aerogenes* *Enterbacter gergoviae* *Klebsiella* spp	*Cedecea* spp *Rahnella* spp *Aeromonas hydrophila* ss *hydrophila* *Enterobacter cloacae* *Providencia* (some)	*Kluyvera* spp
Acidic slant Acidic butt H_2S produced Gas in butt	*Arizona* (some)	*Citrobacter* (some) *Proteus vulgaris*	
Alkaline slant Acidic butt No H_2S No gas	*Obesumbacterium* spp	*Shigella* spp *Providencia* spp *Yersinia pseudotuberculosis* *Xenorhabdus* spp *Pasteurella multocida* (some)	
Alkaline slant Acidic butt No H_2S Gas in butt	*Salmonella choleraesuis* *Salmonella sendai* *Salmonella abortus-equi* *Hafnia alvei*	*Salmonella typhisuis* *Salmonella paratyphi A* *Morganella morganii*	
Alkaline slant Acidic butt H_2S produced No gas	*Salmonella pullorum* (some) *Salmonella gallinarum* *Salmonella typhi*		
Alkaline slant Acidic butt H_2S produced Gas in butt	*Salmonella* serovars (most) *Arizona* serovars (most) *Edwardsiella tarda*	*Citrobacter* spp *Proteus vulgaris* (some) *Proteus mirabilis* *Salmonella typhisuis* (some)	

From Carter GR: Diagnostic procedures in veterinary bacteriology and mycology, Springfield, Ill, 1984, Charles C Thomas.

PRESUMPTIVE IDENTIFICATION OF *E. COLI.*   A variety of tests may be used for quick identification of *E. coli.* The pink colonies (lactose positive) that *E. coli* forms on MacConkey agar may be tested in triple sugar-iron agar and lysine decarboxylase broth. The appearance in triple sugar-iron agar is a yellow slant and yellow butt, with no hydrogen sulfide production but often considerable gas production that can disintegrate the agar slant. Most *E. coli* strains are lysine positive.

Three other test results give a strong presumptive identification of *E. coli:* hydrogen sulfide negative, motility positive, and indole positive in sulfide-indole-motility medium; methyl red positive; and citrate negative.

Organisms from Mastitic Milk Samples

Many organisms, including fungi, may cause mastitis. Milk culture may be used to diagnose clinical mastitis, but its main use is in detecting subclinical mastitis. Subclinical mastitis is difficult to diagnose because no clinical signs exist. Two main tests are employed to detect subclinical mastitis before resorting to culture procedures.

CALIFORNIA MASTITIS TEST.   The California mastitis test (CMT) is a qualitative screening test that can be used as a "cowside" test. The test is based on gel formation when the test reagent reacts with DNA in somatic cells. As the cell count of the milk increases, the gelling action increases. Therefore the test provides an indirect measure of the cell count. The degree of gel formation is scored *negative, trace, 1, 2,* or *3,* and *y* and *t.*

To perform the CMT, about 2 ml of milk are placed in each of the four cups on the CMT paddle and an equal amount of reagent is added. The paddle is gently rotated for about 10 seconds in a circular pattern to mix the milk and reagent. A score is then assigned for each quarter, according to the chart of grading and interpretation (Table 4-9).

Precautions to be considered in this test are as follows:
1. DNA in somatic cells deteriorates upon standing. If the test is to be used as a laboratory test, the milk samples should be kept refrigerated but not for more than 48 hours. Unrefrigerated milk cannot be tested accurately after about 12 hours.
2. White blood cells tend to migrate with milk fat. Therefore thorough mixing of samples just before testing is essential.
3. CMT reaction must be scored 10 to 15 seconds after mixing starts. Weaker reactions fade thereafter.

DIRECT SOMATIC-CELL COUNT.   The direct somatic-cell count may be performed by counting somatic cells using a microscope or with an electronic cell counter (Coulter counter). In either case, the results are reported as the number of cells per milliliter of milk.

MILK CULTURE.   Only positive milk samples identified by CMT or direct somatic-cell count should be cultured. The milk sample is inoculated on blood agar and MacConkey agar and incubated at 37° C for 24 hours. Milk samples also are incubated simultaneously. If the cultures show minimal or no growth after 24 hours of incuba-

TABLE 4-9

Grading of California mastitis test results

Symbol	Meaning	Visible Reaction	Interpretation
−	Negative	Mixture remains liquid with no evidence of a precipitate.	0–200,000 cells/ml 0–25% PMNs
T	Trace	Slight precipitate forms and is seen to best advantage by tipping the paddle back and forth and observing the mixture as it flows over the bottom of the cup. Trace reactions tend to disappear with continued movement of the fluid.	150,000–500,000 cells/ml 30%–40% PMNs
1	Weak positive	A distinct precipitate but no tendency toward gel formation. With some samples the reaction is reversible. With continued movement of the paddle, the precipitate may disappear.	400,000–1,500,000 cells/ml 40%–60% PMNs
2	Distinct positive	Mixture thickens immediately, with some suggestion of gel formation. As the mixture is swirled, it tends to move toward the center, leaving the bottom of the outer edge of the cup exposed. When the motion is stopped, the mixture levels out again and covers the bottom of the cup.	800,000–5,000,000 cells/ml 60%–70% PMNs
3	Strong positive	Gel formation causes the surface of the mixture to become convex. Usually a central peak remains projecting above the main mass after the motion of the paddle has been stopped. Viscosity is greatly increased, so that there is a tendency for the mass to adhere to the bottom of the cup.	Cell number generally >5,000,000/ml 70%–80% PMNs

PMN, Polymorphonuclear leukocyte

Continued

TABLE **4-9**

Grading of California mastitis test results—cont'd

Symbol	Meaning	Visible Reaction	Interpretation
+	Alkaline milk pH 7.0 or over	This notation should be added to the CMT score when the reaction is distinctly alkaline, as indicated by a contrasting deeper purple color.	An alkaline reaction reflects depressed secretory activity as a result of inflammation or in drying-off of the gland.
y	Acidic milk	Bromcresol purple is distinctly yellow at pH 5.2. This notation should be added to the score when the mixture is yellow.	Distinctly acidic milk in the udder is rare. When encountered, it indicates fermentation of lactose by bacterial action within the gland.

tion, a subculture is made on the blood and MacConkey agar plates from the incubated milk samples. The subcultured plates and the original culture plates are incubated for 24 hours at 37° C. A rapid but presumptive identification of the organism may be made on colonial morphology, followed by confirmatory tests:

- *Staphylococcus aureus* forms moderate-size (3-mm) colonies. Colonies of bovine strains are yellow, surrounded by a double zone of hemolysis. This organism does not grow on MacConkey agar.
- *E. coli* forms pink colonies on MacConkey agar and glistening colonies on blood agar, with an unpleasant odor.
- *Klebsiella pneumoniae* colonies become mucoid after 48 hours' incubation. Growth on MacConkey agar is also mucoid.
- *Enterobacter aerogenes* cannot be distinguished from *Klebsiella* species on colony appearance.
- *Streptococcus* forms small (1-mm) colonies resembling dew drops. *Streptococcus agalactiae* strains may produce a clear zone of beta hemolysis. Streptococci are the only bacteria that grow on Edwards' medium. Hence, their growth on Edwards' medium is one of the methods of detecting streptococci associated with mastitis.
- *Pseudomonas aeruginosa* forms large colonies that usually produce a bluish-green pigment on both blood and MacConkey agars. Many strains produce a characteristic and not unpleasant odor.
- *Actinomyces (Corynebacterium) pyogenes* forms small colonies surrounded by a zone of clear hemolysis. At 16 to 24 hours' incubation, the hemolytic effect is often seen before the colonies become visible. No growth occurs on MacConkey agar.
- *Nocardia asteroides* colonies are not usually visible until after 48 to 72 hours' incubation. The colonies become powdery and are intensely white and adherent to the medium. This organism does not grow on MacConkey agar.
- *Pasteurella multocida* forms moderately sized, nonhemolytic colonies that produce a characteristically sweetish odor. The colonies have a superficial resemblance to those of enterobacteria, but no growth occurs on MacConkey agar.

Figure 4-13
Differentiation of streptococci using esculin hydrolysis.

CONFIRMATORY TESTS. *Staphylococcus aureus* appears as Gram-positive cocci, often arranged in clusters resembling "bunches of grapes." The coagulase test is the most definitive test for pathogenicity of staphylococci. It distinguishes *Staphylococcus aureus* from *Staphylococcus epidermidis*, which can occasionally be hemolytic. However, only Gram-positive and catalase-positive cocci should be subjected to the coagulase test. Also, any degree of clotting of the plasma in 3 to 4 hours is regarded as a positive finding. Known coagulase-negative and coagulase-positive staphylococci should be used as controls. Commercial systems, such as ApiStaph-Ident and Minitek (bioMerieux, Hazelwood, MO), can be used to identify staphylococci.

Presumptive identification of *E. coli* and *Klebsiella* and *Enterobacter* species may be made using a few biochemical tests (triple sugar-iron, lysine, sulfide-indole-motility, methyl red, and citrate), as indicated in the previous section. *Serratia marcescens* occasionally causes mastitis. Only a few strains produce the orange-red pigment at 37° C. If, however, the inoculated plates or subcultures are left at room temperature, the pigment may be observed. The API, Enterotube, or Minitek commercial kit system (bioMerieux, Hazelwood, MO) should be used for complete identification of enterobacteriae.

The colony appearance of mastitis-causing streptococci, with their ability to hydrolyze esculin, may be a useful first step in their identification (Figure 4-13). Gram-positive, catalase-negative colonies are streaked on Edwards' medium or esculin blood agar. Browning of Edwards' medium or esculin blood agar, as a sequel to hydrolysis, may be seen with greater clarity if the culture plates are examined under an ultraviolet (Wood's) lamp. A uniform blue glow is evident on uninoculated plates containing esculin and on plates in which the streptococci have not hydrolyzed the esculin. A dark-brown coloration of colonies and the surrounding medium indicates streptococci that attack esculin.

Ruminant red blood cells, partially lysed by the beta-hemolysin of *Staphylococcus aureus* at 37° C, are completely hemolyzed in the presence of Lancefield group-B streptococci, including *Streptococcus agalactiae*. This is the basis of the CAMP test, used to identify *Streptococcus agalactiae*.

The CAMP test uses a blood agar plate prepared with sheep or cattle red blood cells that contain esculin. A thin streak is made down the center of the agar plate using an *S. aureus* strain that produces a good zone of partial hemolysis. Several suspect *S. agalactiae* strains may be tested on one plate. The streptococci to be tested are streaked at right angles to the *S. aureus* streak, bringing them within 1 to 2 mm of the *S. aureus* streak. Include a known *S. agalactiae* streak on every plate as a control. The plates are incubated at 37° C for 24 hours.

An arrow of enhanced, complete hemolysis indicates a positive test for *S. agalactiae* (Figure 4-14). About 5% of *Streptococcus uberis* strains and an occasional strain of *Streptococcus dysgalactiae* produce a small zone of hemolysis close to the S. *aureus* streak, but the reaction is rounded and weak. *S. uberis* may be distinguished from *S. agalactiae* by the color of its colonies and brown discoloration of the medium.

BAGG broth (BBL Microbiology Systems, Cockeysville, MD) is a buffered azide glycerol broth for detection of enteric streptococci, such as *Streptococcus fecalis*. These Lancefield group-D streptococci occasionally may cause mastitis, but they are often present in milk samples as contaminants and must be distinguished from *S. uberis*. BAGG broth is inoculated with the test streptococcus and incubated, in addition to a control broth containing a known *Streptococcus fecalis* culture, for 48 hours at 37° C. Cloudiness in the broth, with a color change from purple to yellow, indicates a positive result. BAGG broth inoculated with *S. uberis* remains clear and purple (negative). Commercial test kits, such as Rapid Strep (bioMerieux, Hazelwood, MO), are available. Figure 4-13 provides a flow chart for identification of some streptococci.

Pseudomonas aeruginosa usually may be identified by the large colonies, blue-green pigment, and characteristic odor it produces. If doubt exists, the tests listed under Primary Identification of Bacteria should be carried out with inoculation of a tube of tech agar (BBL Microbiology Systems, Cockeysville, MD), which is designed to enhance pyocyanin production by *P. aeruginosa* strains. *P. aeruginosa* is the only *Pseudomonas* species that produces the blue-green pigment, pyocyanin.

Figure 4-14
CAMP test for *Streptococcus agalactiae*.

In Gram's stains, *Actinomyces pyogenes* appears as a highly pleomorphic Gram-positive organism, showing all forms, from cocci to rods that tend to occur in palisade and arrangements that resemble Chinese characters. A useful confirmatory test is to inoculate the center of a Loeffler serum slant (Oxoid, Columbia, MD) heavily with the test organism. *A. pyogenes* causes a pit in the serum slant after 24 hours' incubation at 37° C. *Corynebacterium bovis* occurs commonly in milk samples, but the organism's pathogenicity is dubious. It forms small, white, dry, nonhemolytic colonies often confined to the initial streak, where a milk residue is present.

Nocardia asteroides usually may be presumptively identified by its appearance on blood agar. It is a Gram-positive, moderate-sized rod. If the milk sample is centrifuged, modified Ziehl-Neelsen staining reveals a branching, filamentous organism, with some filaments staining red (positive). If a centrifuge is not available, take some material with a Pasteur pipette from the bottom of the tube and make a smear.

Streptomyces is a common, nonpathogenic soil and air organism with colonies quite similar to those of *Nocardia species*. However, most strains of *Streptomyces* have an unmistakable earthy odor, are likely to form filaments in the milk sample, and are negative on modified Ziehl-Neelsen staining.

With experience, a veterinary technician may make a presumptive identification from the characteristic odor of *P. multocida* and from its failure to grow on Mac-Conkey agar. The organism may be identified to the genus level by performance of the tests listed under Primary Identification of Bacteria. In addition, *P. multocida* is a good indole producer. *Pasteurella pneumotropica* also forms indole but is unlikely to be associated with mastitis. If any doubt exists, the organism may be identified using the API or Minitek systems or Enterotube (bioMerieux, Hazelwood, MO).

Organisms from Urine Samples

In contrast to methods used for milk samples, methods of culturing urine samples emphasize procedures for determining the number of bacteria present. However, isolation and identification of pathogenic bacteria also are important when determining the cause of urinary infection.

Fresh urine samples are cultured. Samples that cannot be cultured within 2 hours after collection should be refrigerated. A blood agar plate is streaked with the urine sample using a 0.001-ml calibrated loop (Figure 4-15).

After the plates are incubated at 37° C for 18 to 24 hours, colonies are counted. A bacterial count of less than 10,000 is usually considered insignificant. A commercial Urotube Kit (BBL Microbiology Systems, Cockeysville, MD) method is also available. For positive identification and differentiation of bacteria, the colonies are subjected to Gram's staining, culturing for isolation, and biochemical tests.

Identification of Other Organisms from Routine Cultures

The organisms mentioned here are those commonly isolated from cultures of abscesses and samples from urinary tract, respiratory tract, and other lesions. Several conditions, mentioned in the section on staining, may be diagnosed with some certainty by examination of stained smears only. Confirmatory biochemical tests are

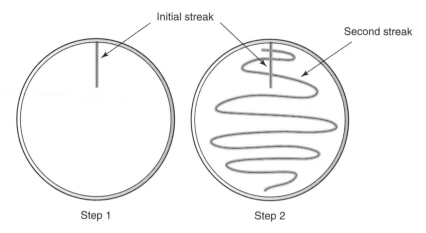

Figure 4-15
Procedure for streaking a urine culture plate. Short, straight initial streak is followed by a second, curved streak covering the remainder of the plate. The loop is not flamed between the first and second streaks.

more conveniently carried out using the API or Minitek systems (bioMerieux, Hazel-wood, MO) in a small laboratory, rather than stocking a large range of conventional biochemical media. Complete information on the methodology of the API and Minitek systems can be obtained from the manufacturer (see Box 4-1). Charts, tables, computerized coding systems, or characterization profiles, designed for use only with the system for which they were produced, are also available. The results of biochemical tests in the miniaturized systems may vary among the systems and may be different from results obtained by conventional test methods.

Most species of *Actinomyces* are anaerobic, except *Actinomyces viscosus,* which may cause granulomatous pleuritis in dogs. This condition must be differentiated from nocardiosis, which has similar clinical signs and gross pathologic changes. These two diseases usually may be diagnosed with the aid of staining.

Actinobacillus species are Gram-negative bacteria that grow on MacConkey agar. They are fermentative, oxidase- and catalase-positive, and nonmotile. *Actinobacillus* species tend to be comparatively species specific: *A. lignieresi* affecting primarily cattle, *A. equuli* foals, *A. suis* pigs and foals, and *A. seminis* causing epididymitis in rams. Epididymitis resulting from *Brucella ovis* may be clinically similar to an *A. seminis* infection, but chronic cases resulting from *A. seminis* are often purulent. The organism is unreactive biochemically and modified Ziehl-Neelsen negative. *Brucella ovis* is seen as clumps of red, modified Ziehl-Neelsen-positive rods in smears from lesions. A few biochemical reactions can be used to differentiate the three main *Actinobacillus* species (Table 4-10).

Aeromonas hydrophila, a Gram-negative, opportunistic pathogen, is most commonly isolated from fish and reptiles but occasionally infects mammals. It is often strikingly hemolytic on blood agar and produces an offensive odor. It grows well on MacConkey agar but is catalase and oxidative positive, whereas the enterobacteria are oxidase negative.

TABLE 4-10

Reactions used to differentiate the three main *Actinobacillus* species

	A. lignieresi	*A. equuli*	*A. suis*
Clear hemolysis on blood agar	−	(−)	(+)
Esculin hydrolysis	−	−	+
Urease production	+	+	+
Salicin (acid)	−	−	+
Mannitol (acid)	+	+	−
Trehalose (acid)	−	+	+

( ), Some exceptions.

Its colonies may resemble those of *Pseudomonas* species. Both genera are motile, but *Aeromonas* species are fermentive and *Pseudomonas* species are oxidative.

The typical clumps of red *Brucella* coccobacilli are seen in smears stained with modified Ziehl-Neelsen or Koster stain from lesions or, with abortions, from fetal stomach contents. *Brucella ovis* and *Brucella abortus* require CO_2 for growth, but *Brucella canis* and *Brucella suis* do not. Other than *B. ovis,* they are rapid urease producers. *B. abortus* gives a positive result in 2 hours and *B. canis* and *B. suis* in a half hour. Selective media are desirable for the brucellae because of the large number of contaminant bacteria present in specimens, as in uterine discharges and cotyledons. Isolation of these organisms is best attempted in a specialized laboratory. A slide agglutination test is available for canine brucellosis (see Chapter 9).

Bordetella bronchiseptica is a respiratory pathogen that may be isolated from pigs with atrophic rhinitis. It may also be a secondary invader in dogs with distemper and a cause of respiratory infections in rabbits and guinea pigs. *B. bronchiseptica* is a small Gram-negative rod that grows on MacConkey agar. It is motile, oxidase and catalase positive, citrate and urease positive, and indole negative. It reduces nitrates and does not attack carbohydrates. Most strains are hemolytic on blood agar.

Many conditions caused by *Campylobacter fetus* subspecies *fetus,* such as abortions in cattle and sheep, may be diagnosed by stained smears. Culture is necessary to confirm the diagnosis. Because these are fastidious organisms, culture is best performed in a specialized laboratory.

Corynebacterium organisms are pleomorphic Gram-positive rods. *Actinomyces pyogenes* is invariably hemolytic, with pinpoint colonies after 24 hours' incubation. A useful identifying feature of *A. pyogenes* is its ability to "pit" a Loeffler's serum slope after 24 hours' incubation. *Rhodococcus equi* is nonhemolytic and unreactive against carbohydrates. However, after 48 hours' incubation, the colonies are characteristically mucoid and salmon pink, both increasing with incubation time. A short list of biochemical reactions for the corynebacteria of veterinary interest is given in Table 4-11. Corynebacteria are rather fastidious, so the sugar reactions should be carried out in cystine trypticase agar (BBL Microbiology Systems, Cockeysville, MD) base medium.

Dermatophilus congolensis is so characteristic in stained smears (see Staining) that it is usually unnecessary to do cultures. Some stains require CO_2 for primary iso-

TABLE **4-11**

Some biochemical reactions for corynebacteria of veterinary interest

	Hemolysis	"Pitting" Loeffler's	Catalase	Urease	NO₃ Red	Glu	Acid in Lact	Malt
Actinomyces pyogenes	+	+	−	−	−	+	+	+
Coryn. renale	V	−	+	V	V	+	V	V
Rhodococcus equi	−	−	+	V	+	−	−	−
C. pseudo-tuberculosis	V	−	+	V	V	+	V	+
C. bovis	−	−	+	−	−	−	−	−
C. kutscheri	−	−	+	V	+	+	−	+
C.. suis (anaerobic)	−	−	−	+	−	V	−	+

Glu, glucose; Lact, lactose; Malt, maltose; V, variable reaction, depending on strain.

lation (a candle jar is satisfactory), but all strains grow aerobically on subculture. Small, rough, hemolytic colonies appear after 48 hours' incubation. The colonies are embedded in the medium.

Erysipelothrix rhusiopathiae and *Listeria monocytogenes,* both moderate-sized, Gram-positive rods, are superficially similar in Gram-stained smears and in culture. They must also be distinguished from nonpathogenic *Erysipelothrix*-like organisms and from nonpathogenic *Listeria* species. The major differentiating characteristics are given in Table 4-12.

On blood agar, colonies of *L. monocytogenes,* beta-hemolytic streptococci, and *Actinomyces pyogenes* have a similar appearance. They form small colonies, surrounded by an entire edge and a clear zone of hemolysis. After 24 hours' incubation, young colonies of *E. rhusiopathiae* usually have a narrow zone of partial hemolysis that progresses to a slight zone of clear hemolysis after 48 hours' incubation.

In Gram-stained preparations from colonies, *L. monocytogenes* has many coccal cells, and care is needed not to mistake it for a streptococcus. Rough colonies of *E. rhusiopathiae* may yield small coccobacilli and short, filamentous forms.

"Tumbling" motility is characteristic of *L. monocytogenes.* This motility may be seen in a wet preparation of a broth culture incubated at room temperature for 2 to 3 hours. Individual cells suddenly tumble over and over before moving off again normally. When grown in a semi-solid medium, *Listeria* produces a characteristic umbrella-shaped growth. The API 20s Kit is available commercially for identification of *L. monocytogenes.*

The hydrogen sulfide production by *E. rhusiopathiae* in triple sugar-iron stab cultures is meager and just along the stab line but is characteristic for the organism. The

TABLE 4-12

Major differentiating characteristics of *Erysipelothrix* and *Listeria* species

	Erysipelothrix Rhusiopathiae	*Erysipelothrix*-like Organisms	Nonpathogenic *Listeria* spp	*Listeria* Monocytogenes
Clear hemolysis	– (24 hr)	–	–	+
Oxidase	–	–	–	–
Catalase	–	–	+	+
Motility	–	–	+	+ (25° C)
Hydrogen sulfide in triple sugar-iron	+ (2–5 days)	+	–	–
Esculin hydrolysis	–	+	+	+
"Bottle brush"in gelatin	+ (3–5 days)	+	–	–

"bottle brush" appearance of colonies in gelatin takes several days to develop and occurs mainly with the rough strains of the organism. Esculin hydrolysis can be tested on esculin blood agar or on esculin slants that are available commercially. Browning of the medium, seen more clearly under ultraviolet light, is a positive reaction. *L. monocytogenes* is isolated easily from abortion specimens and abscesses, but a cold enrichment technique is required to recover the organism from brain specimens (see Bacteriologic Cultures).

Most *Hemophilus* organisms require X and/or V factors for growth. The exceptions are *Hemophilus somnus* and *Taylorella equigenitalis,* though their growth is enhanced by the X factor. Colony growth of *Hemophilus* species is increased in an atmosphere with 5% to 10% CO_2.

Chocolate agar (BBL Microbiology Systems, Cockeysville, MD) is the medium of choice. In an emergency, a fresh blood agar plate, supplying some X factor, and a streak of *S. aureus* (V factor), grows many of the organisms. A greater chance exists of isolating *H. somnus* if generous amounts of tissue are preenriched in brain-heart infusion broth and plated after 24 hours' incubation.

Hemophilus organisms form small, circular colonies, usually needing 48 hours' incubation at 37° C before they are visible. *Actinobacillus pleuropneumoniae* is isolated from swine and is often hemolytic. The other two species of *Hemophilus* isolated from swine include *Hemophilus parasuis* and *Hemophilus suis*. To differentiate between the species, the organism is grown on blood agar and requirements for X and V factors are determined. If the organism requires V factor, it establishes satellite colonies around the *Staphylococcus* species streak. The requirement for both X and V factors may be tested by streaking the suspect organism on trypticase soy agar (with almost

TABLE 4-13

Characteristics of *Hemophilus* species

Species	Factor Required		Required CO$_2$	Principal Host	Disease	Specimen
	X	V				
H. suis	+	+	+	Swine	Glasser's disease	Joint fluid
H. parasuis	−	+	+	Swine	Secondary invader in swine influenza	Lungs
Actinomyces pleuro-pneumoniae	−	+	(+)	Swine	Pleuropneumonia	Lungs, pleura
H. gallinarum	+	+	+	Chickens	Infectious coryza	Nasal discharge and/or trachea
H. paragallinarum	−	+	+	Chickens	Infectious coryza	As above
H. somnus	(+)	−	+	Cattle	Meningoencephalitis, polyarthritis, etc	Brain, joint fluid, lungs
Taylorella equigenitalis	(+)	−	+	Horses	Contagious equine metritis	Cervical swabs

( ), *Not required but enhances growth.*

no X or V factors) and adding discs containing X, V, and combined XV factors (Oxoid, Columbia, MD or BBL Microbiology Systems, Cockeysville, MD) to the surface of the agar. Satellite colonies grow around the disc containing the required growth factor(s).

Table 4-13 summarizes the characteristics of *Hemophilus* species. As shown in Table 4-13, *H. suis* requires both X and V factors, whereas *A. pleuropneumoniae* requires only V factor. A urea test is used to differentiate these two species. *A. pleuropneumoniae* is urease positive, whereas *H. suis* is urease negative.

Moraxella bovis is a small, aerobic, nonmotile, Gram-negative coccobacillus associated with keratoconjunctivitis in cattle. It produces oxidase, and some strains are catalase positive. *M. bovis* does not attack carbohydrates but is weakly proteolytic and slowly liquefies gelatin and pits Loeffler's serum slants. Colony variants are common; hemolytic/nonhemolytic and rough/smooth colonies occur. Subcultures may produce a mixture of colony variants, giving the impression of impure cultures.

Isolation of *M. bovis* is more likely if a swab of lachrymal secretions or discharge is plated directly on blood agar. Failing this, the swab is placed in a little sterile saline and plated out within 2 hours of collection.

When *Nocardia asteroides* is suspected, a smear should be stained from the original specimen with modified Ziehl-Neelsen stain. Observation of modified Ziehl-Neelsen-positive filaments and the characteristic colonies gives a presumptive identification (see Organisms from Mastitic Milk Samples).

Pasteurella organisms have an affinity for the respiratory system, although *P. multocida* may be associated with bovine mastitis and with cat and dog bites. The fermentation of carbohydrates should be tested using CTA-based media (BBL Microbiology Systems, Cockeysville, MD). A few reactions for identification of the *Pasteurella* species are listed in Table 4-14.

P. aeruginosa is the main veterinary pathogen in the *Pseudomonas* genus, with the exception of the exotic species *P. mallei* and *P. pseudomallei*. Identification of *P. aeruginosa* is discussed in the section on bovine mastitis.

TABLE **4-14**

Reactions for identification of *Pasteurella* species

	P. multocida	*P. hemolytica*	*P. gallinarum*	*P. pneumotropica*
Hemolysis (blood agar)	−	+	±	−
Growth: MacConkey agar	−	±	−	−
Indole	+	−	−	+
Urease	−	−		+
Glucose	+	+	+	+
Lactose	−	+	−	+
Sucrose	+	+	+	+
Mannitol	±	+	−	−
Salicin	−	+	−	−
Esculin hydrolysis	−	±	−	−

TABLE 4-15

Differential reactions for Group-c streptococci

	S. equi ss equi	*S. equi* ss zooepidemicus	*S. equi* ss equisimilis
Trehalose	−	−	+
Sorbitol	−	+	−
Lactose	−	+	±
Maltose	+	±	+

TABLE 4-16

Differentiation of three species of staphylococci

	Tube Coagulase Test	Pigmentation of Colony	Purple Agar Base with 1% Maltose
S. aureus	+	+	Diffuse yellow color around colonies in 12–24 hours
S. intermedius	+	−	Yellow to yellow-green under colonies in 48–72 hours*
S. hyicus	+	−	Diffuse alkaline (purple) reaction around colonies

*Not reliable for S. intermedius *strains from species other than dogs.*

Streptococcus species, Gram-positive cocci, form small, circular colonies. On blood agar, a streptococcus species may be beta-hemolytic (total hemolysis), alpha-hemolytic (partial hemolysis), or gamma-hemolytic (no hemolysis). Lancefield grouping can be carried out by the conventional acid-extraction method, or more conveniently using the Streptex latex test (Burroughs Wellcome, Greenville, NC), which covers groups A, B, C, D, F, and G.

Among the most important streptococci are those of group C from horses, which must be differentiated when a decision must be made regarding vaccination against strangles (*Streptococcus equi* subspecies *equi* infection). Table 4-15 lists biochemical tests that can be carried out using CTA-based media (BBL Microbiology Systems, Cockeysville, MD) or peptone water sugars with about 5 drops of sterile serum added per 5 ml of medium.

Coagulase-positive staphylococci have been placed into three biotypes, with *S. aureus* the parent biotype. *S. intermedius* has been isolated from dogs with pyoderma and mastitis and from pigeons, mink, and horses. *S. hyicus* has been recovered from pigs with polyarthritis, the skin of pigs with and without exudative epidermitis ("greasy pig disease"), the intact skin and mange lesions in cattle, and cows with mastitis. Establishing that a *Staphylococcus* species is coagulase positive is probably sufficient because this correlates with pathogenicity (see Organisms from Mastitic Milk Samples). However, a test employing a purple agar base (BBL Microbiology Systems, Cockeysville, MD),

TABLE 4-17

Differential reactions of *Yersinia* species

	Y. pestis	*Y. pseudotuberculosis*	*Y. enterocolitica*
Indole	−	−	±*
Urease	−	+	+
Ornithine decarboxylase		−	+
Esculin hydrolysis	−	+	−
Rhamnose		+	(−)
Sorbitol	−	−	+
Sucrose	−	(−)	+
Salicin	+	+	−

*Most European strains are negative but most American strains are positive.
( ), Some exceptions.

with 1% maltose added, can be used to differentiate the three biotypes (Table 4-16). Also the hyaluronidase test is useful for differentiating the *Staphylococcus* species.

Yersinia species are now members of the family Enterobacteriaceae. The general characteristics of *Yersinia pseudotuberculosis* and *Yersinia enterocolitica* are lactose-negative (colorless) colonies on MacConkey agar, oxidase negative but catalase positive, non–hydrogen-sulfide–producing in triple sugar-iron agar, urease positive but phenylalanine negative, and motile at room temperature but not at 37° C. These two *Yersinia* species are of greatest veterinary interest, but *Y. pestis,* the plague bacillus, is enzootic in wild rodents in 17 western states. *Y. pestis* is urease negative and nonmotile.

Y. pseudotuberculosis usually may be isolated from caseous lesions on primary inoculation of solid media. However, attempted isolation of *Yersinia* species, particularly *Y. enterocolitica,* from feces should employ a cold-enrichment process. Table 4-17 summarizes reactions used to differentiate *Yersinia* species.

◆ Antimicrobial Susceptibility Testing

When bacteria are isolated from a patient, an antimicrobial test is performed to determine the susceptibility or resistance to antimicrobial drugs. The results of this test indicate which antimicrobial to use in treatment. Ideally, the specimen used for antimicrobial susceptibility testing is taken from the animal before treatment begins. The veterinarian may begin treatment before obtaining susceptibility results but then may change to a more appropriate drug when the results are available.

Fresh clinical samples should be used for a direct susceptibility test. First the suspected pathogen should be isolated and then the susceptibility testing done. This ensures that the test is performed on the causative organism rather than on a mixed floral specimen or a contaminant. A Gram's stain is performed on the isolate to determine which antimicrobial discs to use. Some antimicrobials are more effective against Gram-positive or Gram-negative bacteria. Groups of antimicrobials may be tested according to the disease being investigated, such as respiratory disease or mastitis. The organisms typically causing each disease tend to respond to certain groups of antimicrobials.

Agar Diffusion Method

The agar diffusion method for antimicrobial susceptibility testing is most commonly employed and uses paper discs impregnated with antimicrobials. It is quantitative and requires measurement of zone sizes to give an estimate of antimicrobial susceptibility. The concentration of drug in the disc is chosen to correlate with serum and tissue levels of the drug in the treated animal.

Diffusion methods in common use include the U.S. Food and Drug Administration (FDA) method; standardized disc susceptibility method, which is a modified Bauer-Kirby technique and the International Collaborative Study (ICS) standardized disc technique. The FDA susceptibility test, described here, is designed for testing the antimicrobial susceptibility of rapidly growing aerobic pathogens, such as Enterobacteriaceae, staphylococci, and *Pseudomonas* species.

Culture Media for Antimicrobial Susceptibility Testing

Mueller-Hinton agar gives the most reproducible results and is suitable for testing antibiotics and sulfonamides. Veterinary technicians must ensure that no gross moisture is on the agar surface or on the lid before use. Plates may be checked for sterility by incubating two or three from a batch at 37° C for 24 hours.

Some organisms, such as streptococci, do not grow sufficiently well on plain Mueller-Hinton agar for a test to be read. In these cases, Mueller-Hinton agar plus 5% blood must be used. However, having departed from the standardized FDA method, the zone sizes must be interpreted with caution. For example, the zone sizes for novobiocin are smaller if the medium contains blood. Most streptococci are still susceptible to penicillin.

Inoculum Preparation and Inoculation of Plates

A pure culture should be used for susceptibility testing. However, well-spaced colonies on the plate inoculated from an original specimen are usable. With a sterile loop, just the surfaces of three or four of them are touched and placed in saline or broth to make a suspension. If bacteria are taken from just the surface of the colony, less likelihood exists of picking up an unseen contaminant growing at the base of the colony. More than one colony of a bacterial species always should be taken because a single colony may represent a variant that has a susceptibility pattern different from that of the parent strain.

Under no circumstances is it justifiable, with veterinary specimens, to carry out an antimicrobial susceptibility test using the original inoculum because the chance of only one bacterial species being present in the specimen is minimal. Completely erroneous results are obtained if a susceptibility test is carried out with a mixed inoculum containing more than one species.

A correct inoculum density is an important aspect of getting reproducible results. The "lawn" of cells that grows up after inoculation should be evenly distributed. Extremes in inoculum concentration must be avoided. Several methods may be used to obtain a correct inoculum.

The FDA advocates use of a 2- to 8-hour broth culture, incubated at 37° C, to produce a bacterial suspension of moderate turbidity. The culture is prepared by inoculating 4 to 5 ml of nutrient broth, such as trypticase soy broth or brain-heart infusion, with bacteria obtained by touching the surface of three to four similar-appearing colonies. The incubated broth is diluted with sterile saline or distilled water to a controlled density, equivalent to 0.5 McFarland standards attained by adding 0.5 ml of 1.17% $BaCl_2\text{-}2\ H_2O$ solution to 99.5 ml of 0.36-N sulfuric acid. Another method is to dilute an overnight broth culture in saline to the turbidity density described above, which is usually a 1:50 dilution of the overnight broth culture.

A rapid method that gives good results is to make a suspension of three to seven well-spaced colonies in about 2 ml of sterile saline or distilled water. The turbidity thus obtained should be equivalent to 0.5 McFarland barium sulfate turbidity standards.

The Prompt Veterinary Sensitivity Standardizing System (BBL Microbiology Systems, Cockeysville, MD) has been developed to rapidly standardize the inoculum density, making it equivalent in performance to the 0.5 McFarland standard. This precludes the incubation period, periodic checking of the inoculum density, and turbidity adjustment by dilution. Thus the system enables precise, reliable sensitivity results with a more efficient use of time and less chance of human error.

The Prompt System consists of a plastic vial with a snap top containing 1 ml of saline and a separate inoculator wand. The inoculator wand is a polypropylene rod attached to a cap. At the tip of the rod is a cavity for picking up a controlled number of organisms (5 to 10 colonies) from the primary culture plate.

After picking up the colonies, the technician snaps the top off the plastic vial, places the wand firmly into the vial, and mixes the contents. This gives the inoculum density equivalent to the 0.5 McFarland standard.

Inoculation of the plates, using the inoculum prepared by either of the above methods, is carried out by saturation of a sterile cotton swab with the bacterial suspension. Excess moisture is removed from the swab by rotation against the side of the tube above the level of the fluid. The bacterial suspension is streaked evenly over the surface of the agar medium with the swab. The agar medium is streaked successively in three directions and then the swab is run around the circumference of the plate to ensure that the entire surface is covered (Figure 4-16). Inoculated plates should be allowed to dry for 15 to 30 minutes at room temperature before application of the antimicrobial discs.

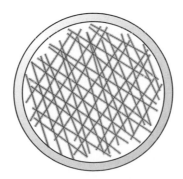

Figure 4-16
In antimicrobial susceptibility testing, the sample is incubated in trypicase soy broth. Then a swab sample is streaked in several directions onto Mueller-Hinton agar.

Antimicrobial Discs

The veterinary technician should use the range of antimicrobial discs that correspond to the drugs most commonly employed in the practice. The antimicrobial content in a disc is indicated in Table 4-18. Only one disc representative each of the tetracyclines and one for the sulfonamides is necessary because of the phenomenon of cross-resistance. For example, if the bacterial species is resistant to one of the tetracyclines, it is usually resistant to all members of the group.

Antimicrobial discs always should be kept in the refrigerator (4° C) when not being used and replaced as soon as possible after use. Outdated discs should never be used. The potency of the antimicrobial discs may be monitored with control organisms of known sensitivity patterns.

The antimicrobial discs are placed on the inoculated agar surface with a disc dispenser or sterile forceps that have been flamed and cooled between each use. The technician gently presses on each disc to ensure contact with the surface. The discs should be no closer than 10 to 15 mm to the edge of the plate and sufficiently separated from each other to avoid overlapping of the zones of inhibition. The spacing can be carried out using sterile forceps with the plate over a template, or by using a disc dispenser. One type of disc dispenser delivers eight different antimicrobial discs onto a standard 100-mm–diameter plate, and another can dispense 12 discs onto a 150-mm Petri dish (BBL Microbiology Systems, Cockeysville, MD and Difco Laboratories, Detroit, MI).

The plates are put in the incubator at 37° C within 15 minutes after placing the discs on the inoculated agar. The plates are placed aerobically and upside down. The plates should be kept in stacks of four or less because plates in the center of a tall stack take longer to reach incubation temperature.

Reading the Zones of Inhibition

The plates should be read after a constant period, most satisfactorily after overnight incubation (18 to 24 hours). Prolonged incubation may alter the size of the zone of inhibition with antimicrobials that are not stable at 37° C or at best make the zones hard to read. If rapid results are imperative, the diameters of the zones of inhibition may be read after 6 to 8 hours' incubation. These results should be confirmed by reading them again after overnight incubation.

The diameter of each inhibition zone (including the diameter of the disc) is measured from the underside of the plate, using calipers, transparent ruler, or template. The zones are measured and recorded to the nearest millimeter. If Mueller-Hinton agar with blood has been used, the zone size must be read from the top surface, with the lid of the plate removed.

Interpretation of Zone Sizes

Table 4-18 lists some of the commonly used antimicrobials and gives the suggested interpretation of zone sizes with the FDA standardized disc method. The zone sizes are divided into two major categories: resistant and susceptible to the particular antimicrobial agent. The latter category is subdivided into intermediate susceptibility and

TABLE 4-18

Interpreting inhibition zone size with the FDA standardized disc method

Antimicrobial	Disc Content	Inhibition Zone Diameter (mm)		
		Resistant Organisms (#)	Susceptible Intermediate	Organisms Susceptible
Ampicillin[a]: for Gram negatives and enterococci	10 μg	≤11	12–13	≥14
Ampicillin[a]: for staphylococci and penicillin G-susceptible organisms	10 μg	≤20	21–28	≥29
Ampicillin[a]: sulbactam for Gram-negative enterobacteria, staphylococci, and *Hemophilus* spp	10 μg	≤19	–	≥20
Bacitracin	10 units	≤8	9–12	≥13
Carbenicillin: for *Proteus* spp, *E. coli*	100 μg	≤17	18–22	≥23
Carbenicillin: for *Pseudomonas aeruginosa*	100 μg	≤13	14–16	≥17
Cephalothin[b]	30 μg	≤14	15–17	≥18
Chloramphenicol	30 μg	≤12	13–17	≥18
Clindamycin	2 μg	≤14	15–20	≥21
Colistin	10 μg	≤8	9–10	≥11
Enrofloxacin	5 μg	≤17	18–21	≥22
Erythromycin	15 μg	≤13	14–17	≥18
Gentamicin	10 μg	≤12	13–14	≥15
Kanamycin	30 μg	≤13	14–17	≥18
Methicillin[c]	5 μg	≤9	10–13	≥14
Nalidixic acid	30 μg	≤13	14–18	≥19
Neomycin	30 μg	≤12	13–16	≥17
Nitrofurantoin	300 μg	≤14	15–16	≥17
Novobiocin[d]	30 μg	≤17	18–21	≥22
Novobiocin[e]	30 μg	≤14	15–16	≥17
Penicillin G for staphylococci[f]	10 units	≤20	21–28	≥29

a – Use for testing susceptibility to ampicillin and hetacillin.

b – Use when susceptibility to cephalothin, cephaloridine, cephalexin, cefazolin, cephacetrile, cephradine, cefaclor, and cephapirin is observed.

c – Use for testing susceptibility to all penicillinase-resistant penicillins.

d – Not applicable to a medium containing blood.

e – Use when the test medium contains blood.

f – Use for testing susceptibility to all penicillinase-susceptible penicillins except ampicillin and carbenicillin.

g – Use for testing susceptibility to all the tetracyclines.

Continued

TABLE 4-18

Interpreting inhibition zone size with the FDA standardized disc method—cont'd

Antimicrobial	Disc Content	Inhibition Zone Diameter (mm)		
		Resistant Organisms (#)	Susceptible Intermediate	Organisms Susceptible
Penicillin G for other bacteria[f]	10 units	≤20	12–21	≥22
Polymyxin B	300 units	≤8	9–11	≥12
Rifampin: for *Neisseria meningitides*	5 μg	≤24	–	≥25
Hemophilus spp		≤16	17–19	≥20
Streptomycin	10 μg	≤11	12–14	≥15
Sulfonamides	250 or 300 μg	≤12	13–16	≥17
Tetracycline[g]	30 μg	≤14	15–18	≥19
Tilmicosin	15 μg	≤11	12–16	≥15
Tobramycin	10 μg	≤12	13–14	≥15
Trimethoprim-sulfa	1.25 μg 23.75 μg	≤10	11–15	≥16
Vancomycin	30 μg	≤9	10–11	≥12

susceptible. For predictive purposes, a resistant organism is not likely to respond to therapy with the drug. A susceptible organism is susceptible to ordinary doses of the antimicrobial. Intermediate susceptibility implies that the organism is susceptible to ordinary doses when the drug is concentrated in the urine or tissues, or the antimicrobial may be used for treatment of systemic infections if a high dosage is safe.

The zone size alone is not indicative of the efficacy of an antimicrobial. Some drugs, such as vancomycin and colistin, do not readily diffuse through agar and give small inhibition zones, even when the test organism is fully susceptible. Therefore direct comparisons of zone diameter, produced by unrelated antimicrobials, are misleading and should not be made.

Control Organisms

Susceptible reference organisms, such as *S. aureus,* American Type Culture Collection (ATCC) 25923, and *E. coli,* ATCC 25922, should be put up regularly, preferably in parallel with each batch of antimicrobial susceptibility tests. These control organisms are used to check such factors as the growth-supporting capability of the medium, potency of antimicrobial discs, and other variable conditions that can affect results.

Limitations of the Test

The FDA method is designed for rapidly growing bacteria. Caution is needed for tests of anaerobes or slow-growing organisms, for which the criteria for interpretation of zone diameters have not yet been established with certainty. In general, the zone diameters are somewhat larger, for an equivalent minimal inhibitory concentration, with slow-growing organisms than with rapid growers.

Some rare strains of staphylococci are resistant to methicillin and other penicillinase-stable penicillins. The routine test cannot be relied on to detect these strains, but they may be detected by incubation of an additional susceptibility test plate, containing a methicillin disc, at 30° C. A reduced zone diameter, or no zone, surrounding the methicillin disc on the plate incubated at 30° C is presumptive evidence of methicillin resistance.

◆ Serologic Examination

Serologic procedures are widely used in veterinary diagnostic laboratories for positive identification of bacteria that are apparently identical in their morphology and physiology. These procedures are faster and more economical than culture methods. Many serologic procedures may be performed without much difficulty at the veterinary clinic.

Sample Collection

Blood samples for serologic testing must be collected in sterile tubes. Samples collected in EDTA, heparin, or sodium citrate are satisfactory. If samples are to be sent to a diagnostic laboratory, they should be freshly collected blood cooled to 4° C when it is clotted. Optimal results are reached when separating the clot from the serum and sending serum samples instead of whole blood. If the serum is to be kept for several days before shipping (waiting for a convalescent sample), the serum must be separated from the clot and stored frozen. Early separation of serum from the clot prevents hemolysis. Hemolyzed blood samples are unsatisfactory because hemolysis makes interpretation of results difficult. If paired serum samples are submitted, they are marked as "acute" and "convalescent" with dates of sample collection.

Serologic Tests

AGGLUTINATION TEST. Agglutination refers to clumping of bacteria caused by a specific antibody. In this procedure, serum containing specific antibodies is added to a standard suspension of antigen, or bacteria. The resulting degree of agglutination, or clumping, or lack of agglutination is then assessed. The agglutination test is one of the most commonly employed tests in diagnosis of bacterial infection. The test may be performed on glass slides or plastic cards or in tubes. The slide and card tests commonly are used as screening tests. In the tube agglutination test, the reagent and serum sample are mixed in a test tube.

The most common serologic test performed in veterinary clinics and at cattle sales is the Brewer card test. The test is performed by mixing stained *Brucella* organisms with serum from an animal. The card is then rocked for a few minutes. A positive reaction is characterized by clumping or agglutination and possibly clearing of the color stain. Clumps may gather around the edge of the card, producing a "ring."

The milk ring test detects antibodies to *Brucella* species in the milk of infected cows. The procedure is performed by adding to the milk sample a suspension of *Brucella* bacteria stained with dye and then thoroughly mixing it. As the cream rises, a mass of agglutinated, dyed bacteria floats upward with the cream and forms a ring. For diagnosis of brucellosis in dogs, a commercial kit is available (see Chapter 9).

PRECIPITATION TEST.   Precipitation is a reaction between a soluble antigen and a soluble antibody, forming an insoluble precipitate. Lancefield classification or grouping of hemolytic streptococci is based on such a precipitation reaction or test. Once streptococci are classified to a particular group by precipitation testing, the species may be identified by using a battery of biochemical tests to detect different sugars. Streptococci of groups B, C, and E are the most frequently encountered streptococci in veterinary medicine.

FLUORESCENT ANTIBODY TECHNIQUE.   The fluorescent antibody technique is used to detect and localize antigens. Almost any antigen, whether fixed in tissues or in live cell suspension, may be detected by this method. In this procedure, a specific antibody is labeled with a fluorescent dye. The labeled antibody is then added to cells or tissues. If the antibody is specific to the antigen being tested for, a stable complex forms and is evident under fluorescent microscopy.

This procedure is useful to detect small numbers of bacteria. It is also useful if two bacterial species are morphologically and physiologically identical, and cultural procedures are time consuming and expensive.

Some bacterial species routinely evaluated with this technique include *Clostridium chauvoei, Clostridium septicum, E. coli* (K99), *Leptospira, Fusobacterium necrophorum,* and *Listeria monocytogenes.* The fluorescent antibody technique is also used for identification of viruses (see Virology).

MYCOLOGY

◆ Supplies and Equipment

A separate room and incubator should be used for fungal culture because spores tend to contaminate plates put up for bacteriologic culture. If an incubator is inadvertently contaminated with fungal spores, the interior should be swabbed thoroughly with 70% ethyl or isopropyl alcohol or a bowl of water and one of alcohol placed at the bottom of the incubator and the incubator left empty of plates for 24 hours, with the door shut, at 37° C.

In addition to those mentioned in the bacteriology section, supplies and equipment required for mycology include 20% potassium hydroxide, lactophenol cotton blue, and India ink. Storage of these reagents in dropper bottles is convenient. A Wood's lamp (ultraviolet light 3650 angstroms), wooden-handled mycology needles, clear cellophane tape, and culture media also are needed.

◆ Fungal Cultures

Fungi that can invade tissue grow at body temperature (37° C). Using this temperature for incubation of primary cultures inhibits many contaminant saprophytic species. The exception to this is examination of specimens for dimorphic fungi, such as *Blastomyces* and *Histoplasma* species. These organisms produce sporulating mycelia at 25° C and in their saprophytic phase but appear as budding yeast cells in 37° C cultures and in animal tissue. Cultures should be incubated, in parallel, at both temperatures.

Cultures for dermatophytes, or ringworm fungi, are incubated at 25° to 30° C. The exception here is the slow-growing *Trichophyton verrucosum*, which can tolerate incubation at 37° C. At this temperature, *T. verrucosum* is less likely to be overgrown by contaminant fungi.

Because many pathogenic fungi, such as *Candida albicans* and *Aspergillus fumigatus*, are ubiquitous, tissue sections showing invasion are mandatory for definitive diagnosis of a mycotic infection. Occasionally, myceliate fungi or yeasts may appear on blood agar plates put up for bacteriology. These fungi or yeasts, of course, may be contaminants, but some of the original specimen, in 10% formalin, should be submitted for histopathologic examination. Examination of a potassium hydroxide (KOH) wet preparation for fungal elements is also useful.

POTASSIUM HYDROXIDE (KOH) PREPARATION. A small amount of material is scraped from the lesion or tissue and placed in a drop of 20% KOH on a microscope slide. A coverslip is placed on the preparation and pressed down gently to spread the preparation. The slide is left to clear in a moist chamber for a few hours or overnight. The chamber can be a Petri dish with a moist filter at the bottom. The slide is placed on a bent glass rod.

Lactophenol cotton blue stain is a mounting medium used to stain fungal preparations on microscope slides. This medium is especially useful for preparing cellophane tape mounts (see Chapter 7). Its components are as follows:
- Liquefied phenol 25.0 ml
- Lactic acid: 20.0 ml
- Glycerol: 40.0 ml
- Cotton blue: 0.05 g
- Distilled water: 15.0 ml

The cotton blue is dissolved in distilled water using a magnetic stirrer. The rest of the ingredients are added and stirred well. The solution is filtered into a stock bottle. The prepared solution has a shelf life of 1 year. It should be refiltered if the dye precipitates.

Fungal Subcultures

Subcultures for identification or referral to another laboratory may be made in several ways.

YEASTS. These organisms may be streaked out on blood agar or Sabouraud's dextrose agar, as for bacteria.

MYCELIATE FUNGI PRODUCING SPORES.   Crosshatches are cut into the center of a Sabouraud's dextrose agar plate with a few shallow cuts from a sterile scalpel. Using the same scalpel, the veterinary technician collects some of the spores from the center of the colony to be subcultured and presses them gently into the crosshatched agar.

MYCELIATE FUNGI NOT PRODUCING SPORES.   A 1 cm² square of agar is cut from the center of a Sabouraud's dextrose agar plate with a sterile scalpel. A square of the same size is taken from the edge of the colony to be subcultured. This square is made to fit snugly into the hole in the agar. Taking material for subculture from the edge of a fungal colony is always advisable because the old mycelia at the center of the colony may not be viable.

Mycology is time consuming and requires experience and rather specialized techniques. Staff members of a small laboratory may prefer to rely on the simplified techniques described in this section, supplemented by referral of specimens to a larger laboratory for histopathologic examination and culture. Table 4-19 contains a list of pathogenic fungi of veterinary importance.

◆ Fungi Causing Deep Mycoses

Specimen Collection

Frozen tissue should be submitted for fungal culture. The tissue containers should be marked "Caution" because fungi-causing mycoses in animals are potential zoonotic agents. Swab samples should not be sent unless a yeast infection is suspected. Such fluids as blood, cerebrospinal fluid, or aspirates should be submitted in screw-cap tubes.

Aspergillus *Species*

These organisms are essentially saprophytes, but some *Aspergillus* species may be opportunistic pathogens, causing both infections and toxicosis. *Aspergillus fumigatus* is estimated to be responsible for 90% to 95% of cases of aspergillosis.

The diagnosis of aspergillosis is based on several observations. Examination of a KOH wet preparation of the original specimen reveals septate hyphae. A colony of *A. fumigatus* grows rapidly, often appearing in 24 to 48 hours. It is flat and at first white and floccose. As conidia develop, the colony rapidly becomes bluish-green and powdery. Old cultures have a characteristic grayish, "smoky" cast.

Some *Aspergillus* colonies bear a strong resemblance to those of certain *Penicillium* species. A cellophane-tape preparation is made to examine the fruiting heads of the suspect colony. This is done by taking about $2^1/_2$ inches of clear cellophane tape and pressing the center of the tape, sticky side down, onto the center of the colony. The tape, with hyphae and fruiting heads adhering to it, is placed with the sticky side down on a microscope slide, with a drop of lactophenol cotton blue on it. The tape acts as its own coverslip. The slide preparation is examined under low power or high dry if necessary.

TABLE 4-19

Summary of pathogenic fungi, species affected, disease or lesions caused, and specimens for diagnosis

Organism	Species Affected	Disease or Lesion	Specimens
Microsporum		Ringworm	Fresh plucked hair and skin scrapings from edges of lesions; send to laboratory in paper envelopes
M. canis	Dogs, cats		
M. distortum	Dogs, cats, horses, pigs		
M. gallinae (T. gallinae)	Chickens, turkeys ("white comb")		
M. gypseum	Horses, cats, dogs, other species		
M. nanum	Pigs		
M. persicolor	Voles, bats, dogs		
Trichophyton			
T. equinum	Horses, donkeys		
T. erinacei	Hedgehogs, dogs, people		
T. mentagrophytes	Most animal species		
T. rubrum	Primarily people, but also dogs, cats		
T. simli	Poultry, monkeys		
T. verrucosum	Primarily cattle		
Candida albicans	Chickens, turkeys, other birds	Infection of mouth, crop, esophagus	Fresh affected tissue or scrapings from affected tissue
Some other *Candida* spp (such as *C. tropicalis*) can cause lesions	Dogs	Mycotic stomatitis	Fixed affected tissue
	Cats	Enteritis of kittens	
	Calves, foals	Infections of oral and intestinal mucosae	
	Cattle	Mastitis	Most common after extensive antibiotic therapy
	Horses	Genital infections—both sexes	
	Pigs	Infection of esophagus and stomach	
Malassezia pachydermatis	Dogs	Chronic otitis externa	Fresh ear swabs

Continued

TABLE 4-19

Summary of pathogenic fungi, species affected, disease or lesions caused, and specimens for diagnosis—cont'd

Organism	Species Affected	Disease or Lesion	Specimens
Cryptococcus neoformans (worldwide distribution)	People, dogs, cats (infection frequently affects nervous systems)	Subacute or chronic affected tissue	Fresh nasal discharge, milk
Cryptococcus neoformans (worldwide distribution)	Cattle	Sporadic cases of mastitis	Fixed affected tissue, brain, lung
Coccidioides immitis (SW USA and South America; occurs in soil)	People, horses, cattle, sheep, dogs, cats, captive feral animals	Disease characterized by granulomas, often in bronchial and mediastinal lymph nodes and lungs; can cause lesions in brain, liver, spleen, kidneys	Fresh and fixed lesions and affected tissue
Histoplasma capsulatum (NE, central, and S central USA; occurs in soil)	People, dogs, cats, sheep, pigs, horses	Disease that generally affects reticuloendothelial system; dogs, cats: ulcerations of intestinal canal; enlargement of liver, spleen, lymph nodes; TB-like lesions	Fresh and fixed lesions or affected tissue
Histoplasma farciminosum (Mediterranean, Asia, Africa, and part of Russia)	Horses, mules, donkeys	Epizootic lymphangitis, African farcy, or Japanese glanders	Fresh pus and discharges from lesions
Blastomyces dermatitidis (USA, Canada, and Africa; occurs in soil)	People, dogs, cats, sea lions	Granulomatous lesions in lungs and/or skin and subcutis	Fresh and fixed lesions and affected tissue
Sporothrix schenckii	People, horses, dogs, pigs, cattle, fowl, rodents	Subcutaneous nodules or granulomas that eventually discharge pus; can include involvement of bones and visceral organs	Fresh and fixed pus, granulomas

Organism	Host	Disease	Specimen
Rhinosporidium seeberi (not yet cultured in vitro)	Horses, dogs, cattle, people	Characterized by polyps on the nasal and ocular mucous membranes	Fresh nasal discharge and polyps; fixed polyps
Aspergillus *A. fumigatus* main pathogen; potentially pathogenic *A. flavus* *A. nidulans* *A. niger*	Many animal species and birds	Fowl: air sac infection; diffuse and nodular forms in lungs; "brooder pneumonia" in chicks and poults; cattle: occasional mycotic abortion and mastitis; horses: guttural pouch mycosis; dog: infection of nasal chambers	Fresh deep scrapings or affected tissue Abortions: see text
A. flavus *A. parasiticus* *A. ochraceus*	Ducklings, domestic birds, pigs, dogs	Aflatoxicosis; affects liver and sometimes kidneys	Suspect food product
A. clavatus	Pigs	Hemorrhagic disease; profuse hemorrhage in many tissues, jaundice, and liver lesions	
	Cattle	Trembling syndrome: *A. flavus* and *A. fumigatus* toxins; abortion; toxins of *A. ochraceus* cause fetal death; hyperkeratosis lesions on muzzle and mouth from *A. clavatus* toxins	
Petriellidium boydii (*Allescheria boydii*)	Cattle Equidae People, other animals	Abortion, mastitis Abortion, metritis, infertility Mycetoma; progressive disease of subcutis	Fresh milk, uterine discharges, affected tissue Fixed affected tissue

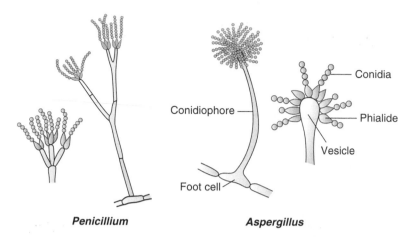

Figure 4-17
Fruiting heads of *Penicillium* and *Aspergillus* species.

A. fumigatus has a vesicle resembling an inverted flask (Figure 4-17). The single row of phialides is borne on the upper half of the vesicle in a crowded parallel fashion. Phialides are produced simultaneously in *Aspergillus* species, whereas with *Penicillium* species successive production occurs.

A tissue sample should be placed in 10% formalin and referred for histopathologic examination. Septate hyphae are seen invading the tissue and causing a tissue reaction.

Candida albicans

This yeast is often a commensal on normal mucous membranes. *Candida* infections most commonly occur after prolonged antibiotic therapy. The diagnosis of candidiasis is based on several findings.

In wet mounts from scrapings from lesions, thin-walled oval and budding yeast cells (2 to 6 μ in diameter) and occasionally pseudohyphae are present. Gram-stained smears disclose intensely Gram-positive oval yeast cells. *C. albicans* grows on blood agar or Sabouraud's dextrose agar as white, smooth colonies with a yeast-like odor. The colonies are not unlike those of micrococci and appear after 24 to 48 hours of incubation.

Presumptive identification of *C. albicans* may be made on its ability to produce germ tubes in bovine serum. A light inoculum of the yeast is made in 0.5 ml of serum incubated at 37° C for 2 hours. In a drop of the inoculated serum examined under the low-power or high-dry objective, the germ tubes appear as small sprouts developing from the yeast cells, without a constriction at their points of origin. Definitive identification is based on fermentation and carbohydrate assimilation tests. Chlamydospore formation on cornmeal agar or chlamydospore agar is also characteristic of *C. albicans*. Histopathologic examination reveals yeast cells and pseudohyphae in tissue, causing an inflammatory reaction. A commercial system, such as API Yeast Ident (bio-Merieux, Hazelwood, MO), can be used to identify *Candida albicans.*

Malassezia pachydermatis

Malassezia pachydermatis (Pityrosporon canis) is one of the most common causes of otitis externa. It is readily observed in Gram-stained smears of exudate as an oval or bottle-shaped, small budding cell. Wet mounts with 10% NaOH show clusters of thick-walled, rounded budding cells. The organism can be cultured on Sabouraud's dextrose agar at 25° C. Addition of olive oil or coconut oil before inoculation enhances growth.

Cryptococcus neoformans

Cryptococcus neoformans is seen most commonly in dogs and cats and occasionally in horses. In all three species the organism usually causes a progressive paranasal infection that does not respond to antibiotic therapy. In such cases, infection resulting from the presence of *Cryptococcus* species or *Aspergillus fumigatus* should be considered.

In clinical cases of cryptococcosis, yeast cells can be seen in wet mounts of the purulent nasal discharge. A little of the discharge is mixed on a slide in a drop composed of distilled water and India ink. The proportion of India ink to water is arbitrary and can be adjusted, but a ratio of 1:2 is usually satisfactory. A coverslip is added and the preparation is examined under low-power and high-dry magnifications. The characteristic and strikingly large capsules of *C. neoformans* show up well by this method. Material should be sent to a reference laboratory for confirmation by culture.

Blastomyces dermatitidis

Blastomycosis is almost always seen in dogs or human beings. It occurs most commonly in the north central and southeastern states of the United States. Granulomatous, discharging ulcers or abscesses usually form in the lungs with subsequent spread to other tissues and organs, including the skin. If material from these lesions, collected by syringe or scalpel, is examined on a wet mount made in 20% KOH, the characteristic yeast form of the organism can be seen. The cells of this dimorphic yeast are large (8 to 15 μ in diameter), oval or spherical, and thick walled. The single bud is connected to the mother cell by a wide base. This characteristic, together with the thick walls of the cells, is typical of *Blastomyces* species. Immunologic tests and mouse inoculation may be used for identification; however, material from the granulomatous nodules should be submitted to a laboratory for confirmation by culture.

Histoplasma capsulatum

In the central United States, histoplasmosis is the most frequently encountered systemic infection in dogs. It is less common in other species, in which the infection can be subclinical. The disease should be suspected in dogs with chronic, intractable coughing and diarrhea. The cells of this dimorphic yeast are small (1 to 3 μ in diameter) and rarely found extracellularly and so are difficult to see in clinical material. Smears from tissue can be stained by the Giemsa or Wright's method and examined under oil immersion. The organisms occur intracellularly, usually in monocytic cells, as small oval cells surrounded by a halo. The exoantigen test is an immunodiffusion test used by some laboratories for rapid identification of *B. dermatitidis, Histoplasma capsulatum,* and *Coccidioides immitis.* Confirmation should be made by submitting material for histopathologic examination and culture.

◆ Dermatophytes

Dermatophytes cause superficial mycoses. Ringworm often may be diagnosed by clinical signs. However, ringworm manifests in several forms: subclinical or inapparent, which is quite common in young kittens and rodents; typical ringed lesions; and nodular or tumorous lesions called *kerions.* Ringworm lesions may have to be differentiated from other conditions that include mite or ectoparasite infestations; *Dermatophilus congolensis* infections in horses, cattle and sheep; pityriasis rosea, of unknown etiology, in pigs; and lesions resulting from hypersensitivity, especially in dogs.

Dermatophytes may be classified as to the habitat in which they are most likely to be found: *anthropophilic,* confined to human beings; *zoophilic,* parasites of animals; and *geophilic,* normally existing as free-living saprophytes in the soil. Of the 15 known geophilic species, 5 may occasionally be opportunist pathogens, and only one, *Microsporum gypseum,* commonly causes lesions in animals. These geophilic species pose a certain difficulty in diagnosis because they must be differentiated from zoophilic species.

Specimen Collection

Hair should be plucked from the periphery of the lesion. A Wood's lamp may help detect hairs that are fluorescent, although not all ringworm organisms cause fluorescence. Hairs cut with scissors give disappointing results because the arthrospores are often at the base of the hairs and remain on the animal. Skin scrapings are taken with a blunt scalpel from the lesion's edge. Scraping should continue until blood is just drawn.

Specimens from pigs, particularly, are often contaminated with saprophytic fungi. Lesions may be swabbed with 70% isopropyl alcohol and allowed to dry before specimens are taken.

Hairs and skin scrapings are collected in paper envelopes. The specimens tend to stay drier and less contaminated in envelopes than when placed in a closed container.

Diagnosis of Ringworm

WOOD'S LAMP EXAMINATION.   Hair samples from dogs and cats, or the animals themselves, should be examined under the Wood's (ultraviolet) lamp. Hairs infected with *Microsporum canis, Microsporum distortum,* or *Microsporum audouinii* (an thropophilic) may fluoresce a clear apple green under the Wood's lamp in a darkened room. About 60% of positive cases involving *M. canis* fluoresce, apparently depending on whether the fungus has reached the right growth stage to produce fluorescence. No fluorescence on Wood's lamp examination does rule out the possibility of ringworm infection.

DIRECT MICROSCOPY. To establish a diagnosis of ringworm, the fungus must be demonstrated in the hairs by direct microscopy. This is particularly essential with geophilic species, such as *M. gypseum.* Its presence in culture alone may simply represent contamination from soil.

A few selected hairs and a little of the skin scrapings are placed in a drop of 20% KOH on a microscope slide. A coverslip is applied with gentle pressure and the preparation is gently heated and allowed to set for 10 to 15 minutes. Another procedure is to leave the preparation in a moist chamber for a few hours or overnight before examination.

The wet preparation is examined under the low-power objective and then under high dry for chains of the highly refractile arthrospores that sheathe infected hairs. These are at the roots of the hairs. The arthrospores of *Trichophyton verrucosum* (cattle) are particularly large (5 to 10 μ), whereas those of *M. canis* are about 2 to 3 μ.

Mange mites also may be observed in the cleared preparations. If scab material is present in samples from cattle, sheep, or horses, make a Gram-stained smear for *D. congolensis.*

CULTURE. *Trichophyton verrucosum* requires thiamin and inositol for growth and *Trichophyton equinum* requires nicotinic acid. These growth factors may be supplied by adding yeast extract to the medium. Phytone yeast extract agar (BBL Microbiology Systems, Cockeysville, MD) is available in dehydrated powder form and supports growth of these two dermatophytes. It contains streptomycin and chloramphenicol, which control bacterial contaminants but not fungi. If the veterinary practice is routinely involved with dermatophyte specimens from horses or cattle, then prepared plates may be used, such as Mycosel agar (BBL Microbiology Systems, Cockeysville, MD) or Mycobiotic agar (Gibco Products, Grand Island, NY), which contain chloramphenicol to suppress bacterial growth and cycloheximide to control saprophytic fungi. Dermatophytes are resistant to both antimicrobial agents.

Sabouraud's dextrose agar is a more conventional medium for culture of dermatophytes. The low pH of about 5.6 inhibits most bacterial contaminants, but many saprophytic fungi grow on it. Prepared plates of Sabouraud's dextrose agar are offered by BBL, Difco, Gibco, and Oxoid. An alternative is to prepare Sabouraud's dextrose agar from dehydrated powder and add Oxoid's SR75 Dermasel supplement, which contains cycloheximide and chloramphenicol. Shallow cuts with a sterile scalpel are made at eight separate sites on the agar plate. A few of the plucked hairs and/or skin scrapings are pushed gently into the agar at these sites.

The temperature of incubation should be 25° to 30° C for optimum growth of dermatophytes. If the temperature is consistently lower than 23° to 24° C, growth is slow and atypical. Although dermatophytes may be grown at a warm ambient temperature, incubating at 28° to 30° C is ideal for growth. For *T. verrucosum*, 37° C is recommended for more rapid growth; this temperature also suppresses growth of saprophytic fungi. Cultures should be incubated for up to 3 weeks for most dermatophytes and up to 6 weeks for the slower-growing species, such as *T. verrucosum.*

To avoid drying of the cultures, tape can be used to seal the plates. The tape should be removed and reapplied every 3 to 4 days because dermatophytes are strict aerobes. The plates are incubated right side (lid) up to prevent spores from being liberated as the plates are opened.

Identification of Dermatophytes

Dermatophytes usually may be identified by colony morphology and by microscopic examination of colonies for macroaleuriospores (old name: macroconidia). Many dermatophytes have characteristically pigmented colonies (Table 4-20).

Suspect colonies should be microscopically examined for macroaleuriospores. A drop of lactophenol cotton blue is placed on a microscope slide. Some material from the center of the colony is teased out in the liquid using flamed mycology needles. The preparation is covered by a coverslip and examined under low-power and high-dry objectives. An easier way to examine for macroaleuriospores is to use the cellophane-tape method (see *Aspergillus fumigatus*).

Some dermatophytes, such as *M. canis* and many *Trichophyton* species, are poor or slow macroaleuriospore producers. Any present are found at the center of the colony. If none are seen on initial examination, reincubating the culture or transferring a piece of thallus aseptically to cereal agar is worthwhile. Growth on this medium usually induces production of macroaleuriospores.

Development of macroaleuriospores may be monitored by preparing a slide culture as follows:

1. A sterile piece of filter paper is placed on the bottom of a sterile Petri dish. The filter paper is wetted with sterile water.
2. A bent glass rod is placed on the filter paper (Figure 4-18).
3. A microscope slide is passed through a flame several times to sterilize it. Then the slide is placed on the glass rod.
4. A 1-cm × 1-cm block of the desired agar is aseptically cut and removed and placed on the flamed slide.
5. The four sides of the agar block are aseptically cut with spores or mycelial fragments of the fungus.
6. The lid is placed on the Petri dish and sealed with masking tape.
7. The slide is incubated at 28° C and checked periodically under the microscope for growth and sporulation. Once sporulation has occurred, forceps are used to carefully remove the coverglass from the agar block (it should be popped off rather than slid off).
8. A drop of 95% ethanol is applied to wet the fungus. A drop of lactophenol cotton blue is placed on a clean slide, the coverslip lowered onto it, and the slide is examined with the microscope.

A dermatophyte test medium in kit form is available from Difco and Pitman-Moore (Mundelein, IL). This is a modified Sabouraud's agar with a pH indicator, phenol red. Any

Continued

TABLE 4-20

Colony characteristics, macroaleuriospores, and main host(s) of some commonly isolated dermatophytes

Dermatophyte and Main Host(s)	Colony Characteristics	Microscopic Characteristics
Microsporum canis Dogs, cats, occasionally other species	Comparatively rapid growth; flat colony; surface white and silky at center, with bright yellow periphery; reverse side is yellow	Some strains are poor producers of macroaleuriospores; when present, 8- to 15-celled, spindle-shaped and older spores ending in a distinct knob
Microsporum gypseum Horses, wild rodents, occasionally other species	Comparatively rapid growth; colony flat, with irregularly fringed border; surface is coarsely powdery, light ochre to cinnamon brown; reverse is brownish yellow	Numerous macroaleuriospores; boat-shaped, 3- to 9-celled, walls rough, shorter, broader than those of *M. canis*
Microsporum distortum Dogs, less common in cats	Growth comparatively rapid; colony flat with tendency to develop radial grooves; surface velvety or fluffy, white to tan; reverse is whitish to yellowish tan	Macroaleuriospores usually numerous and characteristically distorted
Microsporum nanum Pigs, rare in other animals	Growth comparatively rapid; surface at first white and cottony, becoming granular, buff-colored; reverse is brownish red; colonies of some strains have fringed borders	Numerous macroaleuriospores; pear-shaped, 2- to 3 cells with relatively thin walls, characteristic for *M. nanum*

TABLE **4-20**

Colony characteristics, macroaleuriospores, and main host(s) of some commonly isolated dermatophytes—cont'd

Dermatophyte and Main Host(s)	Colony Characteristics	Microscopic Characteristics
Trichophyton mentagrophytes Many species; most commonly dogs, guinea pigs, wild rodents, horses, pigs	Growth rapid; colony type varies from flat, granular, and tan, rather like *M. gypseum*, to heaped and cottony white; reverse is yellowish to orange-brown	Granular colonies have numerous macroaleuriospores, cigar-shaped with 2–6 cells; often no macroaleuriospores from heaped colonies
Trichophyton verrucosum Cattle	Growth very slow, none may be obvious for 2 weeks; colony small, velvety, and white; can later become heaped and folded	Macroaleuriospores are very rare, but at 37° C, thick-walled, rounded chlamydospores can be numerous
Trichophyton equinum Horses, less common in other animals	Growth quite rapid; colony flat, white at first with yellow in peripheral growth, later becoming velvety and cream to tan; reverse can be yellowish in young colony but later becomes dark brown	Macroaleuriospores are rare; if present they are the typical cigar shape of the *Trichophyton* genus

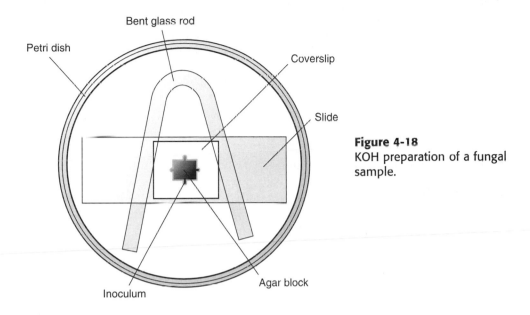

Figure 4-18
KOH preparation of a fungal sample.

dermatophytes present produce alkaline metabolites that change the yellowish medium to red, usually within 14 days.

With veterinary specimens, which contain numerous contaminant fungi, using dermatophyte test medium as the sole culture procedure is unwise. The slant provides too small an area on which to place clinical material. Some contaminant fungi also change the color of the medium, although not to the dark red produced by dermatophytes. However, this color change by dermatophytes masks the characteristic pigmentation of their colonies, which is used for identification.

Dermatophyte test medium may be used as a supplementary identification method, with the suspect dermatophyte subcultured onto the medium. A small hollow is cut in the middle of the dermatophyte test medium slant with a sterile scalpel. Using the same scalpel, the veterinary technician should cut a piece of mycelium from the edge of the colony and fit it snugly into the hollow in the dermatophyte test medium slant. The medium is incubated at 25° to 30° C for 7 to 14 days. A distinct red color in the medium indicates that the fungus may be a dermatophyte.

Nonpathogenic Geophilic Dermatophytes

The following three dermatophytes, which occur in soil, are common contaminants of animal hairs. They are considered nonpathogenic but must be differentiated from dermatophytes capable of causing ringworm:

- *Microsporum cookie:* The surface of the colony is cream colored and powdery, but the reverse is purple-red. Macroaleuriospores are abundant and similar to those of *M. gypseum.*

- *Trichophyton ajelloi:* The surface of the colony is powdery and a rich orange-buff color. The reverse of the colony is violet-black although some strains have a pale yellow reverse. The abundant microaleuriospores are cigar shaped.
- *Trichophyton terrestre:* The colony has a powdery to granular surface, white to cream yellow in color. The reverse is pinkish or yellow. The macroaleuriospores are slender and pencil shaped.

◆ Serologic Diagnosis of Mycoses

Serologic diagnosis of mycoses in animals has received little attention, although in human beings such tests are used to aid diagnosis and prognosis. Unfortunately, serologic diagnosis is not available to veterinarians through most human diagnostic laboratories. Most tests in human medicine are for systemic mycoses and are *in vitro* procedures, including complement fixation, agglutination, and sometimes the precipitin test. Fluorescent antibody techniques have been developed for many fungi, usually to identify isolates rather than to measure antibody.

In vivo skin tests (delayed reaction, 24 to 48 hours) are used in human medicine for diagnosis of histoplasmosis, blastomycosis, coccidioidomycosis, and sporotrichosis. These tests also should be applicable to animals. Skin tests and exoantigen immunodiffusion tests for histoplasmosis have been used in dogs.

Recently, an agar gel immunodiffusion (AGID) test has been used on serum samples from dogs to confirm *Aspergillus fumigatus* infection of the nasal cavity. AGID tests also likely have application in diagnosing fungal upper respiratory infections in horses.

◉ VIROLOGY

Virologic techniques are performed in specialized laboratories. They include histopathologic and serologic examination, electron microscopy, and attempted isolation and identification of the virus. The veterinary technician should contact the diagnostic laboratory to check what facilities are available, what samples are preferred, and whether a transport medium is considered necessary. Table 4-21 indicates the types of specimens usually collected for diagnosis of the more common viral diseases of domestic animals. If an exotic (reportable) disease is suspected, the proper authorities should be notified and no clinical material removed from the farm.

Many of the viral diseases encountered may be diagnosed on clinical and pathologic grounds. Serologic tests are available for most viral diseases. These usually require paired serum samples collected 2 to 3 weeks apart, early in the disease and on recovery. A rising antibody titer indicates recent infection by the virus. Collection of serum samples from contact animals is worth considering because these animals are more likely to have low initial titers to the virus.

Virus isolation is expensive and time consuming and may provide only a diagnosis after the animals have recovered or died. However, in some instances isolation and identification of a virus should be attempted: to establish the identity of a viral disease not previously seen in a practice; to discover the exact agent when serologic and

Text continued on p. 207.

TABLE 4-21

Common viral infections of domestic animals

Virus	Disease or Lesion	Specimens
Bovine herpesvirus 1	Infectious bovine rhinotra-cheitis and infectious pustu-lar vaginitis	Mucosal scrapings; whole aborted fetus or fresh and fixed fetal kidney and liver, paired serum samples
Bovine herpesvirus 2	Bovine mammillitis; dermatitis, often hemorrhagic, of udder and teats, muzzle lesions in sucking calves	Vesicular fluid from early lesions or deep scrapings from older lesions; fixed biopsy; scabs of no value
Alcelaphine herpes-virus 1	Malignant catarrhal fever	Fixed liver, brain, kidney, lymph nodes, adrenals, and lesions from alimentary tract
Flavivirus	Bovine virus diarrhea-mucosal disease	Fresh spleen, lymph nodes and blood clot; serum; fixed por-tions of lesions
Retrovirus	Bovine leukosis	Lesions, fresh and fixed; EDTA blood
Picornaviruses	Enteroviruses: possible involve-ment in neonatal disease	Feces and serum
	Rhinoviruses: upper respiratory tract infection	Nasal mucosal scrapings
	Foot and mouth disease virus: lesions	Vesicular fluid; serum
Parvovirus	Diarrhea in young calves	Feces
Reoviruses	Respiratory and enteric condi-tions in young calves	Nasal mucosal scraping; feces; serum
	Bovine rotavirus: associated with diarrhea in young calves	Feces
Adenoviruses	May cause upper respiratory tract infections	Nasal scrapings
Paramyxovirus	Parainfluenza 3: upper respira-tory tract infections and oc-casionally pneumonia	Nasal scrapings; whole blood; lung
	Rinderpest virus: profuse diar-rhea	Serum
Papilloma virus	Papillomas (warts)	Fixed and fresh excised tumors
Poxviruses	Pseudocowpox (paravacinia, milker's nodules); dermatitis on udder and teats with "horseshoe" scab formation	Deep scrapings of early lesions
	Papular stomatitis: ulcers in buccal cavity and lips, mainly in calves	Deep scrapings of several oral ulcers; fixed tissue from lesion

Continued

TABLE 4-21

Common viral infections of domestic animals—cont'd

Virus	Disease or Lesion	Specimens
Horses		
Herpesvirus	Herpesvirus 1: rhinopneumonitis; abortion	Nasal scraping; fresh, whole aborted fetus or fresh and fixed fetal liver; kidney and lung
	Herpesvirus 2: upper respiratory tract of normal horses; pathogenicity uncertain	Deep scrapings of lesions
	Herpesvirus 3: coital exanthema; venereal vulvitis or balantitis	
Papilloma virus	Papillomas (warts)	Fresh and fixed excised tumors
Orthomyxovirus	Influenza virus: upper respiratory tract infection and occasionally pneumonia	Nasal scrapings; lung; whole blood
Paramyxovirus	Parainfluenza; upper respiratory tract infection	Nasal scrapings from very early cases; serum
Picornavirus	Rhinoviruses: upper respiratory tract infection, mainly in young horses	Nasal scrapings and exudates
Togaviruses	Arteritis; edema of the limbs and eyes; abortion	Nasal or conjunctival exudates in transport medium (Hanks' with antibiotics and 1% bovine albumin; store at $-20°$ C)
	Western, eastern, and Venezuelan equine encephalomyelitis	Fresh and Fixed brain
Sheep		
Herpesvirus	Adenomatosis: chronic progressive lung disease in sheep >4 yr; no metastases	Fixed lung lesion
Paramyxovirus	Parainfluenza 3: signs referable to respiratory tract, with pneumonia in young animals	Nasal scrapings very early in disease; isolation often difficult from pneumonic lesions; serum
Picornavirus	Foot and mouth disease	Vesicular fluid; serum
Togavirus (closely related to BVD virus of cattle)	Border disease of lambs or "hairy shaker" disease: neonatal condition; hairy coat, nervous signs, poor growth	Serum

TABLE 4-21

Common viral infections of domestic animals—cont'd

Virus	Disease or Lesion	Specimens
Poxvirus	Contagious pustular dermatitis; orf; scabby-mouth disease	Scabs and scrapings from young lesions; fixed lesions
Rotavirus	Diarrhea in lambs	Feces and serum
Pigs		
Herpesvirus	Inclusion-body rhinitis (porcine cytomegalovirus): deaths in pigs <2 wk old; subacute in older pigs	Whole, recently dead pig carcass or sick live pig; head of older pigs or fixed nasal mucosa
	Pseudorabies (Aujeszky's disease): respiratory infections and abortions	Lesions from recently dead pigs; serum
	Vesicular disease	Vesicular fluid
Picornavirus	Talfan or Teschen's disease: porcine poliomyelitis	Fresh and fixed whole brain; serum
	Encephalomyocarditis: sudden death in pigs >12 wk old	Recently dead pigs or fresh heart, spleen; fixed heart and brain; serum
	SMEDI viruses: stillbirths, mummification, embryonic deaths, infertility	Aborted fetuses; serum
	Enteroviruses: possible involvement in neonatal diarrhea	Feces; serum
	Foot and mouth disease	Vesicular fluid; serum
Parvovirus	Reproductive failure	Freshly aborted fetuses, especially mummified fetuses; serum
Rotavirus	Acute gastroenteritis in piglets	Feces
Orthomyxovirus	Influenza A: bronchopneumonia and lung edema	Respiratory exudates or lung; serum
Coronaviruses	Transmissible gastroenteritis: vomiting and diarrhea in sows and young pigs	Live affected piglets or fresh and fixed small intestine; serum; feces are valueless
	Hemagglutinating encephalomyelitis: vomiting, wasting, and constipation in young pigs	Live affected piglets or fresh and fixed brain; serum
Cats		
Herpesvirus 1	Herpesvirus serotype 1: rhinotracheitis; occasionally abortion in queens and some fatalities in neonates	Nasal scrapings early in disease

Continued

TABLE 4-21

Common viral infections of domestic animals—cont'd

Virus	Disease or Lesion	Specimens
Herpesvirus 1 —cont'd	Herpesvirus-induced feline urolithiasis	Diagnosis by clinical signs
Parvovirus	Panleukopenia or feline infections enteritis: congenital abnormalities, such as cerebellar hypoplasia	Fresh spleen, fixed portions of intestine, lymph nodes, thymus, bone marrow; EDTA blood
Dogs		
Herpesvirus	Deaths in neonatal pups; may be cause of "fading puppy syndrome"; rhinitis and pharyngitis in pups >6 wk old; vaginitis and abortion	Whole puppy carcass or fresh and fixed kidney, spleen, lungs, liver and nasopharynx; serum
Rhabdovirus	Rabies	Consult with state veterinarian
Papilloma virus	Oral papillomas (warts)	Fixed and fresh excised tumors
Paramyxoviruses	Canine distemper (hard-pad disease)	Fresh whole lung; fixed lung, brain, bladder, kidney, liver, gallbladder
	Parainfluenza: upper respiratory tract infection	Respiratory exudates
Adenoviruses	Infectious canine hepatitis (canine adenovirus 1): Rubarth's disease; hepatitis and death, especially in young pups	Whole puppy carcass or fresh nasopharyngeal scraping, and fresh and fixed lung, kidney, spleen, liver, brain; feces and urine from live pups; serum
	Canine adenovirus 2: upper respiratory tract infection; occasionally causes pneumonia (infectious tracheobronchitis)	Nasal swab and scrapings; fresh and fixed lung
Parvoviruses	Enteritis, myocarditis, leukopenia; closely related to feline panleukopenia virus	Fresh feces; serum; mesenteric lymph nodes; ileum; spleen
Coronavirus	Vomiting, diarrhea	Feces
Reovirus	Reovirus (1 and 2) infection: usually mild upper respiratory infection	Nasal exudates; feces
Rotavirus	Gastroenteritis in young pups	Feces

TABLE 4-21

Common viral infections of domestic animals—cont'd

Virus	Disease or Lesion	Specimens
Birds, Poultry		
Herpesvirus	Infectious laryngotracheitis: severe dyspnea, coughing	Tracheal exudates
	Marek's disease: nervous signs, paralysis	Liver, lungs, tissues, blood, bone marrow
Retrovirus	Avian leukosis: tumorous enlargement of liver and spleen	Spleen, liver
Picornavirus	Encephalomyelitis, paresis, sitting on hock	Brain, gizzard, spinal cord
Reovirus	Infectious bursal disease, swelling of cloacal bursa, edema	Feces, kidney, bursal tissue
Paramyxovirus	Paramyxovirus I: Newcastle disease	Exudate, serum
Poxvirus	Respiratory/nervous signs Fowl pox: Nodules in skin, heavy scabs	Vesicular fluid, scab scrapings

other tests have given equivocal results; to find the immunologic type of a virus in an epizootic; and to verify the etiologic agent if a public health problem is involved.

Isolation of a virus from a diseased animal does not necessarily mean the virus caused the disease, because many viruses can persist in animals without clinical signs of illness. Some other pathogen or condition could have been responsible for the disease. Virus isolation is most successful when specimens are collected early in the active infectious phase of the disease.

Viruses vary greatly in their ability to remain viable in tissues and exudates. Contamination with bacteria greatly decreases the success of attempted virus isolation. Specimens should be:

- Selected based on their likelihood to contain large numbers of virus particles
- Taken from live or very recently dead animals, even if this means sacrificing an affected animal
- Collected aseptically
- Kept at 4° C and taken to a laboratory in the shortest time possible

Collection of Specimens

Viruses are often present in the nasal or pharyngeal secretions early in the acute stage of respiratory diseases. Mucosal scrapings rather than just swabs of the secretions should be taken. Sterile wooden tongue depressors are useful for mucosal scrapings.

Attempted isolation from blood samples may be considered in generalized catarrhal diseases that tend to have a viremic stage. Poxviruses often may be demonstrated by electron microscopy in fluid from early vesicular lesions and sometimes in scabs from early lesions.

Specimens should also be selected for indirect studies, such as serologic, hematologic, histologic, and bacteriologic examinations. Viral diseases often are complicated by pathogenic bacteria acting as secondary invaders, which often can turn a mild viral infection into a serious disease. Specimens for histopathologic examination should consist of thin sections of tissue placed immediately into 10% formalin. Sections for histologic examination must never be frozen because this causes tissue artifacts that may be difficult to differentiate from a pathologic process.

Tissue samples for attempted virus isolation should be 2-inch cubes that contain both diseased and normal tissue, if possible. Mucosal scrapings should be obtained instead of merely swabs. Sterile screw-capped containers should be used for collection, a separate container for each sample. Veterinary technicians must employ strict asepsis and label the containers carefully.

Submission of Samples

Specimens should be refrigerated (4° C) when possible because virus titers decrease as temperature increases. If the specimens are to be delivered to the virology laboratory within 24 hours, they may be stored at 4° C and packed with coolant packs or ice in a polystyrene-insulated carton for shipment. If the time delay will be longer than 24 hours, snap freezing at −70° C and shipping on dry ice is desirable, except for specimens of suspected parainfluenza and influenza virus, in which case the integrity of these viruses is best preserved at −20° C. Specimens must be shipped in airtight containers to prevent entry of CO_2 into the container. CO_2 gas from the dry ice can lower the pH of fluid, killing any pH-labile viruses.

Small pieces of tissue, fecal material, or mucus can be preserved in vials filled with 50% glycol and stored at 4° C. A virus transport medium is available commercially (NCS Diagnostics, Mississauga, Ontario). Because viruses vary in their longevity, a reference laboratory should be contacted for recommendations on the appropriate transport medium and sampling procedure.

Fecal materials and fluids often are submitted for electron microscopic examination. A fixative, such as universal or 10% buffered neutral formalin, should be added to the sample at a maximum of 1:1 fixative to sample to prevent overdilution of virus particles.

For urine samples, approximately 5 ml is sent in a sterile container. Virus transport medium should not be used. The specimen must be kept chilled if it is to arrive at the laboratory within 24 hours of collection; otherwise, it should be frozen at −70° C and shipped frozen.

If blood samples have been collected for serologic examination, they should be left at room temperature and the clot allowed to retract. Then they are refrigerated. Blood samples should not be frozen because freezing causes hemolysis and may render serum samples useless for serologic examination.

Cell Culture

To demonstrate the presence of a virus in a specimen, the virus is grown (isolated) in the laboratory or the virus antigens or antibodies are assayed. Unlike bacteria, which can be grown on nutrient agar, viruses need living cells in which to grow and replicate.

The tissue cells are placed into a suitable glass bottle or chamber containing a medium rich in nutrients. The cells settle and begin to grow in a confluent monolayer across the surface of the container.

Various types of cells have been used for tissue culture of viruses. Most animal cells can be grown *in vitro* for some generations, but some cells divide indefinitely and are used for virus isolation. These cells are called *continuous cell lines* and are of a single type of cell. Continuous cell lines, such as those from fetal kidney, embryonic trachea, skin and other cells, are derived from monkeys, dogs, cattle, pigs, cats, mice, hamsters, rabbits, and other animals. The virus specimen is commonly inoculated into a primary culture of cells derived from the same species of animal from which the specimen was taken.

After the cell culture has been inoculated with the virus specimen and incubated, the cell culture is examined. If the virus is present, cell damage may be visible as the virus particles invade the tissue cells. This damage is referred to as a *cytopathic effect*. Different types of cytopathic effects are used to identify viruses. Some viruses cause cell lysis, whereas others cause the cells to fuse and form syncytiae (sheets) and giant cells. An inclusion body is another type of cytopathic effect that may be seen.

Embryonated Egg Cultures

Embryonated eggs are a valuable medium for cultivation of viruses. Although embryonated eggs are convenient for growing viruses, the range of viruses that can be grown in them is somewhat limited.

Canine distemper virus and poxviruses are grown on chorioallantoic membranes, producing pox lesions visible to the naked eye. Influenza virus grows initially in the amnionic sac and then in the allantoic cavity, causing death of the embryo in 48 to 72 hours. Newcastle disease virus grows in the allantoic cavity, causing death of the embryo in 48 to 72 hours.

◆ Serologic Examination

Clinical signs and cell culture examination may identify the virus to a family level and perhaps to the genus and species level, but definitive identification requires serologic procedures based on immunologic principles. Sometimes these serologic procedures may be used on the specimens directly, which saves the time and expense of cell culture.

Direct Immunofluorescence

In this type of test, an antibody to a specific virus, such as rabies virus, is labeled with a fluorescent dye and is added to the specimen. If virus antigen is present in the specimen, the antibody binds to it (Figure 4-19). If the virus antigen is not present, the

| Antiviral antibody with fluorescent dye | Specimen with antigen | Antibody-antigen-dye complex |

Figure 4-19
With direct immunofluorescence, antiviral antibody labeled with a flourescent dye is added to the specimen, forming an antibody-antigen-dye complex.

| Antiviral antibody | Viral antigen | Antiviral antibody-viral antigen complex | Antirabbit immunoglobulin with fluorescent dye | Antirabbit immunoglobulin bound to antiviral antibody bound to viral antigen |

Figure 4-20
With indirect immunofluorescence, antibody forms a complex with the virus antigen, which then binds with antirabbit immunoglobin and the fluorescent dye.

antibody is washed away in the rinsing step of the procedure. Upon microscopic examination, any antibody-antigen complex is visible as fluorescence.

Indirect Immunofluorescence

An indirect procedure using two antibodies also is used. Antiviral antibodies, called *immunoglobulins,* are produced in an animal, such as a rabbit. The second antibody is an antirabbit immunoglobulin labeled with the fluorescent dye. The second antibody binds to the first antibody, which binds to any virus antigen in the specimen (Figure 4-20). This complex is then detected on microscopic examination.

If no virus antigen is present in the specimen, no binding occurs and the unbound dye is washed away. This technique has some advantages over the direct fluorescent technique, including increased sensitivity. An example of a disease diagnosed by this method is cryptosporidiosis.

Radioimmunoassay

In this procedure, the label is a radioactive element, such as iodine. This radioactive label is attached to an antiviral antibody that combines with virus antigen in the specimen (Figure 4-21). A gamma counter is needed to detect the presence of the antibody-antigen complexes. Thyroid hormone levels are measured by this method.

Antiviral antibody with radioactive iodine

Viral antigen

Antibody-iodine-antigen complex

Figure 4-21
In radioimmunoassay, antiviral antibody labeled with a radioactive element, such as iodine, is added to the specimen, forming an antibody-iodine-antigen complex.

Tray with antiviral antibody-coated wells

Specimen with viral antigens

Tray with bound antibody-antigen

Enzyme-labeled antiviral antibody

Viral antigen bound with both antibodies

Substrate

Substrate reacts with enzyme to produce color change

Figure 4-22
With enzyme-linked immunosorbent assay, viral antigens bind with antibody in the test wells, an enzyme-labeled antiviral antibody is added, and finally a substrate is added to produce a color change.

Enzyme-Linked Immunosorbent Assay

Enzyme-linked immunosorbent assay (ELISA) uses test trays containing antibody-coated wells. The sample is added to the wells and any virus antigen binds to the antibody. A second antiviral antibody is then added; this antibody is enzyme-labeled. If virus was present in the sample and was bound to the antibody that coated the well, the second antibody also binds to the virus. When a substrate that reacts with the enzyme is added, the resultant color change is proportional to the amount of virus antigen present in the sample (Figure 4-22). If no virus was present in the sample, the second antibody is washed away in the rinsing process and no color change is seen. Feline leukemia virus is detected with this method.

Immunodiffusion

With immunodiffusion, antigen in the specimen and antibody are placed into separate wells in agar. They diffuse into the agar and form a visible band of precipitation

Antibody and specimen
with antigen
placed in wells

Diffusion
into agar

Visible band of
precipitation

Figure 4-23
In immunodiffusion, antigen and antibody in separate wells diffuse out into the agar and
form a visible precipitate where they meet.

when they combine (Figure 4-23). If no band forms, no virus antigen is present in the
sample. Bovine leukemia virus is detected by immunodiffusion.

Complement Fixation

Complement is a series of enzymes in normal serum that combine with an antibody-
antigen complex to cause lysis of cells, destruction of bacteria, and other immune responses. In complement fixation, complement becomes "fixed" when it combines
with an antibody-antigen complex. The complement fixation test is used to detect viral antibodies in a serum sample, as in anaplasmosis.

The patient's serum sample is heated to inactivate its complement. A known
amount of complement is added to the serum. A known amount of virus antigen is
then added and this mixture is incubated to allow fixation of the complement if virus
antibodies are present in the serum. Sensitized RBCs (RBCs that have complexed with
anti-RBC antibodies) are then added and the mixture is incubated. If virus antibody is
present in the serum, viral antibody-viral antigen complexes are formed and no lysis
of the RBCs occurs. Complement was "fixed" and was not available to lyse RBCs. If no
virus antibody is present in the serum, complexes of anti-RBC antibody–RBC antigen
and complement are formed, and the RBCs are lysed (Figure 4-24).

Virus Neutralization in Cell Culture

Two types of virus neutralization techniques are used: inhibition of cytopathic effects
and plaque reduction. Before doing these tests, the virus in the sample must be
known to cause cytopathic effects or plaque formation. By using a specific antibody,
the virus can then be identified. Bovine virus diarrhea is diagnosed by virus neutralization.

INHIBITION OF CYTOPATHIC EFFECTS.   A specific antibody to a particular virus
is incubated with a specimen that contains the unidentified virus. Cell culture tubes
are then inoculated with this mixture and checked daily for cytopathic effects. Complete inhibition of cytopathic effects is considered a positive virus neutralization test
and indicates the identity of the virus. The virus in the specimen forms a complex

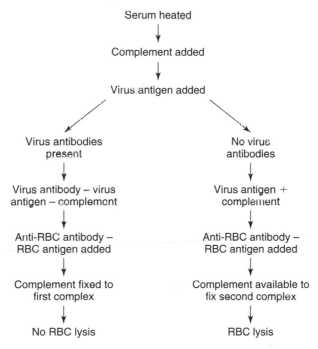

Figure 4-24
Complement fixation test shows no RBC lysis if virus antibody is present.

with the added antibody and was unable to cause cytopathic effects. If cytopathic effects are produced, the particular virus tested is ruled out.

PLAQUE REDUCTION. The specimen containing the unidentified virus is incubated with antibody for a particular virus. Cell culture tubes are then inoculated with this mixture and incubated again. An agar medium containing a dye is added and incubated, and the culture is observed daily for the presence and numbers of plaques, which are necrotic cells surrounded by living cells. Necrotic cells do not pick up the dye and are colorless, whereas living cells are stained by the dye. An 80% or greater reduction of plaque counts is positive and confirms the identity of the virus. In this case, the specific antibody has formed a complex with the virus, preventing it from forming plaques.

Electron Microscopy

The two basic techniques for routine diagnostic use of electron microscopy are negative staining of virus particles and thin-sectioning of virus-infected cells. Electron microscopy may be used to identify viruses to the family level and sometimes to the genus or species level. Parvovirus can be detected by electron microscopy.

NEGATIVE STAINING.   A virus suspension made from a clinical sample is mixed with a heavy-metal stain. The heavy-metal atoms surround the virus particles. The electron beam of the electron microscope passes through the virus particles but cannot pass through the metal atoms. This phenomenon gives the appearance of a "negative stain;" that is, the virus is light and "unstained" and the surrounding background of metallic atoms is dark and appears "stained."

THIN SECTIONING.   This technique uses the intact virus-infected cells, which are examined with the electron microscope. It gives a more reliable diagnosis than simple negative staining of the clinical sample because tissues from the animal or inoculated tissue cell culture are used, and the virus and the cell it is infecting are preserved for examination. This complex procedure consists of several preparatory steps and includes the negative-staining step.

Immunoelectron Microscopy

With this technique, monoclonal or polyclonal antibodies are added to a virus suspension made from the clinical specimen. If the corresponding virus antigens are present in the suspension, antibody-antigen complexes form. The suspension is centrifuged and combined with a heavy-metal stain and then applied to an electron microscope grid for examination using the negative-staining procedure.

Antibody is added to increase the likelihood of seeing virus particles. The complexes or aggregates are more easily seen than a few individual virus particles, especially when virus concentration is low. Coronavirus may be detected by this method.

◆ Direct Detection of Viral Nucleic Acid

In this research technique, DNA strands of a virus are separated and one of the strands is labeled with a radioactive isotope or a nonradioactive label. The labeled "probes" are added to separated strands of viral DNA from cells infected with the unknown virus. Under appropriate conditions, the two strands combine with each other if they are from the same virus. Because one of the strands is labeled, it can be detected and the identity of the virus is confirmed.

Recommended Reading

Carter GR: *Diagnostic procedures in veterinary bacteriology and mycology,* ed 5, San Diego, 1990, Academic Press.

Carter GR, Chengappa MM, Roberts AW: *Essentials of veterinary bacteriology,* ed 5, Philadelphia, 1995, Lippincott, Williams & Wilkins.

Castro AE, Heuschele WP: *Veterinary diagnostic virology,* St Louis, 1992, Mosby.

Cottral: *Manual of standardized methods for veterinary microbiology,* Ithaca, NY, 1978, Comstock Publishing.

Ikram M, Hill E: *Microbiology for veterinary technicians,* St Louis, 1991, Mosby.

Murphy FA et al: *Veterinary virology,* ed 3, Orlando, 2000, Academic Press.

Quinn PJ et al: *Clinical veterinary microbiology,* St Louis, 1994, Mosby.

Urinalysis

JOSEPH G. ZINKL

Urinalysis is a relatively simple, rapid, and inexpensive laboratory procedure. With a minimal investment in laboratory equipment and reagents, the veterinary technician can perform a complete urinalysis that provides a wealth of information about the urinary tract and other body systems.

SPECIMEN COLLECTION

The first step in performance of a urinalysis is proper collection of a urine sample, which must be obtained carefully to ensure meaningful results. Four basic methods exist for collection of a urine sample: cystocentesis, catheterization, expressing the bladder, and natural voiding of the urine (urination). The two preferred methods are cystocentesis and catheterization; these methods provide optimum samples for all aspects of urinalysis by avoiding contamination from the distal genital tract and external areas. Collecting samples by voiding or expression of the bladder may be easier, but urine collected in these ways may be of limited diagnostic value. Except for cytologic examination, performing a urinalysis on preprandial morning samples is best. Morning samples tend to be the most concentrated, which increases the chances of finding abnormalities.

◆ Voided Sample

The simplest sample to obtain is the voided sample, collected as the animal urinates. A sample collected in this manner is not satisfactory for bacteriologic examination because it is often contaminated during urination. Occasionally, voided samples contain increased white blood cell counts because of contamination from inflammatory lesions of the distal genital tract. Results of other evaluations are unaffected.

A voided sample is collected in a clean, although not necessarily sterile, container. If possible, the vulva or prepuce should be washed to decrease contamination of the sample before collection. Animals' owners may not be able to do this because they may be asked to collect a sample when the animal urinates spontaneously. Furthermore, the cleansed tissue in the external orifice area does not remain clean for long. A midurination (midstream) sample is best because it is less likely to be contaminated. However, the initially voided urine is sometimes collected as a precaution against not being able to collect a midurination sample.

Dogs may begin to urinate and then stop when collection is attempted. Chances of successfully obtaining urine may be increased by attaching a paper cup to a long pole and collecting the sample without disturbing the animal. A voided sample from a cat is difficult to obtain. Occasionally, cats urinate into an empty litter pan in a cage devoid of papers. Cows may be stimulated to urinate by rubbing a hand or dry hay ventral to the vulva in a circular fashion. Sheep may be stimulated to urinate by occluding their nostrils. Rubbing a wet, warm cloth on their ventral abdomen may stimulate horses to urinate.

◆ Expressing the Bladder

Urine may be collected in small animals by manual compression of the bladder. Samples obtained in this manner are also unsatisfactory for bacteriologic culturing. As for collection of a voided sample, the external genitalia should be cleaned before bladder expression. With the animal standing or in lateral recumbency, the bladder is palpated and gently gripped in the caudal abdomen. Gentle, steady pressure is applied. Care must be taken not to exert too much pressure and injure or rupture the bladder. Relaxation of the bladder sphincters often takes a few minutes. Bladder expression is recommended because trauma may contaminate the urine with red blood cells (RBCs), or the pressure may force urine back into the ureters and renal pelvis. If bacteria are in the urine, the kidneys may become infected from these bacteria. This method should never be used on animals whose urethra may be obstructed or whose bladder wall may be fragile, because excessive pressure can cause the bladder to rupture. In large animals, urination may be stimulated by maintaining pressure on the bladder through the rectal wall while performing rectal palpation.

◆ Catheterization

Catheterization is the insertion of a catheter into the bladder via the urethra. A variety of catheters exist for different species and sexes. As with the previous two methods of collection, the external genitalia should be cleaned before the procedure. Sterile catheters always should be used and sterile gloves worn. Care must be taken to maintain sterility and prevent trauma to the urinary tract. For female animals a speculum improves visualization of the urethral orifice and thus facilitates the catheterization. The catheter should pass easily through the urethra. A small amount of sterile, water-soluble lubricating jelly, such as K-Y Jelly (Johnson & Johnson, Arlington, Texas), should be placed on the tip of the catheter. Care must be taken to avoid trauma to the sensitive urethral mucosa. The distal end of many catheters is designed for attachment to a syringe so that urine can be collected with gentle aspiration. Collection into a sterile syringe is especially advantageous if bacteriologic culture is anticipated. Often the first portion of the sample obtained is discarded because of possible contamination as the catheter was advanced through the distal urethra (Procedure 5-1).

PROCEDURE 5-1

Methods for catheterization of the urinary bladder

Male Dogs

1. The patient is placed in a standing position, and the operator should stand on the right side of the patient. Catheterization also may be performed with the patient in lateral recumbency. (Left-handed technicians should stand on the left side of the dog. All the activities should be performed with the opposite hand in the directions given below.)
2. Retract the prepuce with the right hand.
3. Gently clean the tip of the penis with a dilute solution of benzalkonium chloride. Dry the tip of the penis with cotton sponges.
4. Apply a small amount of sterile gel (K-Y jelly) to the lead end of a sterile polypropylene urinary catheter (5-, 8- or 10-French). Place the catheter in the external orifice of the penis. The catheter may be wrapped to prevent contamination.
5. Slowly advance the catheter until urine flows from the end or urine can be aspirated with a syringe.
6. Immediately label the syringe or tube with patient identification information using indelible ink.

Female Dogs

1. The patient is placed in a standing position on a table, and the operator should stand behind the patient.
2. An assistant holds the tail up so that it does not interfere with the procedure. The assistant also may support and restrain the patient.
3. Clip or comb any long hair around the vulva so that it will not touch the catheter.
4. Clean and dry the vulva as above.
5. Gently dilate the vulva with a vaginal or nasal speculum to see the urethral orifice.
6. Place the tip of a lubricated, sterile catheter (reusable metal bitch, 10-French, or Foley catheter) in the orifice.
7. Slowly advance the catheter until urine flows from the end or urine can be aspirated with a syringe.
8. Immediately label the syringe or tube with patient identification information using indelible ink.

Male Cats

1. The patient is restrained in dorsal recumbency, and the operator should stand on the right side or behind the patient.
2. With the fingers of the left hand, retract the prepuce and extrude the penis.
3. Clean and dry the penis as described for male dogs.
4. Insert a lubricated, 3.5-French catheter or a tom cat catheter into the external orifice.
5. Gently advance the catheter using a rotary motion until urine flows from the end or urine can be aspirated with a syringe.
6. Immediately label the syringe or tube with patient identification information using indelible ink.

Continued

PROCEDURE 5-1

Methods for catheterization of the urinary bladder—cont'd

Female Cats

1. The patient is restrained in sternal recumbency, and the operator should stand to the rear of the patient.
2. Clean and dry the external surface of the vulva as above.
3. Advance a small bitch catheter or a lubricated, 5-, 8- or 10-French catheter into the vagina while exerting gentle downward pressure on the catheter tip.
4. Because this is a blind procedure, gently advance the catheter and retract it until it enters the urethra.
5. Slowly advance the catheter until urine flows from the end or urine may be aspirated with a syringe.
6. Immediately label the syringe or tube with patient identification information using indelible ink.

Male Horses

1. Both stallions and geldings may be catheterized to obtain urine.
2. The operator, whether right- or left-handed, should stand on the left side of the patient because horses are used to being handled from this side. Foals may be placed in lateral recumbency.
3. Retract the prepuce and expose the tip of the penis.
4. Wash and dry the tip of the penis.
5. Insert into the urethral orifice a lubricated, 22- to 32-French rubber catheter of sufficient length to reach the bladder.
6. Slowly advance the catheter until urine flows from the end of the catheter into an appropriate collecting vessel.
7. Immediately label the vessel or tube with patient identification information using indelible ink.

Female Horses

1. The operator stands to the rear of the patient. For safety the horse should be in a stanchion that allows the operator access to the vulva.
2. Wash and dry the vulva.
3. Guide a metal mare catheter, held under the index finger, into the urethral orifice through the vulva into the vagina.
4. Slowly advance the catheter until urine flows from the end of the catheter into an appropriate collecting vessel.
5. Immediately label the vessel or tube with patient identification information using indelible ink.

Male Cattle

Male cattle are difficult or impossible to catheterize.

Female Cattle

1. The operator stands to the rear of the patient. The cow should be restrained in a head stanchion or a chute. (Calves may be placed in lateral recumbency for ease of catheterization.)

PROCEDURE 5-1

Methods for catheterization of the urinary bladder—cont'd

2. Wash and dry the vulva.
3. Guide a catheter into the urethral orifice using a speculum or by holding it under the index finger.
4. As often as necessary, gently move and probe the urethral orifice to advance the catheter because cows have a urethral diverticulum near the orifice into which the catheter frequently passes.
5. Slowly advance the catheter until urine flows from the end of the catheter into an appropriate collecting vessel.
6. Immediately label the vessel or tube with patient identification information using indelible ink.

◆ Cystocentesis

Cystocentesis is used often to collect sterile urine samples from dogs and cats only when the bladder is distended sufficiently so that it can be easily isolated (Figures 5-1 and 5-2). This eases the procedure and helps avoid damage to other internal organs. Sometimes as much urine as possible is removed from the bladder to prevent pressure on the bladder wall and leakage of urine though the hole created by the needle. However, unless the bladder is markedly extended, a volume sufficient to perform urinalysis and possibly culture (5 to 10 ml) may be removed without damaging the bladder or causing urine to leak through its wall (Procedure 5-2).

Figure 5-1
Cystocentesis in a cat.

Figure 5-2
Cystocentesis in a dog.

PROCEDURE **5-2**

Methods for antepubic cystocentesis

Equipment

No specialized equipment is needed for obtaining urine by cystocentesis.
1. Use sterile 1- or 1.5-inch, 22- or 23-gauge needles (never larger than 20-gauge needles).
2. Use sterile 5- or 10-ml syringes for urinalysis. (Occasionally large amounts of urine may be aspirated for therapeutic reasons.)

Method

The method is similar for dogs and cats and only slightly different for males and females.
1. If the operator is right handed, the patient is placed in a standing position with its head toward the operator's left. (For a left-handed operator, all the activities should be performed with the opposite hand in the directions given below.) Very small animals and most cats may have to be placed in lateral recumbency to provide sufficient space to operate a syringe.
2. In most dogs and cats the caudoventral abdomen is relatively free of hair. Occasionally, a small amount of hair must be clipped from the area into which the needle will be inserted.
3. Clean the area with soap and water and dry with a cotton sponge.
4. Palpate the bladder and gently hold in place against the ventrolateral abdominal wall with the left hand.
5. Insert the needle in a caudodorsal direction toward the midline. For male dogs, insert the needle caudal to the umbilicus and to the side of the sheath. For female dogs and for cats, insert the needle on the ventral midline caudal to the umbilicus.
6. Gently aspirate urine into the syringe. Occasionally it may be necessary to slightly alter the position of the needle by gently turning the syringe to maintain urine flow.

PROCEDURE 5-2

Methods for antepubic cystocentesis—cont'd

7. Immediately label the syringe or tube with patient identification information using indelible ink.
8. If urine is not obtained, completely withdraw the needle and use another sterile needle and syringe to attempt the process again.

All of the above methods of collection are satisfactory for qualitative analysis. However, for quantitative analysis, a 24-hour sample must be collected. Recently, ratios of certain urine constituents, such as protein:creatinine have been used to obtain data that may be interpreted in a similar manner to 24-hour urinary excretions.

QUALITY ASSURANCE

Quality assurance begins with proper specimen identification and handling. All samples should be labeled immediately after collection, and urinalysis should be performed soon after the sample is collected. Reagent strips and tablets must be kept in tightly sealed bottles, and outdated reagents must be replaced with fresh reagents. Reactions for most constituents in urine may be checked against available controls (e.g., Chek-Stix: Miles Laboratories, Terrytown, NY; Uritrol: Harleco, YD Diagnostics, Seoul, Korea, Liquid Urine Control: Kenlor Industries, Inc., Santa Ana, CA). In addition, urine samples with distinct reactions for certain constituents sometimes may be preserved and used as positive controls. The results obtained from control samples and made-up controls should be plotted to determine if observer drift or reagent decomposition is occurring. Technicians gain confidence when they obtain consistent results. Further, veterinarians feel more confident in results generated in a laboratory with a quality assurance program.

SPECIMEN PRESERVATION

Ideally, samples should be analyzed within 30 minutes of collection to avoid postcollection artifacts and degenerative changes. If immediate analysis is not possible, refrigeration preserves most urine constituents for an additional 6 to 12 hours. Crystals may form when the urine cools. Decreased glucose and bilirubin concentrations, increased pH resulting from bacterial breakdown of urea to ammonia, crystal formation with increased sample turbidity, disintegration of casts and RBCs (especially in dilute or alkaline urine), and bacterial proliferation may occur in samples allowed to stand for long periods at room temperature. Many crystals may form in refrigerated samples. Samples should be warmed to room temperature before evaluation, and occasionally crystals that formed during cooling may not dissolve when the sample is warmed. Cells tend to deteriorate rapidly in urine so, if cytologic evaluation is to be performed, the urine should be centrifuged soon after collection and 1 to 2 drops of the patient's serum or bovine albumin added to the sediment to preserve cell morphology.

Refrigerated urine should be warmed to room temperature before determination of the specific gravity and before microscopic evaluation of crystals. Samples to be transported to an outside laboratory or held for longer than 6 to 12 hours may be preserved by addition of one of the following: 1 drop of 40% formalin in 1 oz of urine; toluene sufficient to form a layer on top of the sample; a single thymol crystal; or 1 part 5% phenol to 9 parts urine. If formalin is used as a preservative, chemical tests should be performed before addition of formalin because it interferes with some chemical analyses, especially that for glucose. Formalin, however, is the best preservative for formed elements in urine.

GROSS EXAMINATION

Gross examination includes all of the observations that may be made without the aid of a microscope or chemical reagents (Procedure 5-3).

PROCEDURE 5-3

Routine urinalysis procedure

Reagents and Materials

Refractometer or urinometer
Multistix or other urinalysis strips
3% sulfosalicylic acid
Ictotest tablets and pads
Glass microscope slides (1 × 3 inches) and coverslips (22 × 22 mm)
Microscope with at least 10× and 40× objectives
Automatic pipettes and tips (100 × l)
Calibrated 12-ml, conical centrifuge tubes
Either 10-mm × 75-mm or 12-mm × 75-mm glass test tubes
Test tube rack
Parafilm
Distilled or deionized water
Centrifuge capable of 2000 rpm

Method

1. Prepare a worksheet with patient identification, date, time, and method of urine collection. Worksheets in which data can be recorded next to the test method are extremely helpful for organization, efficiency, and completeness.
2. Record color, appearance, and odor of sample (if any). Record volume of urine obtained for analysis and estimate of total volume if the sample was obtained in a manner so that the bladder was completely emptied. Make sure the sample is at room temperature before proceeding with further evaluation.
3. Label two calibrated centrifuge tubes and pour 5 ml of urine into one tube. Occasionally, it may be necessary to use smaller volumes. However, a standard volume of 5 ml should be used if possible. (Consistency in the volume used will allow comparison and reproducibility in results of sedimentation and microscopic evaluation.) Record on the urinalysis form the volume of urine being used.
4. Centrifuge the sample using a consistent time and speed for reproducibility and adequate sedimentation (generally, 1500 to 2000 rpm [approximately 100 G]

PROCEDURE 5-3

Routine urinalysis procedure—cont'd

for 5 minutes). Record the volume of sediment. Pour the supernatant into the second centrifuge tube for biochemical analysis and refractive index. Leave a small amount of urine in the tube and resuspend the sediment pellet in this urine.

5. Determine and record specific gravity using the refractometer (see Procedure 5-4). Make sure the refractometer is cleaned between samples.

6. Biochemical analysis by reagent strip methods requires timing and proper handling of both the sample and the reagent strips. Reagent strips have buffers and other chemicals on the reaction pads that can be overwhelmed by excess urine, contaminated by flow between pads, and altered by prolonged exposure to oxygen. Make sure the reagent strips are not outdated and close the container tightly immediately after use. Dip the strip quickly into urine supernatant and lightly tap the edge of the strip to remove excess urine without allowing the pads to touch any object or urine to run between pads. Read the reaction pads at appropriate times, comparing color changes to the charts provided. Record the semiquantitative results on the urine worksheet. The remaining supernatant should be retained for further biochemical testing (e.g., tablet tests, sulfosalicylic acid turbidimetry) (see protein determination by sulfosalicylic acid and bilirubin by Ictotest, Procedures 5-5 and 5-6).

7. Using the original tube with sediment, resuspend the pelleted material in the remaining small amount of urine and place one to two drops of unstained urine on a microscope slide for evaluation with reduced condenser lighting or place desired stain in with suspension, mix well, and evaluate stained urine. Place slide on stage of microscope. Record results of low-power findings (10× objective) and high-power findings (40× objective), such as crystal, cells, casts, and bacteria. A thorough and routine slide evaluation allows for consistent and reproducible results.

◆ Urine Volume

The animal's owner often provides information concerning the amount of urine passed. However, owners may mistake frequent urination, or pollakiuria, for increased urine production, or polyuria. Therefore obtaining an estimate of the amount of urine an animal is producing is important. Many factors unrelated to disease influence the amount of urine produced. Some of these factors include water intake, external losses (especially through the respiratory system and the intestinal tract), environmental temperature, amount and type of food, level of physical activity, size of the animal, and species. Observing a single urination is not reliable for estimating urine output of an animal. Ideally, 24-hour urine volume should be determined, although often impractical. Observing an animal in its cage or outdoors may provide a rough estimate of the volume of urine being produced. Table 5-1 lists the approximate daily urine production for common domestic species.

Polyuria, the production of excessive amounts of urine, is usually accompanied by intake of excessive amounts of water (*polydipsia*). Usually, with polyuria the urine is

TABLE 5-1

Normal daily urine production for common domestic species

Species	Daily Urine Output (ml/lb)
Dogs	12–30
Cats	4.5–9
Cattle	8–20
Horses	2–8
Swine	2–14
Sheep, goats	4.5–18

pale and has a low specific gravity. Polyuria occurs in many diseases, including nephritis, diabetes mellitus, diabetes insipidus, pyometra in dogs and cats, and liver disease. It also is seen after administration of diuretics, corticosteroids, or fluids.

Oliguria, a decrease in urine output, may occur when an animal has restricted access to water. It may be severe when the environmental temperature elevation causes excess water loss through the respiratory system or through sweating. Oliguria also occurs with acute nephritis, fever, shock, heart disease, and dehydration. *Anuria,* the complete lack of urine production, could be considered extreme oliguria. Anuria may be seen in complete urethral obstruction and in urinary bladder rupture. Anuria should not be diagnosed unless no urine is voided for about 12 hours and the animal is in a normal state of hydration.

◆ Color

The normal yellow color of urine is due to the presence of pigments called *urochromes.* Often the degree of yellow coloration correlates with the urine's concentration. Colorless urine usually has a very low specific gravity and is often associated with polyuria. Dark yellow to yellow-brown urine generally has a high specific gravity and may be associated with oliguria. Yellow-brown or greenish urine that produces a greenish-yellow foam when shaken is likely to contain bile pigments. Red or reddish-brown urine indicates the presence of RBCs, called *hematuria,* or hemoglobin, called *hemoglobinuria.* Urine that is brown when voided may contain myoglobin (called *myoglobinuria*) excreted during conditions that cause muscle cell lysis, such as exertional rhabdomyolysis in horses. Some drugs may alter the color of urine; red, green, or blue urine may be observed.

◆ Transparency

Urine, except urine of horses, is usually clear when voided. Normal equine urine is cloudy due to a high concentration of calcium carbonate crystals and, rarely, mucus secretion by the kidneys. Transparency is noted as clear, cloudy, or flocculent. Clear samples usually do not have much sediment on centrifugation. Cloudy samples usually contain large particles, and they usually yield a significant amount of sediment on centrifugation. Urine may become cloudy while standing because of bacterial multiplication or crystal formation. Substances that cause urine to be cloudy include RBCs, WBCs, epithelial cells, casts, crystals, mucus, fat, and bacteria. Flocculent samples contain suspended particles that are sufficiently large to be seen with the naked eye.

◆ Odor

The odor of urine is not highly diagnostic but sometimes may be helpful. The urine of male cats, goats, and pigs has a strong odor. An ammonia odor may occur with cystitis caused by bacteria that produce urease (e.g., *Proteus* spp. or *Staphylococcus* spp.) that has metabolized urea to ammonia. Occasionally, samples left standing may develop an ammonia odor resulting from bacterial growth. A sweet, fruity odor indicates ketones and is most commonly found with diabetes mellitus, ketosis in cows, and pregnancy disease in ewes.

◆ Foam

Shaking a sample of normal urine can produce a small amount of white foam. Urine containing large amounts of protein tends to form a greater quantity of foam that remains for some time. Yellow-greenish foam indicates the presence of bile pigments in the sample.

◆ Specific Gravity

Specific gravity is defined as the weight (density) of a quantity of liquid as compared with that of an equal amount of distilled water. The number and molecular weight of dissolved solutes determine the specific gravity of urine. The specific gravity of urine from polyuric patients tends to be low, and that of urine from oliguric patients tends to be high. Table 5-2 lists the reference ranges for urine specific gravity for healthy domestic species.

TABLE 5-2

Urine values for common domestic species

	Dogs	**Cats**	**Horses**	**Cattle**	**Swine**	**Sheep**
Volume (L/day)	0.04–2	0.075–2	3–10	6–25	2–6	0.05–2
Specific gravity	1.025 (1.018–1.045)	1.030 (1.020–1.040)	1.035 (1.020–1.050)	1.015 (1.005–1.040)	1.015 (1.010–1.030)	1.030 (1.020–1.040)
pH	5.2–6.8	6–7	7–8.5	7–8.5	6–8.5	6–8.5
Glucose	None	None	None	None	None	None
Protein	None/ trace	None/ trace	None	None/ trace	None/ trace	None/ trace
Bilirubin	None/ trace	None/ trace	None	None/ trace	None	None/ trace
Ketones	None	None	None	None/ trace	None	None

Figure 5-3
Refractometer or total solids meter. (Courtesy A.O. Corporation, Buffalo, NY.)

Several methods exist to determine the specific gravity of urine. The following details some of these methods.

Refractometer

Specific gravity is most commonly determined by the use of a refractometer or total solids meter (Figure 5-3). Another use for this instrument is estimation of the protein concentration of blood and body fluids. The refractometer determines the refractive index of a fluid: the ratio of the velocity of light in air to the velocity of light in a solution. Light waves bend as they pass through the medium in which they travel. This bending is measured by the refractometer. The refractive index of a fluid is influenced by the same factors that determine specific gravity and therefore provides an estimate of urine specific gravity. Because the density of a fluid is influenced by temperature, refractometers should be temperature corrected to allow accurate and reproducible results. Advantages of the refractometer are that it is easy to use and only a few drops of urine are needed (Procedure 5-4).

Urinometer

Urine specific gravity is less frequently determined by use of a urinometer. The urinometer is a less expensive but less desirable method for determining urine specific gravity. This more cumbersome instrument requires a large volume of urine (approximately 10 ml) and generally provides less reproducible results than a refractometer. The urinometer floats in a vessel containing urine, and the specific gravity is read at the bottom of the meniscus (Figure 5-4). The vessel should be deep enough for the urinometer to float and wide enough so that the urinometer does not cling to the sides of the vessel. The urine should be at room temperature because the urinometer is calibrated at about 20° C (68° F). If the urine is too warm, the reading will be erroneously low; cold urine produces artificially high readings. When the urine volume is insufficient to use the urinometer, it may be diluted with distilled water and the true specific gravity determined in a manner similar to that for more concentrated samples using the refractometer.

PROCEDURE 5-4

Determining urine specific gravity by refractometry

1. Centrifuge the urine at 100 to 200 G for 5 minutes. (Using centrifuged urine is important because suspended materials in the urine cause the line in the refractometer to be indistinct rather than sharp.)
2. Place a drop of urine on the glass plate, close the plastic cover, and determine the specific gravity from an internal scale. (Some older refractometers may have only a scale for refractive index. In this case the specific gravity is determined from charts provided with the instrument.)
3. Occasionally the specific gravity is greater than the upper range of the refractometer. When that occurs, the following steps allow the determination of the specific gravity.
   - Pipette 0.5 ml of urine into a tube.
   - Pipette 0.5 ml of distilled or deionized water into the tube.
   - Gently mix the urine and water.
   - Remove a small portion of the mixture and determine the specific gravity of the mixture.
   - Multiply the numbers after the decimal point by 2 to determine the specific gravity of the urine.
   - Example: Initial reading is above the scale.
     The 1:1 dilution reads 1.036.
     $0.036 \times 2 = 0.072$
     The true urine specific gravity is 1.072.
4. Record the results.

Figure 5-4
Urinometers. The one on the right requires a smaller volume
of urine than the one on the left. (Courtesy Becton-Dickinson,
Franklin Lakes, NJ.)

Reagent Strips

Several reagent strips have been developed to determine urine specific gravity. Reagent strip specific gravity is the least reliable method for determining urine specific gravity. With urine of high specific gravity (higher than 1.030), the strips often show a reaction for a lower specific gravity, or the reaction is inconsistent with those shown on the container label.

Table 5-2 lists the urine specific gravity for normal domestic species. The specific gravity of normal urine varies from one specimen to another, depending on eating and drinking habits, environmental temperature, and when the sample was collected. An early morning sample tends to be the most concentrated.

Causes of Altered Urine Specific Gravity

Increased urine specific gravity is seen with diminished water intake, increased fluid loss through sources other than urination (sweating, panting, or diarrhea), and increased excretion of urine solutes. Decreased water intake in animals with normal renal function rapidly causes increased urine specific gravity. Dehydration increases urine specific gravity. Increased urine specific gravity may occur in acute renal disease. Shock also increases urine specific gravity by decreasing the amount of plasma filtered through the glomeruli.

Decreased urine specific gravity is seen in diseases in which the kidneys cannot resorb water and with increased fluid intake, such as with polydipsia or excessive fluid administration. Pyometra, diabetes insipidus, psychogenic polydipsia, some liver diseases, certain types of renal disease, and diuretic therapy may cause decreased urine specific gravity.

Isosthenuria occurs when the urine specific gravity approaches that of the glomerular filtrate (1.008 to 1.012). Frequently, animals with chronic renal disease produce isosthenuric urine. In animals with kidney disease, the closer the specific gravity is to isosthenuric, the greater the amount of kidney function that has been lost. When these animals are deprived of water, their urine specific gravity usually remains in the isosthenuric range. Animals with decreased renal function that is not completely compromised are often slightly to moderately dehydrated and have urine specific gravity slightly greater than isoshenuric (1.015 to 1.020).

ASSAYS FOR CHEMICAL CONSTITUENTS

Testing for various chemical constituents of urine usually is performed with paper reagent strips impregnated with appropriate chemicals or reagent tablets. Some reagent strips test for numerous constituents simultaneously, and other strips exist for individual tests. Urine is added to these tablets, or the strips are dipped in the urine sample and the color changes are noted at specific intervals (Figures 5-5 and 5-6). The concentration of various constituents is determined by comparison of the resulting colors with color charts on the label of the strip container. The manufacturer's directions must be carefully followed. Reflectance spectrometry instruments are available to automate evaluation and recording of data. These instruments may eliminate the er-

Figure 5-5
Urine being tested with a combination dipstick.

Figure 5-6
After the dipstick is dipped in the urine, the resultant color changes are compared with those on the container, each of which indicates a specific urine constituent.

rors associated with individual differences in color perception; however, they are not widely used in veterinary laboratories.

◆ pH

pH expresses the concentration of hydrogen ion (H^+). Essentially pH is a measure of the degree of acidity or alkalinity of urine. A pH above 7.0 is *alkaline,* whereas a pH below 7.0 is *acidic.* Proper technique must be employed for accurate results. The pH of samples left standing open at room temperature tends to increase resulting from a loss of CO_2, whereas delays in reading the reaction may lead to color changes and false readings. If samples containing urease bacteria (e.g., *Proteus* spp. or *Staphylococcus* spp.) are left standing, the pH is usually increased.

The pH of a healthy animal's urine depends largely on its diet. Alkaline urine usually is found in animals on plant diets, whereas high-protein cereal diets or diets of animal origin cause acidic urine. Therefore herbivores normally have alkaline urine, carnivores acidic urine, and omnivores either acidic or alkaline urine, depending on what was ingested. Many dog foods contain substantial amounts of plant material that may cause the urine to be slightly alkaline. Nursing herbivores have acidic urine from consumption of milk. Table 5-2 lists the normal urine constituents and characteristics, including pH, for common domestic species.

Urine pH is usually measured with reagent strips. Decreased pH (acidity) may be due to several factors, including fever, starvation, high-protein diet, acidosis, excessive muscular activity, or administration of certain drugs. Increased pH (alkalinity) may be caused by alkalosis, infection of the urinary tract with urease bacteria, use of certain drugs, or by urine retention, as occurs with urethral obstruction or bladder paralysis.

◆ Protein

Protein is usually absent or present only in trace amounts in normal urine obtained by catheterization or cystocentesis. In healthy animals, plasma proteins that pass into the glomerular filtrate are resorbed in the renal tubules before the filtrate reaches the renal pelvis. However, voided samples or those obtained by expressing the bladder may contain a small amount of protein resulting from secretions that may contaminate urine during its passage along the urinary tract. Occasionally, trauma to the urinary tract that results from cystocentesis, catheterization, or bladder expression may cause sufficient bleeding to cause a trace of protein in the urine. The relationship of any protein measured in the urine and possible leakage through the renal glomeruli must be interpreted in light of the urine specific gravity, collection method, rate of urine formation, and contributions from any hemorrhage or inflammation noted by sample analysis.

Protein levels in urine may be measured by several methods. The following sections detail some of these methods.

Protein Determination by Reagent Test Strips

Urine dipsticks allow semiquantitative measurement of protein in urine by progressive color changes on the reaction pad. Reagent strip analysis is a rapid, convenient, and reasonably accurate method of determining urinary protein levels. These reactions may be converted to a semiquantitative measurement based on charts provided. The accuracy of these methods is variable. Reagent strips detect primarily albumin and are much less sensitive to globulins. False-positive results also may occur in alkaline urine. Protein measurements considered excessive or pathologic should be confirmed by sulfosalicylic acid turbidimetry or by specific biochemical analysis.

Protein Determination by Sulfosalicylic Acid Turbidimetry

Sulfosalicylic acid turbidity determines urine protein levels by acid precipitation. The resultant turbidity is proportional to the concentration of protein. Results are compared with levels in prepared standards and thus may be reported in semiquantitative units. The advantages of this method are that it is equally sensitive to albumin and globulins, and it is quite useful to confirm strip methods, especially in alkaline urine. Extremely alkaline urine may titrate the acid and decrease the amount of protein precipitated (Procedure 5-5).

PROCEDURE 5-5

Determination of urine protein concentration by the sulfosalicylic acid test

1. Prepare 3% sulfosalicylic acid in distilled or deionized water by dissolving 30 g of sulfosalicylic acid in 1 L of water.
2. Place 1 ml of urine supernatant in two 10 mm × 75-mm glass test tubes.
3. Add 3 ml of 3% sulfosalicylic acid to one of the tubes and 3 ml of water to the other tube. (If the volume of urine is insufficient, the ratio of 1 part urine to 3 parts reagents must be maintained to properly quantitate the reaction.)
4. Mix by inversion.
5. Compare the sulfosalicylic acid tube and the water tube. No turbidity should be in the water tube. Determine the results as follows:

Negative	=	No visible turbity
Trace	=	Barely visible turbity
1+	=	Distinct turbidity but able to read black typing on a white background through the tube
2+	=	Moderate turbidity and unable to read black typing on a white background through the tube
3+	=	Heavy turbidity with fine granulation and cloudiness
4+	=	Heavy and flocculent turbidity

6. Record the results.

Interpretation of Protein in Urine

Very dilute urine may yield a false-negative result because the protein concentration may be below the sensitivity of the testing method. A trace amount of protein in a very dilute sample may be clinically significant because dilute urine often occurs when a large volume of urine is being produced, such as in a patient with chronic renal failure.

Occasionally a small amount of protein is found in the urine of normal animals. Transient proteinuria may be due to a temporary increase in glomerular permeability, allowing excessive protein to enter the filtrate. This condition is due to increased pressure in the glomerular capillaries and may be found with muscle exertion, emotional stress, or convulsions. Occasionally a small amount of urine protein is found after parturition, during the first few days of life, and during estrus. The presence of protein in the urine is usually abnormal and primarily is due to disease of the urinary tract (or possibly the genital system).

In most cases, proteinuria indicates disease of the urinary tract, especially of the kidneys. Both acute and chronic renal diseases lead to proteinuria. Acute nephritis is characterized by marked proteinuria with white blood cells (WBCs) and casts, whereas in chronic renal disease the degree of proteinuria is qualitatively less. However, in chronic renal disease, urine output is usually excessive with low specific gravity; therefore the total protein excreted is actually quite significant. The ratio of urine protein to creatinine is used to determine the degree of protein loss in chronic renal disease.

Multiple myeloma, a cancer of plasma cells, may produce large quantities of protein that may leak through the glomerulus. In patients with myeloma, proteins may be passed in the urine because they have damaged the glomerulus or because they are the so-called "light chains," which freely pass through the glomerular filter. Since these proteins often do not react with the protein pads on dipsticks, the sulfosalicylic acid method is necessary to detect and quantify them.

Mild proteinuria is seen with passive congestion of the kidneys, as in congestive heart failure or any other impediment of blood flow from the kidneys. Proteinuria of renal origin may also be caused by trauma, tumors, renal infarcts, or nephrosis resulting from drugs and chemicals, such as sulfonamides, lead, mercury, arsenic, or ether.

Inflammation of the urinary or genital tract may cause proteinuria of postrenal origin. Proteinuria also may be seen with traumatic catheterization.

◆ Glucose

The presence of glucose in urine is known as *glucosuria* or *glycosuria*. The amount of glucose in the urine depends on blood glucose levels and the rates of glomerular filtration and tubular resorption. Glucosuria usually does not occur in normal animals unless the blood glucose level exceeds the renal threshold (approximately 170 to 180 mg/dl for dogs). At this concentration, tubular resorption cannot keep up with the glomerular filtration of glucose, and glucose passes into the urine.

Glucosuria occurs in diabetes mellitus as a result of a deficiency of insulin or an inability of insulin to function. Insulin is necessary to transport glucose into body cells, and a deficiency causes hyperglycemia and spilling of glucose into the urine. A high-carbohydrate meal may lead to blood glucose levels exceeding the renal threshold and thus glucosuria. Because of this, a period of fasting is recommended before urine glucose concentration is determined. Fear, excitement, or restraint, especially in cats, occasionally causes hyperglycemia and glucosuria as a result of epinephrine release. Glucosuria often occurs after IV administration of fluids containing glucose and occasionally after general anesthesia. Rarely, glucosuria is found in hyperthyroidism, Cushing's disease, and chronic liver disease. A rare condition called *renal glucosuria* may occur when the blood glucose concentration is in the normal range. Renal glucosuria is due to reduced resorption of glucose in the renal tubules. Glucosuria may occur in some cats with chronic disease, possibly as a result of altered proximal renal tubular function.

False positives for glucose may be seen after use of various drugs, including ascorbic acid, or vitamin C; morphine; salicylates, such as aspirin; cephalosporins and penicillin.

Various reagent test strips are available for detecting glucose in urine. Clinitest Reagent Tablets (Bayer Corporation, Terrytown, NY) are also available. These tablets detect any sugar in the urine, whereas the test strips detect only glucose.

◆ Ketones

Ketones include acetone, acetoacetic acid, and beta-hydroxybutyric acid. Ketone bodies are formed during incomplete catabolism of fatty acids. Normal animals have small amounts of ketones in the blood. Conditions characterized by altered carbohydrate metabolism may result in excessive amounts of fat catabolism to provide energy. When fatty acid metabolism is not accompanied by sufficient carbohydrate metabolism, excess ketones spill into the urine, which is called *ketonuria*.

A common cause of ketonuria is ketonemia, or ketosis, in lactating cows and pregnant ewes and cows. In cows, this condition is called *ketosis*. It usually occurs early in lactation (3-6 weeks after freshing) when the energy for milk production exceeds the capacity of the cow to ingest sufficient feed to meet its energy requirements. In ewes, this condition is called *pregnancy toxemia* and is seen when the ewe is carrying twins or triplets. Ketosis is associated with hypoglycemia and is caused by carbohydrate intake insufficient to meet energy requirements. Body fat is then rapidly metabolized, resulting in ketonemia and ketonuria.

Ketonuria frequently occurs in animals with diabetes mellitus. Because the animal lacks the insulin necessary for carbohydrate metabolism, fat is broken down to meet the animal's energy needs and excess ketones are excreted in the urine. Ketones are important sources of energy and are normally produced during fat metabolism. Problems develop, however, when excessive ketones are produced. Ketones are toxic, causing central nervous system (CNS) depression and acidosis. Acidosis resulting from ketonemia is termed *ketoacidosis*.

Ketonemia with ketonuria also occurs with high-fat diets, starvation, fasting, long-term anorexia, and impaired liver function. With a high-fat diet, carbohydrates meet a relatively low percentage of energy needs, so a great amount of fat is used to meet energy needs. In the fasting, starved, or anorexic animal, body fat is used to meet energy needs, producing a greater than normal amount of ketones. With liver damage, impaired carbohydrate metabolism leads to fat serving as the main energy source, especially when the damaged liver cannot store adequate amounts of glycogen.

Measurement of Urine Ketone Content

Urinary ketones are detected using urinary reagent strips with a ketone reagent pad. The color intensity is roughly proportional to the concentration of urine ketones. These methods are most sensitive to acetoacetic acid and less sensitive to acetone and do not detect beta-hydroxybutyric acid.

◆ Bile Pigments

Bile pigments commonly detected in urine are bilirubin and urobilinogen. Only conjugated bilirubin is found in urine because unconjugated bilirubin does not pass through the glomerulus into the renal filtrate, because it is bound to albumin and is not water soluble. Normal dogs, especially males, occasionally have bilirubin in their urine because of a low renal threshold for conjugated bilirubin and the ability of their kidneys to conjugate bilirubin. Many normal cattle also have small amounts of bilirubin in their urine. Bilirubin is usually not found in the urine of cats, pigs, sheep, and horses.

Bilirubinuria is seen in a number of diseases, including obstruction of bile flow from the liver to the small intestine and in some disease of the liver. Bilirubinuria results from accumulation in hepatic cells of conjugated bilirubin regurgitated into the blood and excreted in the urine. Conditions causing biliary obstruction include calculi in the bile duct, tumors in the area of the bile duct, acute enteritis, pancreatitis, and obstruction of the upper intestinal tract. Bilirubinuria also occurs in liver disease. When conjugated, bilirubin enters the bloodstream after being released from damaged liver cells and passes into the urine.

Hemolytic anemia also may cause bilirubinuria, especially in dogs. In hemolytic anemia, the liver's ability to excrete the excess bilirubin may be exceeded, resulting in regurgitation of conjugated bilirubin into the blood and ultimately bilirubinuria. In dogs, unconjugated bilirubin from hemoglobin catabolism in the mononuclear phagocytic system can be conjugated in the kidney and passed in the urine.

Bilirubinuria is detected with the Ictotest (Bayer Corporation, Terrytown, NY) (Procedure 5-6). A diazo compound in the tablet reacts with bilirubin to produce a blue or purple color. The speed with which the color changes and the degree of color change indicate the amount of bilirubin present. Reagent strips are less sensitive than Ictotest tablets. Urine to be tested for bilirubin must not be exposed to light because bilirubin is broken down by short-wave light. False-negative results for bilirubin occur in urine that is exposed to sunlight or artificial light.

In the intestines, bacteria convert bilirubin to *stercobilinogen* and *urobilinogen*. The bulk of these products is excreted in the feces, but some is resorbed into the bloodstream and excreted by the liver into the intestinal tract. A small amount of resorbed urobilinogen is excreted by the kidneys into the urine. Urobilinogen in the urine sample is normal. The reliability of screening tests for detection of urobilinogen is questionable because of the instability of urobilinogen.

PROCEDURE 5-6

Ictotest for bilirubin in urine

1. Place 10 drops of urine supernatant onto the square absorbent test mat supplied with the Ictotest.
2. Place an Ictotest reagent tablet in the center of the mat.
3. Carefully place a large drop of water in the center of the tablet and allow it to bubble for a few seconds.
4. Place a second drop of water on the tablet so that it overflows onto the reagent pad.
5. After 60 seconds, observe the area of the pad around the tablet for color change.
6. Determine the results as follows:

Negative	=	No change or pink to red color
1+	=	Definite blue to purple color
2+	=	Medium blue to purple color
3+	=	Dark purple color after only 30 seconds
4+	=	Dark purple color develops immediately

7. Record the results.

◆ Blood (Hemoprotein)

Tests for blood in urine detect hematuria, the presence of intact RBCs in urine; hemoglobinuria, the presence of free hemoglobin in urine; and *myoglobinuria,* the presence of myoglobin in urine. Hematuria, hemoglobinuria, and myoglobinuria may occur simultaneously. The presence of one does not rule out the others.

Hematuria

Hematuria is usually a sign of disease causing bleeding somewhere in the urogenital tract, whereas hemoglobinuria usually indicates intravascular hemolysis. Some systemic conditions also may cause hematuria. In very dilute or highly alkaline urine, RBCs often lyse to yield hemoglobin. Therefore in dilute or highly alkaline urine, hemoglobinuria may not be due to hemoglobin entering the urine via the glomerulus. Ghost cells (the shells of lysed RBCs) may be seen on microscopic examination of sediment if the source of hemoglobin is lysis of RBCs.

Moderate to large amounts of blood impart a cloudy red, brown, or wine color to urine. Similar colors, but with a transparent appearance that remains after centrifugation, indicates hemoglobinuria. With minute amounts of blood in the urine, a visible color change is usually not evident. Occult, or hidden, blood occurs when the urine is not obviously discolored by blood but blood is detected by chemical analysis. More information on hematuria is found in the section on microscopic examination of urinary sediment.

Hemoglobinuria

Hemoglobinuria usually is due to intravascular hemolysis. Hemoglobin from RBCs broken down intravascularly, or hemoglobinemia, is normally bound to the plasma protein haptoglobin. When hemoglobin is bound to haptoglobin, it does not pass through glomeruli. If intravascular hemolysis overwhelms haptoglobin's binding ability, hemoglobinemia leads to hemoglobinuria because free hemoglobin filters through glomeruli. Hemoglobinuria is indicated by a positive test for hemoglobin without RBCs in the urine sediment, or the degree of the reaction is greater than may be accounted for by the numbers of RBCs in the sediment. When hemoglobin concentration is sufficiently high in the urine to impart red discoloration, the urine remains red after centrifugation. If the discoloration is due to RBCs, the urine is clear above the pellet after centrifugation. Partial clearing after centrifugation indicates both hemoglobinuria and hematuria. The presence of hemoglobin (either as free hemoglobin or in RBCs) must be confirmed by urine dipstick test and further evaluated by microscopic examination.

Hemoglobinuria may be seen with many conditions that cause intravascular hemolysis. Conditions that can cause intravascular hemolysis include immune mediated hemolytic anemia, isoimmune hemolytic disease of neonates, incompatible blood transfusions, leptospirosis, babesiosis, certain heavy metals, such as copper, and ingestion of certain poisonous plants. Other conditions that cause hemoglobinuria include severe hypophosphatemia, postparturient hemoglobinemia in cattle, and hemolysis of cattle that occurs after they drink large quantities of water after being unable to obtain water (e.g., after a long period of low temperatures has frozen the usual water source of the cattle).

If the urine is dilute or very alkaline, hemoglobinuria can originate from lysis of RBCs in the urine. This condition must be considered hematuria because intact RBCs were present initially. Often ghost RBCs may be found when hemoglobinuria is due to release of hemoglobin from RBCs in the urine.

Because the test for blood in the urine detects hemoglobinuria, hematuria, and myoglobinuria, other considerations include urine sediment examination, history, physical examination findings, and additional laboratory procedures to determine the cause of the positive test for blood in the urine.

Myoglobinuria

Myoglobin is a protein found in muscle. Severe muscle damage causes myoglobin to leak from muscle cells into the blood. Myoglobin passes through the glomeruli and is excreted in the urine. Urine containing myoglobin is usually very dark brown to almost black, but at low concentrations the urine may have a similar color to that seen with hemoglobin. Distinguishing myoglobinuria from hemoglobinuria may be difficult. History and clinical features that suggest muscle damage help determine if a positive hemoglobin test is due to myoglobin. Myoglobinuria is frequently seen in horses with exertional rhabdomyolysis (*azoturia*).

Several methods have been used to try to distinguish hemoglobin from myoglobin. None of the methods are completely reliable. They sometimes may be differentiated on the basis of their different molecular weights and different solubility in ammonium sulfate. A method for differentiating hemoglobin and myoglobin is separation of myoglobin by centrifugal-assisted filtration. Because myoglobin has a molecular weight of approximately 16,000 D (daltons) and hemoglobin has a molecular weight of approximately 64,000 D, they may be separated by centrifugal-assisted filtration using special tubes that allow the smaller myoglobin molecules to pass through the filter and prevent passage of hemoglobin molecules. Unfortunately the filters are not entirely selective and hemoglobin often goes through the filter, especially if it is of relatively high concentration. Myoglobin and hemoglobin also may be differentiated by their differences in solubility in an 80% saturated solution of ammonium sulfate. Hemoglobin precipitates in an 80% saturated ammonium sulfate solution, but myoglobin does not. Despite the apparent ammonium sulfate solubility differences this method is not consistent in differentiating hemoglobinuria from myoglobinuria.

Nitrite

Some bacteria contain enzymes that reduce nitrate to nitrite in the urine. The presence of nitrite in urine suggests bacteriuria. However, a negative nitrite test does not indicate that bacteria are absent. To detect nitrate-reducing bacteria, the diet must contain nitrate that can be excreted in the urine, and the urine must be retained in the bladder for sufficient time for organisms to produce detectable concentrations of nitrite. Because animals with urinary tract infections usually urinate frequently, this test is often negative even when bacteria are present. Furthermore, many bacteria do not convert nitrates to nitrites. Microscopic examination remains the best screening test to detect bacteria in urine. Conversely, positive nitrite results should be confirmed with microscopic examination or culture of urine. The nitrite test should be considered a screening test only. It does not substitute for microscopic examination of the urine sediment.

Leukocytes

Presumptive evidence of leukocytes (WBCs) in urine may be obtained with the leukocyte reaction of certain reagent strips. However, many false-negative reactions occur, and microscopic evaluation is necessary to confirm a positive result.

MICROSCOPIC EXAMINATION OF URINE SEDIMENT

Microscopic examination of urine sediment is extremely important, especially for recognizing diseases of the urinary tract. It must be a part of every urinalysis. Many abnormalities in a urine sample cannot be detected with reagent test strips or tablets, but often, more specific information may be obtained by observation of the urine sediment. In addition, urine sediment examination is occasionally an aid in diagnosing systemic disease.

With the exception of horse urine, normal urine of domestic animals does not contain a large amount of sediment. Small numbers of epithelial cells, mucus threads, RBCs, WBCs, hyaline casts, and crystals of various types can be found in the urine of normal animals. The urine of horses usually has large amounts of calcium carbonate crystals. Urine must be collected cleanly because bacteria and aberrant substances may be present in a urine sample that has been contaminated during collection.

The best samples for sediment examination are morning samples or samples collected after several hours of water deprivation. Because such samples are more concentrated, the chances of finding formed elements are increased. Furthermore, sediment examination must be performed on fresh urine. If a voided sample is collected, a midstream sample is preferred because it is less likely to be contaminated by cells, bacteria, and debris from the external genital surfaces. Urine collected by cystocentesis is the best sample for microscopic examination. As discussed previously, changes may occur in a sample as it ages. For example, crystals may form as the sample cools, and casts may dissolve rapidly in alkaline urine. If the sample cannot be examined immediately, it should be refrigerated or preserved.

For semiquantitative measurements of the formed elements in urine, the volume of urine used and the volume of sediment obtained should be recorded. If a sufficient volume has been obtained, 5 ml of a well-mixed sample should be placed in a graduated, conical centrifuge tube and centrifuged for 3 to 5 minutes at approximately 100 G (about 1000 to 2000 rpm, depending on the radius of the centrifuge). Excessive force compacts the sediment and may distort or disrupt formed elements. The procedure should be standardized for a particular centrifuge to yield uniform results. Some centrifuges, such as the Clay-Adams Triac (Becton Dickinson, Franklin Lakes, NJ), are calibrated to provide the proper force over sufficient time to completely sediment the formed elements in the urine. After centrifugation, the volume of sediment is recorded, and the supernatant is gently poured off, leaving about 0.3 ml of urine adhered to the sides of the tube. This remaining urine is allowed to run down the inside of the centrifuge tube, and the sediment is resuspended by gently flicking the bottom of the centrifuge tube.

The sediment may be examined stained or unstained (Procedure 5-7). To examine unstained sediment, a small drop of the suspended sediment is placed on a clean glass slide, covered with a coverslip, and examined immediately. Subdued light that partially refracts the elements must be used to examine unstained urine sediment. Proper lighting is achieved by partially closing the microscope's iris diaphragm and adjusting the condenser downward. With phase-contrast microscopy, formed elements are more easily distinguished than reduced illumination, bright-field microscopy. Microscopes with phase-contrast capabilities are only slightly more expensive than bright-field microscopes and they can also be used for routine microscopy. The illumination of a phase-contrast microscope must be properly adjusted to take full advantage of its capabilities.

Stained sediment may also be examined. Satisfactory stains include Sternheimer-Malbin stain (Sedi Stain: Becton Dickinson, Franklin Lakes, NJ) or 0.5% new methylene blue containing a small amount of formalin. One drop of stain is mixed with the

PROCEDURE 5-7

Microscopic examination of urine sediment

1. Place a small drop of suspended urine sediment on a glass slide and cover with a 22-mm × 22-mm coverslip.
2. Place the slide on the microscope and swing the 10× lens into place.
3. Reduce the light intensity and lower the substage condenser.
4. Focus on the material on the slide.
5. Scan the slide and identify larger elements, such as casts and crystals. Both the center and edges of the slide should be examined.
6. Swing the 40× lens into place and readjust the light, if necessary.
7. Identify formed elements, including RBCs, WBCs, epithelial cells (and their type), casts, crystals, and bacteria.
8. Evaluate the sediment as follows:
   Crystals and casts—numbers per low-power field (LPF)
   Cells (and sometimes casts and crystals)—numbers per high-power field (HPF)
   Bacteria and sperm
Rare	=	Only 2 or 3 seen on scanning several HPF
1+	=	Less than 1/HPF
2+	=	1 to 5/HPF
3+	=	6 to 20/HPF
4+	=	Greater than 20/HPF
9. Record the results.

suspended sediment before placing a drop of sediment on a slide. The amount of illumination is less critical when examining a stained specimen than with an unstained one, although reduced illumination also aids visualization of substances by providing contrast.

The specimen is scanned under low power (10× objective) to gain an impression of what is present and to identify larger elements, such as casts or aggregates of cells. The entire area under the coverslip should be examined because casts tend to migrate toward the edge of the coverslip. Casts and crystals are identified and reported as the number observed per low-power field (LPF). High power (40× objective) is necessary to accurately identify most objects, to detect bacteria, and to differentiate cell types. Epithelial cells, RBCs, and WBCs are reported as the average number observed per high-power field (HPF). Bacteria are reported as few, moderate, or many, and their morphology (cocci, bacilli) is noted.

◆ Constituents of Urine Sediment

Various cells, microorganisms, urinary casts, fat, crystals, and contaminating artifacts may be found in urine sediment.

◆ Erythrocytes

Erythrocytes (RBCs) may have several different appearances, depending on the urine concentration and pH and time elapsed between collection and examination. Red blood cells are small. In a fresh sample, RBCs usually have smooth edges and appear yellow to orange, but they may be colorless if their hemoglobin has diffused during standing (Figure 5-7). In concentrated urine, RBCs shrink and crenate. Crenated RBCs have ruffled edges and are slightly darker. Crenated RBCs may even appear granular as a result of membrane irregularities. In dilute or alkaline urine, RBCs swell and may lyse. Swollen RBCs have smooth edges and are pale yellow or orange. Lysed RBCs may appear as colorless rings (shadow cells or ghost cells) that vary in size. However, lysed RBCs, especially when resulting from marked alkalinity, often dissolve and cannot be

Figure 5-7
Red blood cells in canine urine. (160×)

found on microscopic examination. Normally, urine sediment contains less than 2 to 3 RBCs/HPF (high-power field).

Because mammalian RBCs contain no nucleus, they may be confused with fat globules and yeast. However, their light yellow to orange color usually allows them to be differentiated from these other elements. Furthermore, variation in RBC size is minimal, whereas fat globules vary in size. Erythrocytes in urine usually indicate bleeding somewhere in the urogenital tract or occasionally in the genital system. A voided sample from a female in proestrus or estrus or after parturition may be contaminated with RBCs. Both females and males with inflammatory conditions in the genital system may have RBCs in urine collected by free catch or expression of the bladder. Urine collected by catheterization from females with inflammatory lesions in the genital tract usually are not contaminated, but urine from males with genital tract inflammation may be contaminated. Even the slight trauma that occurs from catheterization, cystocentesis, and manual expression of the bladder may slightly increase the number of RBCs in the sediment. Generally, cystocentesis does not cause much increase in RBC numbers. The veterinary technician should note the method of urine collection on the laboratory report to help determine the significance of RBCs in urine.

◆ Leukocytes

Few leukocytes (WBCs) are found in the urine of animals without urinary or genital tract disease. Leukocytes are spherical and have a granular appearance; they are larger than RBCs and smaller than renal epithelial cells (Figure 5-8). The granular appearance is due to the fact that most WBCs in urine are neutrophils, which contain large numbers of granules. With phase-contrast microscopy and in stained sediment, the polymorphic nucleus of neutrophils often may be seen. Leukocytes are usually in low numbers in urine (0 to 1/HPF). Finding more than 2 to 3 WBCs/HPF indicates inflammation somewhere in the urinary or genital tracts. The term for excessive WBCs in the urine is *pyuria*. Pyuria is indicative of nephritis, pyelonephritis, cystitis, urethritis, or ureteritis. Urine with increased numbers of leukocytes should be cultured for bacteria even if organisms are not observed by microscopic examination.

Figure 5-8
White blood cells in canine urine. (500×)

◆ Epithelial Cells

Three types of epithelial cells may be found in urinary sediment.

Squamous Epithelial Cells

Squamous epithelial cells, derived from the distal urethra, vagina, vulva, or prepuce, are occasionally found in voided samples. Usually their presence is not considered significant. These flat cells with a homogeneous appearance are the largest cells found in urine sediment. They often have straight edges and distinct corners. They may show a small, round nucleus (Figures 5-9 and 5-10). Squamous epithelial cells are not normally found in samples obtained by cystocentesis or catheterization.

Transitional Epithelial Cells

Transitional epithelial cells come from the bladder, ureters, renal pelvis, and proximal urethra. They are usually round, but they may be pear shaped or caudate. They are granular, have a small nucleus, and are larger than WBCs (Figures 5-10, 5-11, and 5-12). Occasional transitional cells (0 to 1/HPF) may be found in urinary sediment as a result of sloughing of old cells, but an increased number suggests cystitis or pyelonephritis. Increased numbers also may be seen if catheterization was used to obtain the sample.

Renal Epithelial Cells

Renal epithelial cells are the smallest epithelial cells seen in urine. They originate in the renal tubules, are only slightly larger than WBCs, and are often confused with them. Renal epithelial cells are generally round and contain a large nucleus and non-granular cytoplasm (Figures 5-10 and 5-13). They are rarely found (0 to 1/HPF). Increased numbers of these cells occur in diseases of the kidney parenchyma.

Figure 5-9
Squamous epithelial cells in canine urine. (400×)

Red blood cells

Intact   Ghost   Crenated

Epithelial cells

Renal   Squamous   Transitional   Caudate

WBC (pus cells)   Yeast bodies   Sperm

Figure 5-10
Cell types that may be found in urine.

Figure 5-11
Transitional epithelial cells in canine urine. (1000×)

A

B

Figure 5-12
Cluster of bladder epithelial cells and numerous RBCs. **A,** Bright-field microscopy. **B,** Phrase-contrast microscopy. (160×)

Figure 5-13
Renal epithelial cells in canine urine. (1000×)

◆ Microorganisms

A variety of microorganisms may be found in urine sediment, including bacteria, fungi, and protozoa. Normal urine is free of bacteria, but it may be contaminated by bacteria residing on the epithelium of the vagina, vulva, or prepuce during urination. Normal urine collected by cystocentesis or catheterization does not contain bacteria. Because bacteria often proliferate in urine that has been left standing for some time, especially at room temperature, the urine must be immediately examined or refrigerated until it can be examined. Bacteria are minute and can be identified only at higher magnifications (Figure 5-14). They may be round (cocci) or rod shaped

Figure 5-14
Bacteria and leukocytes. **A,** Bright-field microscopy. **B,** Phase-contrast microscopy. (400×)

(bacilli), usually refract light, and appear to be quivering as a result of Brownian movement. They are reported as few, moderate, or many. A large number of bacteria accompanied by a large number of WBCs indicate infection and inflammation of the urinary tract (e.g., cystitis, pyelonephritis) or genital tract (e.g., prostatitis, metritis, vaginitis, or balanitis).

Yeast are often confused with RBCs or lipid droplets, but they usually display characteristic budding, and may have double refractile walls (Figure 5-15). Yeast usually are contaminants in urine samples because yeast infection of the urinary tract is rare in domestic animals. Yeast infection of the external genitalia may cause yeast to be present in voided samples. Fungi also may be found in urine. Fungi are filamentous and usually branching. Septa may be seen when the microscope is optimally adjusted. Fungal infections of the urinary tract are uncommon, but they are very serious when they occur.

◆ Casts

Casts are formed in the lumen of the distal and collecting tubules of the kidney, where the concentration and acidity of urine are greatest. In the renal tubules, secreted protein precipitates in acidic conditions and forms casts shaped like the tubules in which they form. All casts are cylindric, with parallel sides. Cells in the area also may be incorporated into casts, imparting the morphologic features that allow them to be identified specifically. Casts dissolve while in alkaline urine, so cast identification and quantitation are best performed in fresh samples that have not become alkaline with standing. Because casts dissolve quickly in alkaline urine they are rarely seen in the sediment of herbivores, which characteristically have alkaline urine. Casts may be disrupted with high-speed centrifugation and rough sample handling. A few hyaline casts or granular casts (0 to 1/HPF) may be seen in normal urine, but larger numbers of casts indicate a lesion in the renal tubules. The number of casts observed is not a reliable indicator of the severity of the urinary disease.

Figure 5-15
Yeast. (400×)

Hyaline Casts

A few hyaline casts may be seen in urine from normal animals. These are clear, colorless, and highly refractile (Figures 5-16 and 5-17). They are difficult to see and usually are only identified using dim light. Hyaline casts are cylindric, with parallel sides and usually rounded ends. They are easier to identify in stained sediment and with phase-contrast microscopy than in unstained sediment. Increased numbers of hyaline casts indicate the mildest form of renal irritation. Their numbers also are increased with fever, poor renal perfusion, strenuous exercise, or general anesthesia.

Granular Casts

Granular casts are the most common type of cast seen in animals. These are simply hyaline casts containing granules (Figures 5-16, 5-17, and 5-18). The granules are from tubular epithelial cells and WBCs that became incorporated in the cast and then degenerated. Granular casts are seen in large numbers with acute nephritis and indicate more severe kidney damage than do hyaline casts.

Epithelial Casts

Epithelial casts comprise epithelial cells from the renal tubules. Epithelial cells in casts are always of the renal epithelial type because this is the only epithelial cell present at the site of cast formation. Granular casts usually accompany them. These casts are seen in acute nephritis or other conditions that cause degeneration of the renal tubular epithelium.

Leukocyte Casts

Leukocyte casts contain WBCs (see Figure 5-17). Usually they are accompanied by free WBCs. The presence of WBCs and leukocyte casts indicates inflammation in the renal tubules.

Figure 5-16
Hyaline and granular casts. **A,** Bright-field microscopy. **B,** Phase-contrast microscopy. (100×)

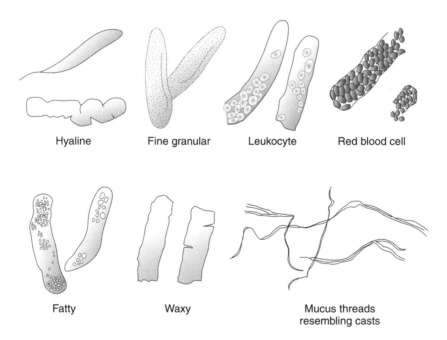

Figure 5-17
Various types of casts that may be found in urine.

Erythrocyte Casts

Erythrocyte casts are deep yellow to orange. The RBC membranes may or may not be visible (see Figure 5-17). Erythrocyte casts indicate renal bleeding. Bleeding may be strictly from hemorrhage resulting from trauma or bleeding disorders, or it may occur as part of an inflammatory lesion.

Figure 5-18
Granular cast in canine urine. (500×)

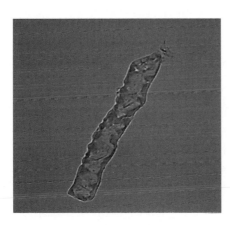

Figure 5-19
Waxy cast. (400×)

Waxy Casts

Waxy casts resemble hyaline casts but are usually wider, with square ends rather than round ends and a dull, homogeneous, "waxy" appearance. They are more opaque than hyaline casts (Figures 5-17 and 5-19). They indicate chronic, severe degeneration of the renal tubules.

Fatty Casts

Fatty casts contain many small droplets of fat that appear as refractile bodies (see Figure 5-17). They are frequently seen in cats with renal disease because cats have lipid in their renal parenchyma. They are occasionally seen in dogs with diabetes mellitus. Large numbers of fatty casts suggest degeneration of the renal tubules.

Mucus Threads

Mucus threads are often confused with casts, but they do not have the well-delineated edges of casts. They resemble a twisted ribbon more than a cast (see Figure 5-17). A large amount of mucus is normally present in equine urine because horses have mucus glands in the renal pelvis and ureter. In other animals, mucus indicates urethral irritation or contamination of the sample with genital secretions.

◆ Spermatozoa

Spermatozoa are occasionally seen in the urine sediment of intact male animals. They are easily recognized and have no clinical significance (Figures 5-10 and 5-20).

◆ Parasite Ova, Microfilariae

Parasite ova may be seen in the urine sediment of animals with urinary parasites or because of fecal contamination at the time of collection of the urine sample. Para-

Figure 5-20
Spermatozoa in canine urine. (400×)

Figure 5-21
An egg of *Capillaria plica,* the bladder worm of dogs. (400×)

sites of the urinary tract include *Capillaria plica,* a bladder worm of dogs and cats; *Dioctophyma renale,* a kidney worm of dogs; and *Stephanurus dentatus,* a kidney worm of pigs (Figure 5-21). Microfilariae (e.g., *Dirofilaria immitis*) may be seen in the urine sediment of dogs with adult heartworms and circulating microfilariae, if hemorrhage into the urine occurs either from disease or as a result of trauma during collection.

◆ Fat Droplets

In urine sediment, fat droplets are lightly green-tinged, highly refractile, spherical bodies of varying sizes (Figure 5-22). Because they vary in size, they can be distinguished from RBCs and yeast, which tend to be of uniform size. If a sediment smear is allowed to sit for a few moments before it is examined, fat droplets rise to a plane just beneath the coverslip, while other formed elements settle to the top of the slide. Therefore fat droplets are often not in the plane of focus of other formed elements. Small, round structures found under the coverslip are usually fat globules. Uniformly sized, round structures found in a lower plane are usually RBCs. In sediment stained with Sudan III stain, fat droplets appear orange or red. Frequently, fat droplets from catheter lubricants or from oily surfaces of collecting vials and pipettes may contaminate urine. Fat in the urine, called *lipuria,* is seen to some degree in most cats. Lipuria also is seen with obesity, diabetes mellitus, and hypothyroidism, and rarely after a high fat meal.

◆ Crystals

The presence of crystals in the urine is termed *crystalluria.* Crystalluria may or may not be of clinical significance. Certain crystals form as a consequence of their elements being secreted into the urine by normal renal activity. Some crystals form as a consequence of metabolic diseases. Conditions that lead to crystal formation may also cause formation of urinary calculi. The type of crystals formed depends on the urine pH, concentration and temperature, and the solubility of the elements (see Figure 5-22). If a urine sample is allowed to stand and cool before examination, the number of crystals in the sample increases because the materials that make up crystals are less soluble at lower temperatures. Refrigerated samples often have many more crystals than warm, fresh samples. Sometimes crystals dissolve when a refrigerated sample is warmed to room temperature. Crystals are generally reported as occasional, moderate, or many.

Triple Phosphate

Triple phosphate (struvite) crystals are found in alkaline to slightly acidic urine. Generally triple phosphate crystals are eight-sided prisms, with tapering sides and ends. Triple phosphate crystals typically are described as resembling coffin lids, although they may assume other shapes. Occasionally they may assume a fern-leaf shape, especially when the urine contains a high concentration of ammonia (Figures 5-22 and 5-23).

Figure 5-22
Various types of crystals that may be found in urine.

Figure 5-23
Triple phosphate crystal in canine urine, resembling a coffin lid. (200×)

Figure 5-24
Amorphous phosphates in canine urine. (400×)

Amorphous Phosphate

Amorphous phosphate crystals are common in alkaline urine and appear as a granular precipitate (Figures 5-22 and 5-24).

Calcium Carbonate

Calcium carbonate crystals, commonly seen in the urine of horses, are round, with many lines radiating from their centers (Figures 5-22 and 5-25). They also may have a "dumbbell" shape.

Amorphous Urates

Amorphous urates appear as a granular precipitate similar to amorphous phosphates. But amorphous phosphates are found in alkaline urine (see Figure 5-22), whereas amorphous urates are seen in acidic urine.

Ammonium Biurate

Ammonium biurate crystals are round and brownish, with long spicules (thorn apple shape) (Figures 5-22 and 5-26). Often the spicules fracture and the remaining crystal

Figure 5-25
Calcium carbonate crystals in urine of a horse. (400×)

Figure 5-26
Ammonium biurate crystals in urine of a dog. (160×)

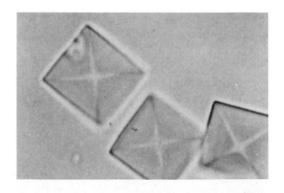

Figure 5-27
Calcium oxalate dihydrase crystals, resembling a square envelope. (400×)

is brown, with fine radiating lines. They are most common in animals with severe liver diseases, such as portacaval shunts.

Calcium Oxalate

Calcium oxalate dihydrate crystals generally appear as small squares, containing an X across the crystal, resembling the back of an envelope (Figures 5-22 and 5-27). Calcium oxalate monohydrate crystals may be small and dumbbell shaped or they may be elongated and pointed at each end (resembling a slat from a picket fence). Calcium dihydrate crystals are found in acidic and neutral urine and are commonly seen in small numbers in dogs and horses. The urine of animals poisoned with ethylene glycol (antifreeze) often contains large numbers of calcium oxalate crystals, especially calcium monohydrate crystals. Animals with oxalate urolithiasis may have large numbers of calcium oxalate crystals in their urine, and large numbers of oxalate crystals may indicate predisposition to oxalate urolithiasis.

Sulfonamide

Sulfonamide crystals may be seen in animals being treated with sulfonamides. Sulfonamide crystals are round, usually dark, with individual crystals radiating from the center. They are less likely to be observed in alkaline urine because these crystals are more soluble in alkaline urine. Prevention of precipitation of these crystals in the renal tubules is assisted by maintenance of alkaline urine and encouraging the animal to drink.

Leucine and Tyrosine

Animals with liver disease may have leucine and tyrosine crystals in their urine. Tyrosine crystals are dark and needlelike (see Figure 5-22). They often are found in small clusters.

Cystine

Cystine crystals appear as six-sided (hexagonal), flat plates and can be associated with renal tubular dysfunction or cystine urolithiasis (Figure 5-22).

◆ Artifacts

Many artifacts may enter the urine sample during collection, transportation, or examination. Recognition of these structures as irrelevant and not a normal part of the sediment is important. These contaminants may be a source of great confusion.

Air bubbles, oil droplets (usually resulting from lubricated catheters), starch granules (from surgical gloves), hair, fecal material, plant spores, dust, bacteria, and fungi may contaminate urine. Ova of intestinal parasites may be observed as a result of fecal contamination of the urine sample.

◉ UROLITHIASIS

Uroliths are calculi (stones) composed of various minerals, found anywhere in the urinary tract; their occurrence is termed *urolithiasis.* They may cause blockage of urine outflow from the bladder into the urethra, they may lodge in the urethra causing severe, acute inability to urinate, or they may remain in the bladder and cause inflammation and bleeding. Determining the composition of calculi is critical because their prevention and the animal's prognosis depend on identification of their composition. Once composition is determined, proper therapy may be initiated to remove them and prevent their reoccurrence. Urolithiasis may be a particular problem in castrated male ruminants. Lodging of calculi in the urethra obstructs the outflow of urine, which is a major problem in lambs and steers, particularly those that are fed high-concentrate rations. The most common calculi in these species are composed of calcium, magnesium, and ammonium carbonate, or calcium, magnesium, and ammonium phosphate.

Analysis of the mineral composition of uroliths may be determined by submitting it intact to a reference laboratory for quantitative analysis (Urinary Stone Laboratory, Department of Medicine and Epidemiology, School of Veterinary Medicine, University of California, Davis, CA or Urolithiosis Laboratory, College of Veterinary Medicine, University of Minnesota, St. Paul, MN). Occasionally, a reasonable idea about the composition of a urolith may be made by its gross and radiographic appearance and the crystal types found in the sediment.

Triple Phosphate (Struvite)

In dogs and cats, one of the most common uroliths observed is triple phosphate uroliths. They are composed of salts of magnesium, ammonium, and calcium (i.e., the anions), and phosphate (i.e., the cation). These are generally radioopaque, hard, white or yellow, and powdery when crushed and are common in alkaline urine. Alkaline urine often occurs in urinary tract infection in carnivores, especially with *Streptococcus* urinary tract infections.

Urate

Urate uroliths are composed of ammonium urate and are usually radiolucent, yellow, and brittle. These uroliths are seen mostly in Dalmatians because this breed excretes much uric acid. They sometimes may be found in other dog breeds.

Cystine

Cystine uroliths are usually yellow, smooth, easily pulverized, and radiolucent.

Oxalate

Oxalate uroliths are composed of calcium oxalate and are radioopaque and hard. They do not crush easily, have sharp protrusions on their surface, and may severely traumatize the bladder.

Recommended Reading

Chew DJ, DiBartola SP: *Interpretation of canine and feline urinalysis,* Wilmington, Del, 1998, The Gloyd Group, Inc.

Ling GV: *Lower urinary tract diseases of dogs and cats: diagnosis, medical management, prevention,* St Louis, 1995, Mosby.

Modern urine chemistry, Elkhart, Ind, 1993, Miles Laboratories.

Osborne CA, Finco DR, editors: *Canine and feline nephrology and urology,* Baltimore, 1995, Lippincott, Williams & Wilkins.

Osborne CA, Stevens C: *Handbook of canine and feline urinalysis,* St Louis, 1981, Ralston Purina.

CHAPTER 6

Internal Parasites

CHARLES M. HENDRIX

This chapter discusses the roles that veterinary technicians play in assisting the veterinarian in diagnosing endoparasites (internal parasites) of domestic animals such as dogs, cats, cattle, horses, sheep, and poultry. Diagnosis of endoparasitism is one of the most frequently performed procedures in the veterinary clinical setting. As such, diagnoses must be performed accurately and efficiently so that the information may be related to the client and appropriate treatment initiated.

An accurate diagnosis of endoparasitism is based primarily upon the veterinarian's and the technician's awareness of parasites that are prevalent in the immediate geographic area or ecosystem. However, because of the mobility of clients during their lifetime, residence in or travel to another region also should be considered when endoparasitism is among several differential diagnoses.

Heavily parasitized animals often show clinical signs suggestive of the infected organ system. Depending on the system, these signs may include diarrhea or constipation, anorexia, vomiting, blood in the stool, or fat in the stool. Parasitized animals are frequently lethargic and display an unthrifty appearance characterized by weight loss or stunted growth, dull haircoat, dehydration, or anemia. The animal also may experience coughing or difficulty in breathing.

Internal parasites of domestic animals comprise several types of organisms that live internally in animals, feed on their tissues or body fluids, or compete directly for their food. These organisms range in size from too small to be seen with the naked eye, or microscopic, to more than 1 m in length. Parasites also vary in their location within the host and in the means by which they are transmitted from one host to another. Because of these diverse variations, no single diagnostic test can identify all endoparasites.

The veterinary technician may be asked to perform a wide variety of diagnostic procedures to diagnose endoparasitism. These procedures usually detect the adult stages of a parasite or their eggs or larval stages in the animal's feces, urine, or blood. Mature parasites are seldom found because they are generally hidden within the body

257

of the animal. The only way to detect their presence is by necropsy, or postmortem dissection. An assorted battery of diagnostic procedures may not be in common use in veterinary practices but are described in this chapter because they may be useful to veterinary technicians working in research or diagnostic laboratories.

This chapter includes illustrations and brief descriptions of some of the eggs, larvae, and adult parasites that may be diagnosed in common domesticated animals. Sometimes eggs of certain groups of parasites are quite similar; differentiation of individual species or genera based on their morphologic characteristics may be difficult or impossible. Parasites with similar eggs usually are differentiated by fecal culture (procedure to be described later) and larval identification. This chapter does not provide descriptions of parasite larval cultures; those descriptions and methodologies are found in the reference texts listed at the end of this chapter.

The technician must remember that the diagnostic tests used to detect endoparasitism may be unreliable. An animal may be infected with endoparasites; however, if the infection is slight, no eggs or larvae may be observed in the specimens tested. If an inappropriate test is used, it is also possible that no parasites may be detected. Another common problem is trying to diagnose endoparasitism before the parasite completely develops. Many parasites can produce clinical disease before they become reproductively mature.

The time elapsed between initial infection with a parasite until the infection can be detected using common diagnostic procedures is called the *prepatent period*. The best example of this concept is trying to diagnose hookworm disease *(Ancylostoma caninum)* in a 1-week–old puppy by observation of eggs on fecal flotation. This attempted diagnosis is a waste of time because the minimum time for infection until adult hookworms are present in the bowel and begin to produce eggs (prepatent period) is 12 days. The astute veterinary practitioner uses fecal flotation results but also the puppy's history, clinical signs, and other laboratory tests (e.g., blood values) to arrive at a specific diagnosis of ancylostomiasis (infection with hookworms).

COMMON TYPES OF PARASITES

Complete coverage of the discipline of veterinary parasitology is beyond the scope of this textbook. Only the general types of parasites of domestic animals and their life cycle stages that may be recovered using commonly employed diagnostic procedures are described. The reference textbooks listed at the end of this chapter provide more detailed coverage of veterinary parasitology and specific parasites.

Internal parasites, called *endoparasites,* live within an animal. These parasites derive their nutrition and protection at the expense of the infected animal, which is called the *host.* The various internal parasites have many different life cycles. Each parasite's life cycle is distinctive and comprises various developmental stages, which may occur all within the same host or separately within sequential hosts.

The host that harbors the adult, mature, or sexual stages of a parasite is called the *definitive host.* The dog is the definitive host for *Dirofilaria immitis;* adult male and female heartworms are found in the right ventricle and pulmonary arteries of the dog's heart. The host that harbors the larval, immature, or asexual stages of a parasite is called the *intermediate host.* The mosquito is the intermediate host for *D. immitis;* first, second, and third larval stages of *D. immitis* are found within the mosquito intermediate host.

The life cycle of most parasites has at least one stage at which the parasite may be passed from one host to the next. Diagnostic procedures frequently detect this stage; therefore it is referred to as the *diagnostic stage.* The diagnostic stage of a parasite may leave the host through excreta, such as feces or urine, or it may be transmitted via the blood to its next host by an arthropod, such as a mosquito. The microfilarial stage is the diagnostic stage of *D. immitis;* the female mosquito takes in the microfilariae during a blood meal.

◆ Protozoa (Unicellular Organisms)

Protozoa are unicellular, or one-cell, organisms, some of which may be parasitic in domestic animals. These protozoans can infect a variety of tissue sites within the definitive host. The most common sites for their detection are in blood samples, in which they are called *blood protozoa* or *hemoprotozoa,* or within fecal samples, in which they are called *intestinal protozoa.* The protozoan's life cycle may be either simple or complex.

Most hemoprotozoa seen in the United States are found in erythrocytes (red blood cells, RBCs) within a stained blood smear. Ticks usually serve as intermediate hosts and transmit the RBCs containing the hemoprotozoa from one animal to the next. *Babesia bigemina* is a tear-shape or pear-shape hemoprotozoan found within the RBCs of infected cattle. It is transmitted by *Boophilus annulatus,* a tick described in Chapter 7.

Trypanosomes are another group of hemoprotozoans occasionally found in the United States. Rather than being found within RBCs, trypanosomes are extracellular and "swim" within the blood. They are 3 to 10 times as long as an RBC is wide and are banana shape. They have a lateral undulating membrane and a thin, whiplike tail (flagellum) that is used for swimming. These parasites are also transmitted by blood-feeding arthropods (see Reduviid bugs in Order: Hemiptera in Chapter 7).

◆ Trematodes (Flukes)

The trematodes (also called *flukes*) are flatworms with unsegmented, leaf-shape bodies. In domestic animals in the United States, most adult flukes are found in the intestinal tract, the liver, or the lungs. In these sites, the hermaphroditic (having male *and* female sex organs) flukes lay eggs that are passed with the feces. The end portion of many fluke eggs has a small cap, lid, or door; this structure is called an *operculum* and is common among the flukes.

Within each fluke egg is a larval stage known as a *miracidium,* which hatches and exits the egg through the operculum. This stage penetrates the *first intermediate host,* which is usually a snail. Within the snail, the miracidium develops into a sporocyst, which then produces many tiny structures called *rediae.* Each redia may produce many cercariae. The cercaria exits the snail and may take one of three pathways to enter the definitive host: it may develop into a metacercaria and encyst upon vegetation, whereby it is ingested by the definitive host; it may be ingested by a second intermediate host and become encysted within that host, which is subsequently ingested by the definitive host; or it may directly penetrate the skin of the definitive host.

Flukes of veterinary importance include the liver flukes of cattle and sheep (*Fasciola hepatica, Fascioloides magna, Dicrocoelium dendriticum*) and the lung fluke of dogs and cats (*Paragonimus kellicotti*).

◆ Cestodes (Tapeworms)

Like trematodes, cestodes (tapeworms) are also flatworms. They differ, however, in that cestodes are ribbon-like and divided into a long chain of proglottids, which are segments connected like train cars behind a *scolex* or "head," by which the tapeworm attaches to the wall of the host's intestine. Most tapeworms release their proglottids one at a time or in short chains into the feces. Proglottids in the feces can be observed with the naked eye. A few tapeworms release eggs directly from the worm's uterus.

Tapeworm proglottids have muscles that enable them to move about. Pet owners often observe these tapeworms as "little white worms" crawling on the pet's feces, haircoat, or bedding. These fresh proglottids are said to resemble "cucumber seeds." When the proglottids dry out, they resemble uncooked grains of rice.

Tapeworm proglottids often contain eggs when they are passed into the feces. These eggs contain hexacanth embryos, which are embryos with an internal structure with six hooks.

An intermediate host, usually a mammalian host, such as a rabbit, ingests these hexacanth embryos. The hexacanth embryo grows within the tissues of the intermediate host to a "bladderworm" stage, which is a fluid-filled larval stage. The definitive host becomes infected by ingesting the intermediate host, which contains the bladderworm larval stage. Examples of tapeworms that develop into the bladderworm stage in the intermediate host is the canine Taeniid tapeworm (*Taenia pisiformis*) and the coenurus tapeworm (*Multiceps multiceps*). In some tapeworms (*Echinococcus granulosus, Echinococcus multilocularis*), the larval stage within the vertebrate host is a hydatid cyst.

When the intermediate host is an arthropod, such as a flea or a grain mite, the hexacanth embryo develops into a microscopic larval stage known as a *cysticercoid.* The cysticercoid stage is tiny and contains a small fluid-filled space. The definitive host becomes infected by ingesting the intermediate host, which contains the cysticercoid larval stage. The cysticercoid stage develops in the fringed tapeworms of cattle (*Thysanosoma actinoides*) and the double-pore tapeworm of dogs and cats (*Dipylidium caninum*).

◆ Nematodes (Roundworms)

Nematodes often are referred to as *roundworms* and are the most important group of parasites in veterinary parasitology. They may be found in almost any tissue of domestic animals, including the intestines, skin, lungs, kidneys, urinary bladder, nervous tissue, and blood.

Nematodes as a group have diverse, complicated life cycles. Their eggs or larvae are most commonly recovered from the feces. The eggs of nematodes infecting the kidney or urinary bladder may be recovered from the urine.

Examples of intestinal nematodes include large roundworms (*Toxocara canis, Toxascaris leonina*), hookworms (*Ancylostoma caninum, Uncinaria stenocephala*), and whipworms (*Trichuris vulpis*). Urinary roundworms include canine kidney worms (*Dioctophyma renale*). Respiratory roundworms include the lungworms of cattle and sheep (*Dictyocaulus* species and *Muellerius capillaris*). Nematodes of the blood vasculature are a special group, of which the heartworm of dogs (*Dirofilaria immitis*) is an example. Adult female heartworms give birth to small, wormlike prelarval (embryonic) stages called *microfilariae.* The microfilariae often are observed in a peripheral blood smear and are approximately 310 μ long. These microfilariae can be transmitted to other animals by mosquitoes.

◆ Acanthocephalans (Thorny-Head Worms)

Acanthocephalans (thorny-head worms) are uncommon parasites with complicated life cycles. On the cranial end of these helminths is a spiny proboscis, which is used to attach to the lining of the intestine wall. Thorny-head worms do not have a true gut; they absorb nutrients through their body wall. Acanthocephalans usually are recovered at necropsy.

The most "famous" acanthocephalan is *Macracanthorhynchus hirudinaceus,* a parasite of pigs. This parasite has the dubious honor of possessing the longest scientific name among the parasites of domestic animals. *Oncicola canis* is the acanthocephalan of dogs.

COMMON ENDOPARASITES OF DOMESTIC ANIMALS

Following are descriptions of most of the common endoparasites in domestic animals in the United States. Information is given on the organ or organ system parasitized in the host; prepatent period, or time from initial infection until the diagnostic stage may be recovered, where appropriate; description of the diagnostic stage, or life cycle stage commonly used to make a diagnosis, such as *eggs* or *larvae,* and diagnostic stage most commonly identified.

◆ Endoparasites of Dogs and Cats

Parasites of the Gastrointestinal Tract

NEMATODES (ROUNDWORMS). *Spirocerca lupi,* the esophageal worm, is a nematode that often forms nodules in the esophageal wall of dogs and cats. Occasionally it may be found in gastric nodules in cats. Adult worms reside deep within these nodules and expel their eggs through fistulous openings in the granuloma. Eggs are passed through the host animal's esophagus and out in the feces. The thick-shelled eggs are 30 to 37 μ by 11 to 15 μ and contain a larva when they are laid. These eggs have a unique "paper clip" shape. Figure 6-1 shows the characteristic ovum of *S. lupi.* Eggs usually may be observed on fecal flotation and may be recovered when vomitus has been subjected to a standard fecal flotation procedure. Radiographic or endoscopic examination may reveal characteristic granulomas within the esophagus or within the stomach. The prepatent period is 6 months.

Physaloptera species are stomach worms of dogs and cats. Although they occasionally are found in the lumen of the stomach or small intestine, *Physaloptera* species usually are firmly attached to the mucosal surface of the stomach, where they suck blood. At this site, these nematodes may be viewed with an endoscope. Their diet consists of blood and tissue derived from the host's gastric mucosa. Their attachment sites continue to bleed after the parasite detaches. Vomiting, anorexia, and dark, tarry stools may be observed in affected animals.

The adults are creamy white, sometimes tightly coiled, and 1.3 to 4.8 cm long. They are often recovered in the pet's vomitus and may be confused with ascarids, or roundworms. A quick way to differentiate the two parasites is to break open an adult specimen and (if that specimen happens to be female) examine the egg type microscopically. The eggs of *Physaloptera* species are small, smooth, thick-shelled, and em-

Figure 6-1
Characteristic ovum of *Spirocerca lupi.* The thick-shell eggs contain larvae and measure 30 to 38 μ by 11 to 15 μ. Eggs usually may be observed on fecal flotation and may be recovered when vomitus has been subjected to a standard fecal flotation procedure.

Figure 6-2
Characteristic ovum of *Physaloptera* species. The oval, thick-shell eggs contain larvae and measure 49 to 58 μ by 30 to 34 μ. Eggs usually may be recovered on a standard fecal flotation, using solutions with a specific gravity above 1.25.

bryonated when passed in the feces. Eggs are 30 to 34 μ by 49 to 59 μ and contain a larva when they are laid. Figure 6-2 shows the characteristic ovum of *Physaloptera* species. Eggs usually may be recovered on a standard fecal flotation, using solutions with a specific gravity above 1.25. The prepatent period is 56 to 83 days.

Aonchotheca putorii is commonly referred to as the gastric capillarid of cats. It was once known by a former name, *Capillaria putorii.* This capillarid frequently parasitizes mustellids, such as mink, but it also has been reported in cats. These nematodes are rarely reported in North America. The eggs of *A. putorii* easily are confused with other trichinelloid nematodes (see the section on feline whipworms). Their eggs are 53 to 70 μ by 20 to 30 μ and exhibit a netlike surface similar to that of the eggs of *Eucoleus aerophilus,* an upper respiratory capillarid. The eggs of *A. putorii* are dense, less delicate than those of *E. aerophilus,* and organized in a longitudinal formation. They have flattened sides and contain a one- or two-cell embryo, which fills the egg.

Ollulanus tricuspis is "the feline trichostrongyle." This parasite usually is associated with vomiting in cats. It is most commonly identified by examination of the cat's vomitus with a dissecting or compound microscope. Feline vomitus also may be examined using a standard fecal flotation procedure. The best flotation solution for identification is a modified Sheather's flotation solution. Adult female *O. tricuspis* are 0.8 to 1.0 mm long and have three major tail cusps, which are the origin of the name *tricuspis.* Adult males are 0.7 to 0.8 mm long and have a copulatory bursa. The female worms are viviparous (bear live young). The infective third-stage larvae (500 by 22 μ) mature to adults in the cat's stomach. Free-living stages are not required for completion of the life cycle. Transmission occurs through ingestion of vomitus from infected cats.

Toxocara canis, Toxocara cati, and *Toxascaris leonina* are the ascarids of dogs and cats. These roundworms are found in the small intestine of dogs and cats in most areas of the world. All young puppies and kittens presented to a veterinary clinic should be examined for these large, robust nematodes. Adult ascarids may vary from 3 to 18 cm in length and when passed are usually tightly coiled, much like a coiled bedspring. The eggs of *Toxocara* species are spherical, with a deeply pigmented center and a rough, pitted outer shell. Eggs of *T. canis* are 75 to 90 μ in diameter (Figure 6-3), whereas

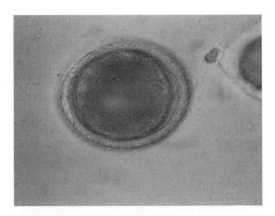

Figure 6-3
Characteristic ovum of *Toxocara* species. These eggs are spherical, with a deeply pigmented center and a rough, pitted outer shell. Eggs of *T. canis* are 75 to 90 μ in diameter.

those of *T. cati* are smaller, only 65 to 75 μ in diameter (Figure 6-4). The eggs of *Toxascaris leonina* are spherical to ovoid, with dimensions of 75 μ by 85 μ. These eggs have a smooth outer shell and a hyaline or "ground glass" central portion. Figure 6-5 shows the characteristic ovum of *Toxascaris leonina*. The prepatent period for *T. canis* is 21 to 35 days, whereas that of *T. leonina* is 74 days.

    Ancylostoma caninum, a canine hookworm; *Ancylostoma tubaeforme,* a feline hookworm; *Ancylostoma braziliense,* a canine and feline hookworm; and *Uncinaria stenocephala,* a northern canine hookworm, are small intestinal nematodes. Hookworms are found throughout the world and are common in tropical and subtropical areas of North America. Hookworm infection, which can produce severe anemia in young kittens and puppies, can be a serious problem in kennels and catteries. The prepatent period depends on the species of hookworm and the route of infection.

    Eggs of all hookworm species are oval or ellipsoid, have thin walls, and contain 8 to 16 cells when passed in the pet's feces. Because these eggs larvate rapidly in the external environment (as early as 48 hours after feces are passed), fresh feces are needed for diagnosing hookworm infections. Eggs of *A. caninum* are 56 to 75 μ by 34 to 47 μ (Figures 6-6 and 6-8). Those of *A. tubaeforme* are 55 to 75 μ by 34.4 to

Figure 6-4
Characteristic ovum of *Toxocara cati.* These eggs are smaller than those of *T. canis,* measuring only 65 to 75 μ in diameter.

Figure 6-5
Characteristic ovum of *Toxascaris leonina.* These eggs are spherical to ovoid, with dimensions of 75 by 85 μ. They have a smooth outer shell and a hyaline or "ground glass" central portion.

44.7 μ. Those of *A. braziliense* are 75 μ by 45 μ and those of *U. stenocephala,* 65 to 80 μ by 40 to 50 μ. These eggs usually may be recovered on a standard fecal flotation.

Strongyloides stercoralis and Strongyloides tumefaciens are often referred to as "intestinal threadworms." These nematodes are unique: only a parthenogenetic female (female that can lay eggs without copulation with a male) is parasitic in the host. Parasitic males do not exist. These females produce eggs, but in dogs these eggs hatch in the intestine, releasing first-stage larvae. Figure 6-7 shows the parasitic adult females, eggs, and first-stage larvae of *Strongyloides* species. The larvae are 280 to 310 μ long and have a rhabditiform esophagus, with a club-shape cranial corpus, a narrow median isthmus, and a caudal bulb. The prepatent period is 8 to 14 days.

Trichuris vulpis, the canine whipworm, and *Trichuris campanula* and *Trichuris serrata,* the feline whipworms, reside in the cecum and colon of their respective hosts. Canine whipworms are common, but feline whipworms are rare in North America and diagnosed only sporadically throughout the world. Whipworms derive their name from the fact that the adults have a thin, filamentous cranial end (i.e., the lash of the whip) and a thick caudal end (i.e., the handle of the whip). The

Figure 6-6
Characteristic hookworm ovum. The eggs of *Ancylostoma caninum* are 56 to 75 μ by 34 to 47 μ, those of *A. tubaeforme,* 55 to 75 μ by 34.4 to 44.7 μ, those of *A. braziliense,* 75 by 45 μ, and those of *U. stenocephala,* 65 to 80 μ by 40 to 50 μ.

Figure 6-7
Parasitic adult females, eggs, and first-stage larvae of *Strongyloides* species. These larvae are 280 to 310 μ long and have a rhabditiform esophagus, with a club-shape cranial corpus, a narrow median isthmus, and a caudal bulb.

egg of the whipworm is described as *trichinelloid* or *trichuroid*. It has a thick, yellow-brown, symmetric shell with polar plugs at both ends. The eggs are unembryonated (not larvated) when laid. Eggs of *T. vulpis* are 70 to 89 μ by 37 to 40 μ. Figure 6-8 shows the characteristic egg of *T. vulpis*. The prepatent period for *T. vulpis* is 70 to 90 days.

The eggs of *T. campanula* and *T. serrata* may be easily confused with those of *Aonchotheca putorii*, *Eucoleus aerophilus*, and *Personema felis cati*, parasites of the feline stomach, respiratory tract, and urinary system, respectively. The eggs of *T. campanula* average 63 to 85 μ by 34 to 39 μ. When examining a cat's feces for feline trichurids, the veterinary technician should be aware of pseudoparasites, which are eggs of trichurids or capillarids that parasitize such hosts as mice, rabbits, or birds (an outdoor cat's prey). The eggs of these trichurids or capillarids may pass unaltered through the cat's gastrointestinal system, remaining intact and unembryonated.

Enterobius vermicularis is the human pinworm and *does not* parasitize dogs or cats. Nevertheless, the family pet is often falsely incriminated by family practitioners or pediatricians as a source of pinworm infection in young children. The veterinary technician should remember this rule: *Pinworms are parasites of omnivores (mice, rats, monkeys, people) and herbivores (rabbits, horses) but never carnivores (dogs, cats).*

CESTODES (TAPEWORMS).   *Dipylidium caninum* is often called the "double-pore" or "cucumber seed" tapeworm. This tapeworm is the most common tapeworm found in the small intestine of the dog and cat because the dog or cat becomes infected by ingesting the flea intermediate host. Fleas often contain this parasite's infective cysticercoid stage. This tapeworm has motile, terminal, gravid proglottids, which usually are found on the feces (Figure 6-9), on the pet's haircoat, or in the bedding of the host. In the fresh state, these proglottids resemble cucumber seeds. This resemblance is the origin of the common name, the "cucumber seed" tapeworm. These terminal proglottids have a lateral pore located along the midpoint of each of their long edges, the origin of the second common name, the "double-pore" tapeworm.

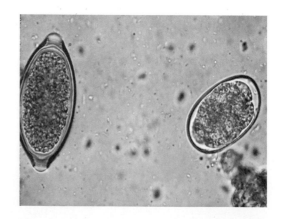

Figure 6-8
Characteristic ovum of *Trichuris vulpis*. Eggs of *T. vulpis* are 70 to 89 μ by 37 to 40 μ (*left*). Characteristic ovum of *A. caninum*, 56 to 75 μ by 34 to 47 μ (*right*).

If fresh proglottids are teased or broken open, they may reveal thousands of unique egg packets, each containing 20 to 30 hexacanth embryos. Figure 6-10 shows the unique egg packet of *D. caninum*. The proglottids of *D. caninum* often dry out in the external environment. As they lose moisture, they shrivel up and resemble uncooked grains of rice. If reconstituted with water, the dried proglottids usually assume their former cucumber-seed appearance. The prepatent period for *D. caninum* is 14 to 21 days.

Taenia pisiformis, Taenia hydatigena, and *Taenia ovis* are the canine taeniids. As with *D. caninum, Taenia* tapeworms appear as motile, terminal, gravid proglottids on the feces, on the pet's haircoat, or in the bedding of the host. In the fresh state, these proglottids have a single lateral pore located along the midpoint of either of their long edges (as opposed to the "double-pore" tapeworm).

As with *D. caninum,* if these fresh proglottids are teased or broken open, they may reveal thousands of hexacanth embryos. The proglottids of *Taenia* species also dry out in the external environment and resemble uncooked grains of rice. If reconstituted with water, they too usually assume their former single-pore appearance. If gravid proglottids of *Taenia* species are recovered from a dog's or cat's feces, the proglottid should be torn open or macerated in a drop of saline solution on a glass slide to reveal the characteristic eggs under the compound microscope.

Figure 6-9
Characteristic motile, terminal, gravid proglottids of *Dipylidium caninum* on canine feces. In the fresh state, these proglottids resemble cucumber seeds; hence the common name, the "cucumber seed" tapeworm.

Figure 6-10
Characteristic egg packet of *Dipylidium caninum.* Each egg packet may contain up to 30 hexacanth embryos.

The eggs of taeniid tapeworms are slightly oval and are 43 to 53 μ by 43 to 49 μ in diameter (*T. pisiformis*), 36 to 39 μ by 31 to 35 μ in diameter (*T. hydatigena*), and 19 to 31 μ by 24 to 26 μ (*T. ovis*). Eggs of *Taenia* species contain a single *oncosphere* with three pairs of hooks. The oncosphere is often called a *hexacanth embryo*. Figure 6-11 shows the unique features of this taeniid tapeworm. The eggs are similar to those of *Echinococcus* and *Multiceps* species.

Taenia taeniaeformis, or *Hydatigera taeniaeformis,* is called the "feline tapeworm" or the "feline taeniid." This tapeworm is observed infrequently in cats allowed to roam and prey upon house and field mice and rats. The egg of this tapeworm is 31 to 36 μ in diameter and contains a single oncosphere with three pairs of hooks. The oncosphere is often called a *hexacanth embryo.* As with the eggs of the canine taeniids, the eggs are similar to those of *Echinococcus* species (see Figure 6-11).

Multiceps multiceps and *Multiceps serialis* also are tapeworms of the small intestine of canids. The eggs of *M. multiceps* are 29 to 37 μ in diameter, whereas those of *M. serialis* are elliptic and measure 31 to 34 μ by 29 to 30 μ. Both contain a single oncosphere with three pairs of hooks. As with the eggs of the canine and feline taeniids, the eggs of *Multiceps* species are similar to those of *Echinococcus* species (see Figure 6-11).

Echinococcus granulosus and *Echinococcus multilocularis* are tapeworms associated with unilocular and multilocular hydatid disease. *E. granulosus* is the hydatid cyst tapeworm of dogs, whereas *E. multilocularis* is the hydatid cyst tapeworm of cats. These are important parasites because of their extreme zoonotic potential. The egg of *E. granulosus* is ovoid and 32 to 36 μ by 25 to 30 μ. It contains a single oncosphere with three pairs of hooks. The egg of *E. multilocularis* is ovoid and 30 to 40 μ. It contains a single oncosphere with three pairs of hooks. These eggs are very similar in appearance to those of *Taenia* and *Multiceps* species (see Figure 6-11).

Figure 6-11
Characteristic ova of the taeniid tapeworms are slightly oval and 43 to 53 μ by 43 to 49 μ in diameter (*Taenia pisiformis*), 36 to 39 μ by 31 to 35 μ in diameter (*Taenia hydatigena*), and 19 to 31 μ by 24 to 26 μ (*Taenia ovis*). Eggs of *Taenia* species contain a single oncosphere with three pairs of hooks. The oncosphere is often called a *hexacanth embryo.* The eggs are similar to those of *Echinococcus* and *Multiceps* species. The dissimilar ovum is that of *A. caninum,* the hookworm.

The adult *Echinococcus* is a tiny tapeworm, only 1.2 to 7.0 mm in length. The entire tapeworm has only three proglottids: immature, mature, and gravid. When passed, the tiny gravid proglottids are often overlooked by the client, the veterinary technician, and the veterinarian. Definitive diagnosis of *Echinococcus* infection is best achieved by identifying adult tapeworms taken from the host's intestinal tract. In the rare instances in which *Echinococcus* infection is suspected, antemortem diagnosis is accomplished by purging the dog or cat using arecoline hydrobromide PO at 3.5 mg/kg and collecting the feces. This procedure usually is performed only when this infection is strongly suspected. Entire worms or their proglottids may be collected from the final clear mucus. Because of the severe zoonotic potential, all evacuated material should be handled with caution. *Rubber gloves should be worn.* After the feces have been examined, they should be incinerated.

Spirometra species are often referred to as "zipper tapeworms" or *sparganosis tapeworms* (Figure 6-12). These tapeworms are often found in the small intestine of both the dog and cat. These tapeworms are often found in pets in Florida and along the Gulf Coast of North America. This tapeworm is a clinical oddity because it produces an operculated egg. Each proglottid of *Spirometra* species has a central spiral uterus and an associated uterine pore through which eggs are released. These tapeworms characteristically release eggs until they exhaust their uterine contents. Gravid segments usually are not discharged into the pet's feces.

The tapeworm is unique because while it is attached to the host's jejunum, the mature proglottids often separate along the longitudinal axis for a short distance. The tapeworm appears to "unzip," which is the origin of its common name, the "zipper tapeworm." Spent "zipped" and "unzipped" proglottids often appear in the feces of the pet.

Figure 6-12
Spent proglottids of *Spirometra mansonoides,* the "zipper tapeworm." This tapeworm is unique because while it is attached to the host's jejunum, the mature proglottids often separate along the longitudinal axis for a short distance. The tapeworm appears to "unzip," which provides the origin for its common name, the "zipper tapeworm." Spent "zipped" and "unzipped" proglottids often appear in the feces of the pet.

The egg of *Spirometra* species resembles that of a fluke, or digenetic trematode (Figure 6-13). The egg has a distinct operculum at one end of the pole of the shell. The eggs are oval and yellowish-brown. They average 60 by 36 μ, have an asymmetric appearance, and are rather pointed at one end. When the eggs rupture, a distinct operculum is visible. The eggs are unembryonated when passed in the feces.

Diphyllobothrium species are often referred to as "broad fish tapeworms." This tapeworm may be 2 to 12 m long; however, it probably does not grow as large as 12 m in dogs and cats. Each proglottid of this tapeworm has a central rosette-shape uterus and an associated uterine pore through which eggs are released. These tapeworms continually release eggs until they exhaust their uterine contents. The terminal proglottids become senile rather than gravid and detach in chains rather than individually.

The egg of *Diphyllobothrium* species also resembles that of a fluke (digenetic trematode). The egg is oval and has a distinct operculum at one end of the shell. The eggs are light brown, averaging 67 to 71 μ by 40 to 51 μ. They tend to be rounded on one end. The operculum is present on the end opposite the rounded end. The eggs are unembryonated when passed in the feces.

TREMATODES (FLUKES).   *Platynosomum fastosum* is the "lizard poisoning fluke" of cats (Figure 6-14). The adult flukes inhabit the liver, gallbladder, bile ducts, and less commonly the small intestine. The brownish, operculated eggs are 34 to 50 μ by 20 to 35 μ.

Nanophyetus salmincola is the "salmon poisoning fluke" of dogs in the Pacific Northwest region of North America. The adult fluke inhabits the small intestine and serves as a vector for rickettsial agents, which produce "salmon poisoning" and "Elokomin fluke fever" in dogs. The eggs are unembryonated when laid and measure 52 to 82 μ by 32 to 56 μ (Figure 6-15). They have an indistinct operculum and a small, blunt point at the end opposite the operculum.

Alaria species are intestinal flukes of dogs and cats and are found throughout the northern half of North America. Their ova are large, golden brown, and operculated (Figure 6-16). They are 98 to 134 μ by 62 to 68 μ.

Figure 6-13
Characteristic ovum of *Spirometra mansonoides.* The egg of *Spirometra* species resembles that of a fluke (digenetic trematode). The egg has a distinct operculum at one end of the shell. The eggs are oval and yellowish-brown. They average 60 by 36 μ and have an asymmetric appearance. They tend to be rather pointed at one end.

PROTOZOANS (UNICELLULAR ORGANISMS). *Isospora* species (coccidians) are protozoan parasites of the small intestine of both dogs and cats. They produce a clinical syndrome known as *coccidiosis*, one of the most commonly diagnosed protozoan diseases in puppies and kittens. Coccidiosis is rarely a problem in mature animals. The oocyst is the diagnostic stage observed in a fecal flotation of fresh feces. It is un-

Figure 6-14
Characteristic ovum of *Platynosomum fastosum,* the "lizard poisoning fluke" of cats. The brownish, operculated eggs are 34 to 50 μ by 20 to 35 μ.

Figure 6-15
Characteristic ovum of *Nanophyetus salmincola.* The eggs are unembryonated when laid and measure 52 to 82 μ by 32 to 56 μ. They have an indistinct operculum and a small, blunt point at the end opposite the operculum.

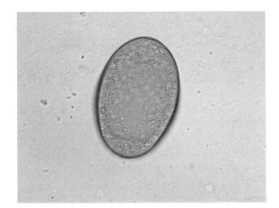

Figure 6-16
Characteristic ovum of *Alaria* species, the "intestinal flukes" of dogs and cats. They are found throughout the northern half of North America. The eggs are large, golden brown, and operculated. They measure 98 to 134 μ by 62 to 68 μ.

sporulated in fresh feces and varies in size and shape among the common *Isospora* species (Figures 6-17 and 6-18).

The canine coccidians and their oocyst measurements are *Isospora canis,* 34 to 40 μ by 28 to 32 μ; *Isospora ohioensis,* 20 to 27 μ by 15 to 24 μ; and *Isospora wallacei,* 10 to 14 μ by 7.5 to 9 μ. The feline coccidians and their measurements are *Isospora felis,* 38 to 51 μ by 27 to 29 μ, and *Isospora rivolta,* 21 to 28 μ by 18 to 23 μ. The prepatent period varies among species but is usually 7 to 14 days.

Toxoplasma gondii is another intestinal coccidian of cats. Its oocysts usually are diagnosed using a standard fecal flotation. Oocysts of *T. gondii* are unsporulated in fresh feces and measure 10 by 12 μ. Several immunodiagnostic tests using whole blood or serum are available for diagnosis of *T. gondii* infection. The prepatent period is highly variable, ranging from 5 to 24 days, and depends on the route of infection.

Cryptosporidium is another coccidian parasite that parasitizes the small intestine of a wide variety of animals, including dogs and cats. The sporulated oocysts in the feces are oval to spherical and measure only 4 to 6 μ. Diagnosis is by a standard fecal flotation. The oocysts are extremely small and may be observed just under the coverslip, not in the same plane of focus as other oocysts and parasite

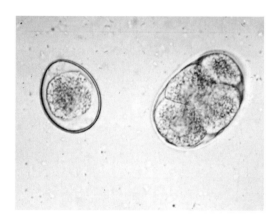

Figure 6-17
Unsporulated oocyst of *Isospora* species. Oocysts vary greatly in size. Also see Figure 6-18. *Ancylostoma caninum (right).*

Figure 6-18
Sporulated oocyst of *Isospora* species. The canine coccidians and their measurements are *Isospora canis,* 34 to 40 μ by 28 to 32 μ; *Isospora ohioensis,* 20 to 27 μ by 15 to 24 μ; and *Isospora wallacei,* 10 to 14 μ by 7.5 to 9 μ. The feline coccidians and their measurements are *Isospora felis,* 38 to 51 μ by 27 to 29 μ, and *I. rivolta,* 21 to 28 μ by 18 to 23 μ. *Ancylostoma caninum (right).*

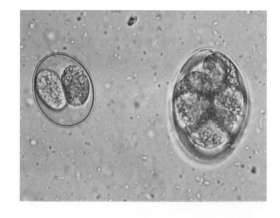

ova (Figure 6-19). Examination of fresh fecal smears using special stains (modified acid-fast stain) is also helpful. Because people may become infected with *Cryptosporidium* species, feces suspected of harboring this protozoan should be handled with great care.

Sarcocystis is another coccidian parasite found in the small intestine. Several species infect dogs and cats. Identification of an individual species may be quite difficult. The oocysts of *Sarcocystis* species are sporulated when passed in the feces. Each oocyst contains two sporocysts, each with four sporozoites. These individual oocysts measure 12 to 15 μ by 8 to 12 μ and may be recovered in a standard fecal flotation of fresh feces.

Giardia species are flagellated protozoans often recovered from the feces of dogs and cats with diarrhea, but they also may be recovered from animals with normal stools. This parasite occurs in two morphologic forms: a motile feeding stage (the *trophozoite,* Figure 6-20) and a resistant cyst stage. The motile stage is pear-shape and dorsoventrally flattened, and contains four pairs of flagella. It measures 9 to 21 μ by 5 to 15 μ. Two nuclei and a prominent adhesive disc are present on the cranial portion of the cell, resembling a pair of eyes staring back at the observer.

Figure 6-19
Oocysts of *Cryptosporidium* species.

Figure 6-20
Motile trophozoite of *Giardia* species.

The mature cysts are oval and are 8 to 10 μ by 7 to 10 μ. They have a refractile wall and four nuclei. Immature cysts, which represent recently encysted motile forms, contain only two nuclei (Figure 6-21). In dogs, diarrhea may begin as early as 5 days after exposure to *Giardia,* with cysts first appearing in the feces at 1 week.

Diagnosis is by a standard fecal flotation. Zinc sulfate (specific gravity 1.18) is considered the best flotation medium for recovering cysts. Cysts are often distorted, with a semilunar appearance. The motile trophozoite occasionally may be found on a direct smear of fresh feces using isotonic saline. Lugol's iodine may be used to visualize the internal structures of cysts and trophozoites. Fecal immunodiagnostic tests are also commonly employed.

Parasites of the Circulatory System

NEMATODES (ROUNDWORMS).   *Dirofilaria immitis* is often referred to as the *canine heartworm;* however, this nematode also has been known to parasitize cats and ferrets. Adult heartworms are found within the right ventricle, the pulmonary artery, and the fine branches of that artery. This parasite is often recovered in a variety of aberrant sites, such as the brain, the anterior chamber of the eye, and within subcutaneous sites. The prepatent period in dogs is approximately 6 months.

In microfilaremic dogs, diagnosis is by observing microfilariae in blood samples using one of several concentration techniques (modified Knott's test) or the commercially available filter techniques (Figures 6-22 and 6-23). For infected dogs with no circulating microfilariae, infection also may be diagnosed using commercially available immunodiagnostic tests.

A subcutaneous filariid of dogs, *Dipetalonema reconditum,* also produces microfilariae in the peripheral blood. The microfilariae of this nonpathogenic nematode must be differentiated from those of *D. immitis* (see Figures 6-22 and 6-23).

TREMATODES (FLUKES).   *Heterobilharzia americanum,* the canine schistosome, is a blood fluke that parasitizes the mesenteric veins of the small and large intestines and portal veins of the dog. This fluke is enzootic in the mud flats of the Mississippi delta and the coastal swampland of Louisiana. Although this fluke inhab-

Figure 6-21
Cysts of *Giardia* species. The mature cysts are oval and measure 8 to 10 μ by 7 to 10 μ. They have a refractile wall and four nuclei. Immature cysts, which represent recently encysted motile forms, contain only two nuclei.

its the vasculature, its presence is manifested by bloody diarrhea. Infected dogs also exhibit emaciation and anorexia. Diagnosis is by identification of the thin-shelled egg, about 80 by 50 μ, which contains a *miracidium*. Figure 6-24 shows the morphologic features of the egg of *H. americanum*. The prepatent period is approximately 84 days.

Figure 6-22
Microfilariae of *Dirofilaria immitis* from a peripheral blood sample subjected to the modified Knott's test. The microfilariae of *D. immitis* average 310 μ long. In contrast, the microfilariae of *Dipetalonema reconditum* average 285 μ long.

Figure 6-23
An individual microfilaria of *Dirofilaria immitis* from a peripheral blood sample subjected to the modified Knott's test. Note the tapered cranial end and straight tail. Microfilariae of *Dipetalonema reconditum* have a blunt (rounded) cranial end and may exhibit a shepherd's crook (hooked) tail.

Figure 6-24
Characteristic thin-shell ovum of *Heterobilharzia americanum*. These ova are approximately 80 by 50 μ and contain a miracidium.

PROTOZOANS (UNICELLULAR ORGANISMS). *Babesia canis* is an intracellular parasite found within the erythrocytes of dogs, also referred to as a *piroplasm* (pear-shape body) (Figure 6-25). Diagnosis is by observing basophilic, pear-shape trophozoites in RBCs on stained blood smears.

Cytauxzoon felis is another intracellular parasite sporadically reported in the RBCs of cats in sites (Missouri, Arkansas, Georgia, Texas) throughout the United States. It also produces piroplasms, which have been described as shaped like a "bejeweled ring" and are referred to as the *ring form* in stained blood smears. Cytauxzoonosis is a rapidly fatal disease, and its prognosis is poor.

Hepatozoon canis is an intracellular parasite found within the dog's neutrophils and monocytes (rather than the erythrocytes). These intracellular inclusions are oblong and average 11.4 by 5.3 μ in size. These stages are infrequently found on peripheral blood smears. For cystic stages of this parasite, see Parasites of the Musculoskeletal System.

Figure 6-25
Basophilic, pear-shape trophozoites of *Babesia canis* within canine RBCs in a stained blood smear.

Figure 6-26
Adult female *Linguatula serrata,* the "canine pentastome" or "canine tongueworm." This parasite of the nasal and respiratory passages of dogs resembles a helminth, but it is actually a type of arthropod (it has a mitelike larval stage).

Parasites of the Respiratory System

PENTASTOMIDS (TONGUEWORMS). Pentastomids (tongueworms) resemble helminths but are actually an arthropod. *Linguatula serrata* is the "canine pentastome" or the "canine tongueworm" (Figure 6-26). Pentastomes are usually parasites of snakes and reptiles, but this tongueworm parasitizes the nasal and respiratory passages of dogs. It resembles a helminth but is a type of arthropod (it has a mite-like larval stage). The pentastome eggs measure 70 by 90 μ (Figure 6-27). On the inside of the egg, the mitelike larval stage with jointed claws is visible.

NEMATODES (ROUNDWORMS). *Aelurostrongylus abstrusus* is the feline lungworm. The adults live in the terminal respiratory bronchioles and alveolar ducts, where they form small egg nests or nodules. The eggs of this parasite are forced into the lung tissue, where they hatch to form characteristic first-stage larvae, approximately 360 μ long. Each larva has a tail with an S-shape bend and a dorsal spine (Figure 6-28). Characteristic larvae on fecal flotation or the Baermann

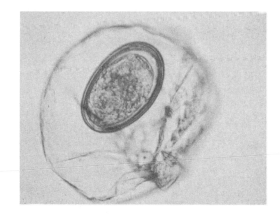

Figure 6-27
Characteristic ovum of *Linguatula serrata.* The pentastome eggs measure 70 by 90 μ. In the interior of many pentastome eggs, one may observe a mitelike larval stage with jointed claws.

Figure 6-28
Characteristic first-stage larva of *Aelurostrongylus abstrusus,* the "feline lungworm." The larva is approximately 360 μ long and has a tail with an S-shape bend and a dorsal spine. Diagnosis is accomplished by finding these characteristic larvae on fecal flotation or by using the Baermann technique.

technique can determine their presence. Recovering the larvae on tracheal washing is also possible (Figure 6-29). The prepatent period is approximately 30 days.

Filaroides (oslerus) osleri, Filaroides hirthi, and *Filaroides milksi,* the canine "lungworms," are found in the trachea, the lung parenchyma, and the bronchioles, respectively. The larva is 232 to 266 μ long and has a short, S-shape tail. *Filaroides* species are unique among the nematodes in that their first-stage larvae are immediately infective for the canine definitive host. No period of development is required outside the host. Diagnosis is by finding these characteristic larvae on fecal flotation or by using the Baermann technique. Figure 6-30 shows the unique infective larvae of *F. osleri.* Nodules of *F. osleri* are usually found at the bifurcation of the trachea, where they can be observed via endoscopic examination. The prepatent period for *F. osleri* is approximately 10 weeks.

Eucoleus aerophilus (Capillaria aerophila) is a capillarid nematode found in the trachea and bronchi of both dogs and cats. The prepatent period is approximately 40 days. In standard fecal flotations, eggs of *Eucoleus* species are often confused with those of *Trichuris* (whipworms). Eggs of *E. aerophilus* are smaller than whipworm

Figure 6-29
Numerous first-stage larvae of *Aelurostrongylus abstrusus,* recovered on tracheal washing.

Figure 6-30
Characteristic, infective first-stage larva of *Filaroides osleri,* a canine "lungworm." The larva is 232 to 266 μ long and has a short, S-shape tail.

eggs (59 to 80 μ by 30 to 40 μ), more broadly barrel shape, and lighter in color. The egg also has a rough outer surface with a netted appearance.

Eucoleus böehmi is found in the nasal cavity and frontal sinuses of dogs. Its eggs are smaller and have a smoother outer surface than those of *E. aerophilus*. Its shell has a pitted appearance. This parasite can be detected using a standard fecal flotation.

TREMATODES (FLUKES). *Paragonimus kellicotti* is the "lung fluke" of dogs. Adult hermaphroditic flukes occur in cystic spaces within the lung parenchyma of both dogs and cats. These cystic spaces connect to the terminal bronchioles. The eggs are found in sputum or feces. They are yellowish brown with an operculum and measure 75 to 118 μ by 42 to 67 μ (Figure 6-31). Fluke eggs usually are recovered using fecal sedimentation techniques; however, the eggs of *P. kellicotti* may be recovered using standard fecal flotation solutions. The eggs of *P. kellicotti* also may be recovered in the sputum via tracheal washing. The adult flukes within the cystic spaces of the lung parenchyma can also be observed using thoracic radiography. This fluke's prepatent period is 30 to 36 days.

Parasites of the Urogenital System

NEMATODES (ROUNDWORMS). *Dioctophyma renale* is the "giant kidney worm" of dogs. This largest of parasitic nematodes frequently infects the right kidney of dogs and gradually ingests the renal parenchyma, leaving only the capsule of the kidney. Eggs may be recovered by centrifugation and examination of the urine sediment. They are characteristically barrel shape, bipolar, and yellow brown. The egg's shell has a pitted appearance. Eggs measure 71 to 84 μ by 46 to 52 μ. Figure 6-32 shows the characteristic ovum of *D. renale*. *D. renale* also may occur freely within the peritoneal cavity. When it is in this location, eggs are not passed to the external environment. The prepatent period is approximately 18 weeks.

Capillaria plica and *Capillaria (personema) felis cati* are nematodes of the urinary bladder of dogs and cats, respectively. Their eggs may be found in urine or in

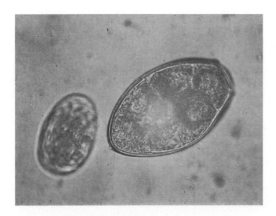

Figure 6-31
Characteristic ovum of *Paragonimus kellicotti,* the "lung fluke" of dogs recovered using a standard fecal flotation. The eggs may be found in either sputum or feces but often are recovered on fecal flotation. The yellowish-brown, operculated eggs measure 75 to 118 μ by 42 to 67 μ. *Ancylostoma caninum* egg *(left).*

Figure 6-32
Characteristic ovum of *Dioctophyma renale* recovered from urine sediment. These eggs are characteristically barrel-shape, bipolar, and yellow brown. The egg shell has a pitted appearance. Eggs measure 71 to 84 μ by 46 to 52 μ.

feces contaminated with urine. Eggs are clear to yellow in color, measure 63 to 68 μ by 24 to 27 μ, and have flattened bipolar end plugs. Their outer surface is roughened. These eggs may be confused with those of the respiratory and gastric capillarids and with those of the whipworms.

Parasites of the Eye and Adnexa

NEMATODES (ROUNDWORMS). *Thelazia californensis* is the "eyeworm" of dogs and cats. Adult parasites can be recovered from the conjunctival sac and lachrymal duct. Examination of the lachrymal secretions may reveal eggs or first-stage larvae. As mentioned previously, *D. immitis* may be recovered from a variety of aberrant sites, such as the anterior chamber of the eye.

Parasites of the Musculoskeletal System

PROTOZOANS (UNICELLULAR PARASITES). In the United States, canine hepatozoonosis is most commonly diagnosed by muscle biopsy rather than by examination of peripheral blood smears for infected leukocytes. Muscle lesions consist of large cysts, pyogranulomas, and myositis. The cysts produced are round to ovoid and range from 250 to 500 μ in diameter. The center of the cyst demonstrates a basophilic nucleus surrounded by small basophilic bodies. Surrounding the nucleus and the basophilic bodies are concentric layers of fine multilaminated membranes, giving an "onion-skin" appearance. In most cases, no inflammatory response is associated with the cyst. Roughening and thickening of bone surfaces also may be apparent.

◆ Endoparasites of Cattle and Other Ruminants

Parasites of the Gastrointestinal Tract

NEMATODES (ROUNDWORMS). The "bovine trichstrongyles" comprise several genera of nematodes within the abomasum and small and large intestine of cattle and

A

B

C

Figure 6-33
Characteristic "trichostrongyle-type" ova of the bovine trichostrongyles. These oval, thin-shell eggs contain four or more cells. They measure 70 to 120 μ long. Some of these ova can be identified by their respective genus; however, identification is usually difficult because mixed infections are common.

other ruminants. Genera that produce "trichostrongyle-type eggs" are *Bunostomum, Cooperia, Chabertia, Haemonchus, Oesophagostomum, Ostertagia,* and *Trichostrongylus.* These seven genera (and others) produce oval, thin-shell eggs. They contain four or more cells and are 70 to 120 μ long. Some of these ova may be identified to their respective genus; however, identification is usually difficult because mixed infections are quite common.

Upon identification of the characteristic eggs, the veterinary technician should record the finding as "trichostrongyle-type egg" (Figure 6-33). They should not be recorded as individual genus names. Identification to genus and species usually is performed by fecal culture and larval identification.

Nematodirus species and *Marshallagia* species are also "bovine trichostrongyles;" however, their eggs are much larger than those of the genera mentioned previously.

Their eggs are the largest in the trichostrongyle family. Figure 6-34 shows the large eggs of *Nematodirus* species. In a standard fecal flotation, the eggs of *Nematodirus* species are large (150 to 230 μ by 80 to 100 μ) and have tapering ends and 4 to 8 cells. The eggs of *Marshallagia* species also are large (160 to 200 μ by 75 to 100 μ), have parallel sides and rounded ends, and contain 16 to 32 cells.

Strongyloides papillosus is often referred to as the "intestinal threadworm." These nematodes are unique in that only a parthenogenetic female (female that lays eggs without copulating with a male) is parasitic in the host. Parasitic males do not exist. These females produce larvated eggs measuring 40 to 60 μ by 20 to 25 μ. Eggs usually are recovered in flotation of fresh feces. The prepatent period is 5 to 7 days (see Figure 6-7 for the parasitic adult females, eggs, and first-stage larvae of *Strongyloides* species).

Trichuris ovis is commonly called the "whipworm," infecting the cecum and colon of ruminants. The section on nematode parasites of the gastrointestinal tract of dogs and cats contains details regarding the gross morphology of adult whipworms. The egg of the whipworm is described as trichinelloid or trichuroid. It has a thick, yellow-brown, symmetric shell with plugs at both ends. The eggs are unembryonated (not larvated) when laid. Eggs of bovine whipworms measure 50 to 60 μ by 21 to 25 μ.

CESTODES (TAPEWORMS).   *Moniezia* species are tapeworms found in the small intestine of cattle, sheep, and goats. These tapeworms produce eggs with a characteristic square or triangular shape. Two species are common, *Moniezia benedini* in cattle and *Moniezia expansa* in cattle, sheep, and goats. The eggs of both species can be easily differentiated using standard fecal flotation procedures. Figure 6-35 shows representative eggs of *Moniezia* species. The eggs of *M. expansa* are triangular or pyramidal and 56 to 67 μ in diameter. The eggs of *M. benedini* are square or cuboidal and approximately 75 μ in diameter. The prepatent period for these tapeworms is approximately 40 days.

Thysanosoma actinoides is the "fringed tapeworm," found in the bile ducts, pancreatic ducts, and small intestine of ruminants. Eggs of this tapeworm occur in packets of 6 to 12 eggs, with individual eggs measuring 19 by 27 μ.

Figure 6-34
Characteristic large ova of *Nematodirus* species. In standard fecal flotation, the eggs of *Nematodirus* species are larger than those of other bovine trichostrongyles (150 to 230 μ by 80 to 100 μ), have tapering ends, and four to eight cells.

TREMATODES (FLUKES). "Rumen flukes" are comprised of two genera, *Paramphistomum* and *Cotylophoron*. These adult flukes reside in the rumen and reticulum of cattle, sheep, goats, and many other ruminants. The eggs of *Paramphistomum* species measure 114 to 176 μ by 73 to 100 μ, whereas the eggs of *Cotylophoron* species measure 125 to 135 μ by 61 to 68 μ. The prepatent period of *Paramphistomum* species is 80 to 95 days.

Fasciola hepatica is the "liver fluke" of cattle, sheep, and other ruminants. The hermaphroditic adult flukes are found in the bile ducts of the liver. The eggs measure 140 by 100 μ and are yellowish-brown, oval, and operculated (Figure 6-36). The prepatent period for *F. hepatica* is approximately 56 days.

Dicrocoelium dendriticum is the "lancet fluke" of sheep, goats, and oxen. These tiny flukes reside within the fine branches of the bile ducts. The brown eggs have an indistinct operculum and measure 36 to 45 μ by 20 to 30 μ. Eggs of this and the above-mentioned trematodes may be recovered from feces using fecal sedimentation or a commercially available fluke egg recovery test.

Figure 6-35
Characteristic ova of *Moniezia* species. The eggs of *Moniezia expansa* are triangular or pyramidal and 56 to 67 μ in diameter. The eggs of *Moniezia benedini* are square or cuboidal and approximately 75 μ in diameter.

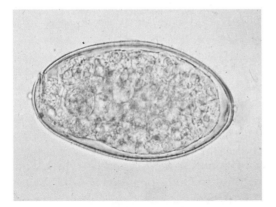

Figure 6-36
Characteristic operculated ovum of *Fasciola hepatica*, the "liver fluke" of cattle, sheep, and other ruminants. The eggs measure 140 by 100 μ and are yellowish-brown and oval.

PROTOZOANS (UNICELLULAR ORGANISMS). Ruminants serve as host to many species of *Eimeria*. It is often difficult to identify individual species of coccidia because their oocysts are so similar in size and shape. The two most common species of coccidia in cattle, *Eimeria bovis* and *Eimeria zurnii,* can be differentiated on a standard fecal flotation. Oocysts of *E. bovis* are oval, have a micropyle, and measure 20 by 28 μ, whereas those of *E. zurnii* are spherical, lack the micropyle, and measure 15 to 22 μ by 13 to 18 μ. When oocysts are recovered on fecal flotation, the observation is usually noted as "coccidia."

Cryptosporidium is another coccidian parasite that parasitizes the small intestine of a variety of animals, including cattle, sheep, and goats. The sporulated oocysts in the feces are colorless and transparent and measure only 5.0 to 4.5 μ. Diagnosis is by standard fecal flotation and stained fecal smears. Because people may become infected with *Cryptosporidium* species, feces suspected of harboring this protozoan should be handled with great care (see Figure 6-19 for features of the oocysts of *Cryptosporidium* species).

Parasites of the Circulatory System

NEMATODES (ROUNDWORMS). *Elaeophora schneideri,* the "arterial worm," is found in the common carotid arteries of sheep in the western and southwestern United States. Microfilariae are 270 μ long and 17 μ thick, bluntly rounded cranially, and tapering caudally. They are found in the skin, usually in the capillaries of the forehead and face. Filarial dermatitis is seen on the face, poll region, and feet of sheep.

Diagnosis is by observation of characteristic lesions and identification of microfilariae in the skin. The most satisfactory means of diagnosis is to macerate a piece of skin in warm saline and examine the material for microfilariae after about 2 hours. In sheep, microfilariae are rare and may not be found in the skin of infected animals. Postmortem examination may be necessary to confirm the diagnosis. The prepatent period is 18 weeks or longer.

PROTOZOANS (UNICELLULAR ORGANISMS). *Babesia bigemina* is an intracellular parasite found within the RBCs of cattle. This parasite is a large piroplasm, 4 to 5 μ long by about 2 μ wide. It is characteristically pear-shape and occurs in pairs, forming an acute angle within the erythrocyte. The intermediate host for this protozoan parasite is the tick, *Boophilus annulatus.*

Parasites of the Respiratory System

NEMATODES (ROUNDWORMS). *Dictyocaulus* species are lungworms of cattle (*Dictyocaulus viviparus*), sheep, and goats (*Dictyocaulus filaria*). Adults are found in the bronchi. The prepatent period varies with the species but is approximately 28 days. Eggs usually are coughed up and swallowed and hatch in the intestine, producing larvae that may be recovered in the feces.

Larvae of *D. filaria* have brownish food granules in their intestinal cells, a blunt tail, and a cranial cuticular knob. They are 550 to 580 μ long. Larvae of *D. vivipa-*

rus also have brownish food granules in their intestinal cells but have a straight tail; they lack the cranial cuticular knob. These larvae are 300 to 360 μ in length (Figure 6-37).

Muellerius capillaris often is called the "hair lungworm." Adults are found within the bronchioles, mostly in nodules in the lung parenchyma of sheep and goats. The eggs develop in the lungs of the definitive host and the first-stage larvae are coughed up, swallowed, and passed out with the feces. They are 230 to 300 μ long. The larval tail has an undulating tip and a dorsal spine (Figure 6-38).

Protostrongylus species adults occur in the small bronchioles of sheep and goats. Again, the eggs develop in the lungs of the definitive host and the first-stage larvae are coughed up, swallowed, and passed out with the feces. These larvae are 250 to 320 μ long. This nematode's larval tail has an undulating tip but lacks the dorsal spine. The Baermann technique is used to diagnose lungworm infection in ruminants.

Figure 6-37
Representative eggs and larvae of *Dictyocaulus* species, cattle "lungworms."

Figure 6-38
First-stage larva of *Muellerius capillaris,* the "hair lungworm" of sheep and goats. First-stage larvae are 230 to 300 μ long. The larval tail has an undulating tip and a dorsal spine.

Parasites of the Eye and Adnexa

NEMATODES (ROUNDWORMS).   *Thelazia rhodesii* and *Thelazia gulosa* are the "eyeworm" of cattle, sheep, and goats. Adult parasites may be recovered from the conjunctival sac and lachrymal duct. Examination of the lachrymal secretions may reveal eggs or first-stage larvae. Figure 6-39 shows adult *Thelazia* in the conjunctival sac of a cow.

Parasites of the Abdominal Cavity

Setaria cervi is the "abdominal worm" of cattle. Adults are found free within the peritoneal cavity. The sheathed microfilariae are approximately 250 by 7 μ. Diagnosis is by demonstration of microfilariae in blood smears.

◆ Endoparasites of Horses

Parasites of the Gastrointestinal Tract

ARTHROPODS (LARVAL FLIES).   These parasites are unusual: their adult form is an ectoparasite and their larval form is an endoparasite. Larval *Gasterophilus* species or "horse bots" parasitize the stomach of horses. Because these stages are larval or immature stages of nonparasitic adult flies, no demonstrable egg stage may be recovered from horse feces. The third larval stage exits the gastrointestinal tract via the feces; therefore this stage may be recovered from the feces. The brown larvae are up to 20 mm in length and have dense spines on the cranial border of each segment. A pair of distinct mouth hooks is found on the cranial end of the first segment and a spiracular plate on the caudal end. The veterinary technician should be able to grossly identify horse bots as *Gasterophilus* species.

NEMATODES (ROUNDWORMS).   *Habronema* species and *Draschia megastoma* are nematodes found in the stomach of horses. *Habronema microstoma* and *H. muscae* occur on the stomach mucosa, just beneath a thick layer of mucus; *D. megastoma* is often associated with large, thickened fibrous nodules within the stomach mucosa. Larvae of both may parasitize skin lesions, causing a condition known as "summer

Figure 6-39
Adult *Thelazia* species, the "eyeworm," in the conjunctival sac of a cow.

sores" (see Chapter 7 for a description of this condition and the larvae). The prepatent period is approximately 60 days. Larvated eggs or larvae may be recovered on a standard fecal flotation. The eggs of both genera are elongated, have thin walls, and measure 40 to 50 μ by 10 to 12 μ.

Trichostrongylus axei is another nematode that may infect the stomach of horses. They are unusual: they also can infect cattle and sheep. Their eggs are classified as "strongyle-type" eggs.

Parascaris equorum often is called the "equine ascarid" or "equine roundworm." It is found in the small intestine of horses, particularly young foals. The prepatent period is 75 to 80 days. Eggs recovered from the feces of young horses are oval and brown. The shell is thickened, with a finely granular surface. The eggs measure 90 to 100 μ in diameter. The center of the egg contains one or two cells (Figure 6-40). Eggs may be recovered easily on standard fecal flotation.

Strongyles are nematodes that parasitize the large intestine of horses and are typically divided into two types: large strongyles and small strongyles. The small strongyles comprise several genera that vary in pathogenicity. The large strongyles are the most pathogenic of the strongyles. *Strongylus vulgaris, Strongylus edentatus,* and *Strongylus equinus* are the large strongyles (Figure 6-41).

Figure 6-40
Characteristic ovum of *Parascaris equorum,* the "equine ascarid" or the "equine roundworm." The shell is thickened, with a finely granular surface. The eggs measure 90 to 100 μ in diameter. The center of the egg contains one or two cells.

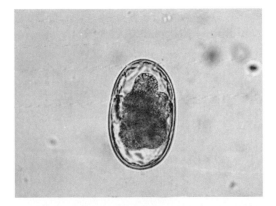

Figure 6-41
"Strongyle-type ovum" of horses. These eggs contain an 8- to 16-cell morula and measure approximately 70 to 90 μ by 40 to 50 μ. When these characteristic eggs are found on fecal flotation, the observation is recorded as "strongyle-type" ova, rather than as a particular species of strongyle.

Regardless of whether these endoparasites are a small strongyle or a large strongyle, their eggs are virtually identical. Identification to the species level is accomplished by fecal culture and identification of larvae. Strongyle eggs are most often observed in a standard fecal flotation. They contain an 8- to 16-cell morula and measure approximately 70 to 90 μ by 40 to 50 μ. When these characteristic eggs are found on fecal flotation, the observation is recorded as "strongyle-type" ova, rather than as a particular species of strongyles.

Strongyloides westeri is often referred to as the "intestinal threadworm" of horses. These nematodes are unique: only a parthenogenetic female (one that can lay eggs without copulating with a male) is parasitic in the host. Parasitic males do not exist. These females produce larvated eggs measuring 40 to 52 μ by 32 to 40 μ. Eggs usually are recovered on flotation of fresh feces. The prepatent period is 5 to 7 days (see Figure 6-7 for the parasitic adult females, eggs, and first-stage larvae of *Strongyloides* species).

Oxyuris equi is the "pinworm" of horses. The adult worms are found in the cecum, colon, and rectum. Adult worms are often observed protruding from the horse's anus. The adult female worms attach their eggs to the anus with a gelatinous, sticky material that produces anal pruritus in infected horses. Eggs also may be recovered from the feces. The eggs are 90 by 40 μ, with a smooth, thick shell. They are operculated, slightly flattened on one side, and may be larvated (Figure 6-42). The prepatent period is approximately 4 to 5 months. Diagnosis is by finding the characteristic eggs on microscopic examination of cellophane tape impressions or by scraping the surface of the anus.

CESTODES (TAPEWORMS). *Anoplocephala perfoliata, Anoplocephala magna,* and *Paranoplocephala mamillana* are the "equine tapeworms." *A. perfoliata* is found in the small and large intestine and cecum. *A. magna* is found in the small intestine and occasionally the stomach. *P. mamillana* also is found in the small intestine and occasionally the stomach. The eggs of *A. perfoliata* have thick walls, with one or more flattened sides, and measure 65 to 80 μ in diameter. Those of *A. magna* are similar but slightly smaller, measuring 50 to 60 μ. The eggs of *P. mamillana* are oval and have thin walls, measuring 51 to 37 μ. Eggs of all three species have a three-layer egg shell, with the innermost lining called the *pyriform apparatus,* which is pear-shaped. Eggs of all equine tapeworms can be recovered using a standard fecal flotation. The prepatent period of all three species ranges from 28 to 42 days.

PROTOZOANS (UNICELLULAR ORGANISMS). *Eimeria leuckarti* is a coccidian found in the small intestine of horses. This protozoan demonstrates unique, large

Figure 6-42
Characteristic ovum of *Oxyuris equi,* the "pinworm" of horses. The eggs are 90 by 40 μ, with a smooth, thick shell. They are operculated and slightly flattened on one side. The eggs may be larvated.

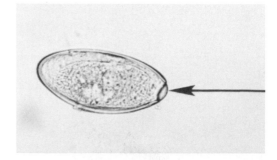

oocysts (80 to 87 μ by 55 to 60 μ), with a thick wall, a distinct micropyle, and a dark brown color. These oocysts can be recovered on fecal flotation and are the largest coccidian oocysts. They are frequently observed on histopathologic examination. The prepatent period ranges from 15 to 33 days.

Parasites of the Circulatory System

PROTOZOANS (UNICELLULAR ORGANISMS).   *Babesia equi* and *Babesia caballi* are intracellular parasites found within the RBCs of horses. They are also referred to as the "equine piroplasms." Diagnosis is by observing basophilic, pear-shape trophozoites in RBCs on stained blood smears. Trophozoites of *B. equi* may be round, amoeboid, or pyriform. Four organisms may be joined, giving the effect of a Maltese cross. Individual organisms are 2 to 3 μ long. Trophozoites of *B. caballi* are pyriform, round, or oval and 2 to 4 μ long. They occur characteristically in pairs at acute angles to each other.

Parasites of the Respiratory System

NEMATODES (ROUNDWORMS).   *Dictyocaulus arnfieldi*, the "equine lungworm," is found in the bronchi and bronchioles of horses, mules, and donkeys. Its eggs are ellipsoid and embryonated, measuring approximately 80 to 100 m by 50 to 60 μ. Eggs can be recovered on fecal flotation of fresh (less than 24 hours old) feces. Larvae hatch from the eggs within a few hours after feces are passed. The prepatent period for the equine lungworm is 42 to 56 days.

Parasites of the Eye and Adnexa

Thelazia lacrymalis is the "eyeworm" of horses throughout the world. Adult parasites may be recovered from the conjunctival sac and lachrymal duct. Examination of the lachrymal secretions may reveal eggs or first-stage larvae.

   The unsheathed microfilariae of *Onchocerca cervicalis* have been incriminated as causing periodic ophthalmia and blindness in horses. These may be detected by ophthalmic examination.

Parasites of the Abdominal Cavity

Setaria equina is the "abdominal worm" of horses. Adults are found free within the peritoneal cavity. The sheathed microfilariae are 240 to 256 μ long. Diagnosis is by demonstration of microfilariae in blood smears.

◆ Endoparasites of Swine

Parasites of the Gastrointestinal Tract

NEMATODES (ROUNDWORMS).   *Ascarops strongylina* and *Physocephalus sexalatus* are the "thick stomach worms" of the porcine stomach. Both of these nematodes produce thick-wall, larvated eggs that may be recovered on fecal flotation. The eggs of both species are similar. The eggs of *A. strongylina* are 34 to 39 μ by 20 μ and have thick shells surrounded by a thin membrane that produces an irregular outline. The eggs of *P. sexalatus* are 34 to 39 μ by 15 to 17 μ. The prepatent period for both species is approximately 42 days.

Hyostrongylus rubidus is referred to as the "red stomach worm" of swine. The eggs are "trichostrongyle type;" that is, they are oval, thin-shell eggs. They contain four or more cells and measure 71 to 78 μ by 35 to 42 μ. These eggs may be recovered on fecal flotation. As with bovine trichostrongyles, definitive diagnosis can be made only by fecal culture and larval identification. The prepatent period is approximately 20 days.

Ascaris suum, the "swine ascarid" or the "large intestinal roundworm," is the largest nematode found within the small intestine of pigs. The eggs may be recovered on standard fecal flotation. They are oval and golden brown, with a thick albuminous shell bearing prominent projections. These eggs measure 70 to 89 μ by 37 to 40 μ (Figure 6-43).

Strongyloides ransomi, the "intestinal threadworm" of pigs, is unique in that only a parthenogenetic female is parasitic in the host. Parasitic males do not exist. These females produce larvated eggs measuring 45 to 55 μ by 26 to 35 μ. Eggs are usually recovered in flotation of fresh feces. The prepatent period is 3 to 7 days (see Figure 6-7).

Oesophagostomum dentatum, the "nodular worm of swine," is found in the large intestine of swine. The prepatent period is 50 days. Their eggs are "trichostrongyle type;" that is, they are oval, thin-shell eggs. They contain 4 to 16 cells and measure 40 by 70 μ. These eggs may be recovered on a standard fecal flotation. As with bovine trichostrongyles, definitive diagnosis may be made only by fecal culture and larval identification.

Trichuris suis is commonly called the "whipworm," infecting the cecum and colon of swine. (See the section on nematode parasites of the gastrointestinal tract of dogs and cats for details on gross morphology of adult worms.) The egg of the whipworm is described as *trichinelloid* or *trichuroid*. It has a thick, brown, barrel-shape shell with plugs at both ends. The eggs are unembryonated (not larvated) when laid. Eggs of porcine whipworms measure 50 to 60 μ by 21 to 25 μ. The prepatent period is 42 to 49 days.

Figure 6-43
Characteristic ovum of *Ascaris suum,* the "swine ascarid" or the "large intestinal roundworm" of pigs. The eggs are oval and golden brown, with a thick, albuminous shell bearing prominent projections. They measure 70 to 89 μ by 37 to 40 μ.

ACANTHOCEPHALANS (THORNY-HEAD WORMS). *Macracanthorhynchus hirudinaceus* is the "thorny-head worm" of the small intestine of swine. It is called "thorny-head" because of its spiny proboscis, which it embeds as an anchor into the small intestinal mucosa of the host. The eggs have a triple-layer shell, are oval, and measure 67 to 100 μ by 40 to 65 μ (Figure 6-44). The eggs may be recovered on a standard fecal flotation. The prepatent period is 60 to 90 days.

PROTOZOANS (UNICELLULAR ORGANISMS). *Balantidium coli* is the "ciliated protozoan" found in the large intestine of swine. Although commonly observed during microscopic examination of fresh diarrheic feces, it is generally considered to be nonpathogenic. Two morphologic stages may be found in feces: the "cyst" stage and the motile "trophozoite" stage. Both stages may vary in size. This is a large protozoan parasite. The trophozoites may be 150 by 120 μ, with a sausage- to kidney-shape macronucleus. It is covered with numerous rows of cilia and moves about the

A
 B

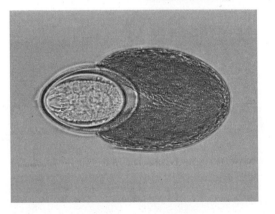 C

Figure 6-44
Ova of *Macracanthorhynchus hirudinaceus,* the "thorny-head worm" of the small intestine of swine. The eggs have a triple-layered shell, are oval, and measure 67 to 100 μ by 40 to 65 μ.

microscopic field with lively motility. The cyst is spherical to ovoid and 40 to 60 μ in diameter, with a slight greenish-yellow color. Both of these stages may be easily recognized by microscopic examination of the intestinal contents or fresh, diarrheic feces. Figure 6-45 shows the trophozoite stage of *B. coli* recovered on fecal flotation. Figure 6-46 shows *B. coli* in histopathologic section.

Cryptosporidium is another coccidian parasite that parasitizes the small intestine of a wide variety of animals, including swine. The sporulated oocysts in the feces are colorless and transparent and measure only 4.5 to 5.0 μ. Diagnosis is by standard fecal flotation and stained fecal smears. Because people may become infected with *Cryptosporidium* species, feces suspected of harboring this protozoan should be handled with great care (see Figure 6-19).

Isospora suis is the coccidian that parasitizes the small intestine of swine, especially young piglets. Oocysts are usually found on flotation of fresh feces. They are subspherical, lack a micropyle, and measure 18 to 21 μ (Figure 6-47). Postmortem

Figure 6-45
Trophozoite stage of *Balantidium coli,* the "ciliated protozoan" found in the large intestine of swine. The trophozoites may be 150 by 120 μ, with a sausage- to kidney-shape macronucleus. They are covered with numerous rows of cilia and move about the microscopic field with lively motility. The cyst is spherical to ovoid and 40 to 60 μ in diameter, with a slight greenish-yellow color.

A

B

Figure 6-46
Balantidium coli in a histopathologic section. This is a large protozoan parasite.

diagnosis in piglets exhibiting clinical signs, but not shedding oocysts, can be achieved by direct smear of the jejunum stained with Diff-Quik. Diagnosis is by observation of the banana-shape merozoites. The prepatent period is 4 to 8 days.

Parasites of the Respiratory System

NEMATODES (ROUNDWORMS). *Metastrongylus apri,* the "swine lungworm," is found within the bronchi and bronchioles of pigs. The oval, thick-wall eggs measure 60 by 40 µ and contain larvae. Eggs can be recovered on fecal flotation using a flotation medium with a specific gravity above 1.25 or by using the fecal sedimentation technique. The prepatent period is approximately 24 days.

Parasites of the Urinary System

NEMATODES (ROUNDWORMS). *Stephanurus dentatus,* the "swine kidney worm," is found in the kidney, ureters, and perirenal tissues of pigs (Figure 6-48). Their eggs are "strongyle-type;" that is, they are oval, thin-shell eggs, containing 4 to 16 cells, and measuring 90 to 120 µ by 43 to 70 µ. Eggs may be recovered from the urine using urine sedimentation. The prepatent period is extremely long, approximately 9 to 24 months.

Figure 6-47
Oocyst of *Isospora suis.*

Figure 6-48
Egg of *Stephanurus dentatus,* the "swine kidney worm." These eggs are "strongyle type," that is, they are oval, thin-shell eggs, containing 4 to 16 cells and measuring 90 to 120 µ by 43 to 70 µ. Eggs can be recovered from the urine using urine sedimentation.

DIAGNOSIS OF ALIMENTARY PARASITISM

Parasites can infect the oral cavity, esophagus, stomach, small and large intestines, and other internal organs of animals. Detection of these parasites involves collection and microscopic examination of feces. Diagnosis is usually by finding life cycle stages of the parasite within the feces. These stages include eggs, oocysts, larvae, segments (tapeworms), and adult organisms. Veterinary technicians may perform the following procedures to detect parasitic infections.

◆ Collection of Fecal Samples

Fecal samples collected for routine examination should be as fresh as possible. Specimens that cannot be examined within a few hours of excretion should be refrigerated or mixed with equal parts of 10% formalin. The need for fresh feces stems from the fact that eggs, oocysts, and other life cycle stages may be altered by development, making diagnosis extremely difficult.

Small Animal Fecal Samples

Several methods are used for collecting feces from companion animals. An owner may collect a fecal sample immediately after the animal has defecated. The feces may be stored in any type of container, such as a zippered plastic bag or a clean, small jar. Veterinary hospitals may dispense containers to their clients for this purpose. In either case, only a small amount of feces (1 teaspoon) is required for proper examination. All specimens should be properly identified with the owner's name, animal's name, and species of animal.

Fecal samples also may be collected directly from the animal at the veterinary hospital, using a gloved finger or fecal loop. If a glove is used, the feces may remain in the glove, with the glove turned inside out, tied and labeled. Samples collected with a fecal loop should be used for direct examination only, as the amount collected is relatively small.

Large Animal Fecal Samples

Fecal specimens collected from livestock may be obtained either directly from an individual animal's rectum or from a number of animals to make up a pooled sample. Samples collected directly from an individual animal using a gloved hand can remain in the glove, with the glove turned inside out, tied, and labeled.

Pooled samples are collected from a number of animals housed together and then commingled in a single container. These samples are used to get an idea of the degree of infection within the group. Pooled samples can be collected in any type of container, as long as it is clean and can be tightly sealed. These samples should be labeled with the species, pen or group number, owner, and time of collection.

◆ Examination of Fecal Samples

Several precautions should be taken during fecal examination:

- Fecal samples are handled with care. *The feces may contain parasites, bacteria, or viruses that are zoonotic (i.e., hazardous to people). Appropriate clothing and gloves should be worn. If gloves are not worn, hands should be frequently washed with soap and water. No food or drink should be allowed in the examination area.*
- The laboratory area is cleaned thoroughly after the examinations are completed. *Spilled materials create a hazardous area in which to work and could pose a serious threat to staff members' health.*
- Accurate and thorough records are maintained. *Records should contain the date, owner's name, and any parasites found in the sample. If the sample is negative, it should be recorded as such.*

Gross Examination of Feces

Several characteristics of the feces also should be recorded and reported to the veterinarian. They are as follows:

- Consistency: Fresh feces should be somewhat formed, depending on the species of animal. Diarrhea or constipation could be the result of a parasitic infection.
- Color: Fecal color may be affected by the food an animal eats. Also malabsorption or a parasitic infection may alter the color of feces.
- Blood: Blood may impart a dark reddish-brown color to feces or it may appear as bright red streaks in the feces. In either case, blood may indicate a severe parasitic infection or other serious intestinal diseases. Blood in the feces is an important clinical finding and should be brought to the attention of the veterinarian. Digested blood has a dark, tarry appearance.
- Mucus: Mucus in the feces can be a result of digestive disorders or a parasitic infection. In either case, its presence should be reported to the veterinarian.
- Parasites: Adult parasites or tapeworm segments can be found in the feces. Adult roundworms resemble strings of spaghetti, whereas tapeworm segments look more like pieces of rice. Tapeworm segments may be identified by microscopic examination. The segments of two common tapeworms infecting dogs and cats are shown in Figure 6-49. Figure 6-50 shows the segments found in livestock feces.

Occasionally, a client may submit a dried tapeworm segment. To identify the tapeworm species, the dried segments must be soaked in saline for 1 to 4 hours. Once the segments are rehydrated, they may be identified by size, shape, and the eggs contained within.

Segments of some tapeworm species do not contain eggs, and some segments may have expelled their eggs before the examination was conducted. In either case, a tapeworm segment may be identified as such by finding small mineral deposits (*calcareous bodies*) within the segment (Figure 6-51). This is done by crushing the tapeworm-like segment between two glass slides and examining the material with a microscope.

Microscopic Examination of Feces

Microscopic examination of feces is the most reliable method to detect parasitic infections. A microscope with 4×, 10×, and 40× objectives is required for proper examination of a fecal specimen (see Chapter 1). A mechanical stage is helpful. A micrometer is also useful but not required (Procedure 6-1).

Figure 6-49
Mature segments of the most common tapeworms of dogs and cats. *Left, Taenia* species. *Right, Dipylidium caninum.*

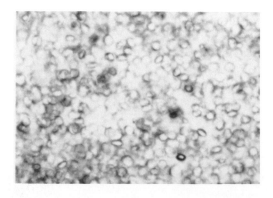

Figure 6-50
Chains and individually mature segments of tapeworms of cattle, *Moniezia* (*left*) and horses, *Anoplocephala* (*right*).

Figure 6-51
Microscopic calcium deposits (calcareous bodies) in tapeworm tissue.

PROCEDURE **6-1**

Examination of tapeworm segments

Materials

Thumb forceps
Dissection needles (hypodermic needles work well)
Microscope slides and coverslips
Saline
Wooden applicator sticks

Procedure

1. Remove the segment from the feces with thumb forceps and place in a drop of saline on a slide.
2. Using the dissection needles, pull the segment into several small pieces. Crush the pieces with a wooden applicator stick.
3. Remove the large pieces. Add more saline, if needed, and place a coverslip on the slide.
4. Examine the slide with the microscope (described later) for tapeworm eggs.

Fecal specimens should be examined routinely with the 10× objective. The examination should begin at one corner of the slide and end at the opposite corner, moving over the slide in a systematic pattern (Figure 6-52). The microscope should be focused continually with the fine-tuning knob during the examination. The initial plane of focus should be that of air bubbles because most eggs are found in this plane. Any material found during the initial scan, including parasite eggs, may be more closely examined using the more powerful objectives.

CALIBRATION OF THE MICROSCOPE. The size of the various stages of many parasites is often important for correct identification. Some examples are *Trichuris* vs. *Capillaria* eggs and *Dipetalonema* vs. *Dirofilaria* microfilariae. Accurate measurements are obtained easily with the use of a calibrated eyepiece on the microscope. Calibration must be performed on every microscope to be used. Each objective (lens) of the microscope must be individually calibrated. Calibration of the microscope is described in Chapter 1.

Figure 6-52
Diagram of a scheme of movement of the microscopic field to thoroughly examine the area under the coverslip.

The *stage micrometer* is a microscope slide etched with a 2-mm line marked in 0.01-mm (10-μ) divisions (Figure 6-53). The veterinary technician should remember that

1 micron (μ) = 0.001 mm

The *eyepiece scale* is a glass disc that fits into and remains in one of the microscope eyepieces. This disc is etched with 30 hash marks spaced at equal intervals (see Figure 6-53). The number of hash marks on the disc may vary with different manufacturers, but the calibration procedure is the same for all.

The stage micrometer is used to determine the distance in microns between the hash marks on the eyepiece scale for each objective lens of the microscope being calibrated. This information is recorded and labeled on the microscope for future reference.

To begin the calibration procedure, the veterinary technician should start on low power (10×) and focus on the 2-mm line of the stage micrometer.

2 mm = 2000 μ

The eyepiece is rotated so that the hash-mark scale is horizontal and parallel to the stage micrometer scale (see Figure 6-53). The zero (0) point is aligned on both scales.

The point on the stage micrometer aligned with the "10" hash mark is determined on the eyepiece scale. In Figure 6-53, this point is at 0.125 mm on the stage micrometer. This number is multiplied by 100. In the above example,

0.125 μ × 100 = 12.5 μ

This means that at this power (10×), the distance between each hash mark on the eyepiece scale is 12.5 μ.

These steps are repeated at each magnification (10×, 40×, 100×). The information is recorded on a label and attached to the calibrated microscope. For example,

Objective	Distance Between Hash Marks (μ)
10×	12.5
40×	2.5
100×	1.0

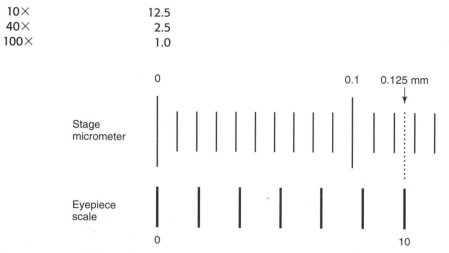

Figure 6-53
Stage micrometer and eyepiece scale used to calibrate a microscope.

To measure an object, such as a parasite egg, one end of the egg is placed on the zero mark and the number of divisions to the other end of the egg is counted. The number of divisions counted is multiplied by the calibration factor for the objective being used. For example, a trichostrongyle egg is 24 divisions long and 13.5 divisions wide when measured with the 40× objective. The calibration factor for the 40× objective is 2.5. Therefore the egg is:

24× 2.5 = 60 μ long

and

13.5 × 2.5 = 33.75 μ wide

To measure a microfilaria, the head is aligned with the zero mark and the number of divisions to the end of the tail is counted. To measure round parasite eggs, the technician should measure through the middle of the egg. For more accurate measurements, the higher objective is used (40× instead of 10×).

EXAMINATION OF DIRECT SMEARS. A direct smear of feces is used to rapidly estimate an animal's parasite burden. This procedure also is used to detect some of the motile protozoa found in feces.

Advantages of direct smears include short preparation time and minimal equipment required to run the procedure. Disadvantages include the small amount of feces examined, which may not be enough to detect a low parasite burden, and the amount of fecal debris on the slide, which could be confused with parasitic material.

A fecal sample for a direct smear preparation may be obtained from an animal using a fecal loop or a rectal thermometer (after measuring the animal's temperature). Either way, only a very small amount of feces is needed (Procedure 6-2).

PROCEDURE 6-2

Direct smear procedure

Materials

Microscope slide and coverslip
Applicator stick or toothpick
Optional: Lugol's iodine or new methylene blue

Procedure

1. Place a drop of saline or water on the microscope slide with an equal amount of feces. A drop of stain may be added at this time.
2. Thoroughly mix the feces and saline or water with the applicator stick to form a homogeneous emulsion.
3. Make a smear on the slide. Be sure the smear is thin enough to see newspaper print through it.
4. Remove any large pieces of feces. Add more saline or water if needed and apply a coverslip.
5. Examine the smear using the 10× objective for parasite eggs and larvae or the 40× objective for motile protozoal organisms.

Concentration Methods for Fecal Examination

The following methods are used to concentrate parasitic material in feces. A concentration technique makes it possible to examine a large amount of feces in a relatively short time. Also, a low parasite burden can easily be identified. Two types of procedures are most often used in veterinary hospitals: *flotation* and *sedimentation*.

FLOTATION SOLUTIONS. Fecal flotation methods are based on the specific gravity of parasitic material and fecal debris. *Specific gravity* refers to the weight of an object as compared with the weight of an equal volume of water. The specific gravity of most parasite eggs is between 1.100 and 1.200 g/ml, whereas the specific gravity of water is 1.000 (Procedure 6-3).

To allow for flotation of parasite eggs, oocysts, and other life cycle stages, the flotation solution must have a higher specific gravity than that of the parasitic material. Several salt and sugar solutions work well for flotation. Most have a specific gravity of

---

PROCEDURE 6-3

Preparation of flotation solutions

Sugar Solution (Sheather's Solution)

1. Pour 355 ml of warm water into a beaker. Add a stir bar and place on a hot plate. Heat the water on high, but not to the boiling point.
2. Slowly add 1 lb of granulated sugar to the water, stirring constantly. Allow the sugar to dissolve completely before removing from the heat source.
3. Add 6 ml of 40% formalin or liquid phenol after the solution has completely cooled.
4. Check the specific gravity of the solution with a hydrometer before using (Figure 6-54). (Hydrometers are available from scientific supply houses.)
5. If the specific gravity is below the desired range, heat the solution and add more sugar.
6. If the specific gravity is above the desired range, add water and stir.

Sodium Nitrate Solution

1. Add about 315 g of sodium nitrate to 1 L of water while stirring. Heating is not necessary, but it hastens the dissolution process.
2. Check the specific gravity and adjust as needed.

Zinc Sulfate Solution

1. Add about 386 g of zinc sulfate to 1 L of water while stirring. Heating is not necessary, but it hastens the dissolution process.
2. Check the specific gravity and adjust as needed.

Saturated Sodium Chloride Solution

1. Add table salt to water until the salt no longer dissolves but tends to settle to the bottom of the container. The specific gravity of this solution cannot go any higher than 1.200.

1.200 to 1.250. In this range, heavy fecal debris sinks to the bottom of the container, while parasitic material rises to the top of the solution.

Sodium nitrate solution is the most common fecal flotation solution used in veterinary hospitals today. This solution is efficient for floating parasite eggs, oocysts, and larvae. It may be purchased with commercial diagnostic test kits or in individual aliquots. The major disadvantage of using sodium nitrate is the expense. Sodium nitrate also forms crystals and distorts eggs if allowed to sit longer than 20 minutes.

Another solution commonly used for flotation is sugar solution. Sugar solution is inexpensive and does not crystallize or distort eggs. Sugar solution may be made anywhere and has a long shelf life. Although sticky to work with, spilled sugar solution may be removed with warm, soapy water.

Zinc sulfate solution is more commonly used in diagnostic laboratories. Zinc sulfate floats protozoal organisms with the least amount of distortion. It generally is used in combination with one of the previously mentioned solutions.

The least desirable solution used is saturated sodium chloride solution. This solution corrodes laboratory equipment, forms crystals, and severely distorts parasite eggs. Saturated sodium chloride solution is also a poor flotation medium, as the maximum specific gravity obtainable is 1.200, allowing heavier eggs to remain submerged. A number of choices in flotation techniques exist (Procedure 6-4).

STANDARD FECAL FLOTATION. The standard or simple fecal flotation is one of the most common flotation techniques used in veterinary hospitals. This technique

Figure 6-54
Measuring the specific gravity of a flotation solution with a hydrometer.

PROCEDURE 6-4

Standard flotation procedure

Materials

Flotation solution
Shell vial or test tube and test tube rack
Waxed paper cups
Cheesecloth cut into 6-inch × 6-inch squares
Wooden tongue depressor
Microscope slides and coverslips

Procedure

1. Take about 2 g (½ tsp) of feces and place it in the cup. Add 20 ml of flotation solution. Using a tongue depressor, mix the feces and flotation solution until no large fecal pieces remain.
2. Wrap cheesecloth around the lip of the cup, while bending the cup to form a spout. Pour the mixture through the cheesecloth, into a vial. Fill the vial so that a meniscus is formed (Figure 6-56). If the cup does not have enough fluid, fill the vial with as much mixture as is available and then fill the remainder with flotation solution.
3. Gently place a coverslip on top of the vial.
4. Allow the unit to remain undisturbed for 10 to 20 minutes (sugar solution requires a longer waiting time than does sodium nitrate). If the preparation is not allowed to sit this long, some eggs will not have time to float to the surface. If allowed to sit for more than an hour, some eggs might become waterlogged and sink, or the eggs may become distorted.
5. Carefully remove the coverslip by picking it straight up and placing it on a microscope slide, with the wet side adjacent to the slide.
6. Examine the area of the slide under the coverslip, as described earlier in this chapter, using the 10× objective. Record any parasitic material found in the sample.

uses a test tube or vial, in which feces and flotation solution are mixed. A coverslip or microscope slide is placed on top of the test tube and the unit is allowed to sit undisturbed. Any parasite eggs in the feces float to the top and stick to the underside of the coverslip or microscope slide. The coverslip or slide is then removed and microscopically examined for parasitic material. Although the standard flotation technique is easy to perform, it is less efficient at floating parasitic material than the centrifugal technique, described later in this chapter.

Commercial flotation kits use the same principle as the standard flotation technique. These kits contain a vial with a filter; some also include prepared flotation solution. Examples of commercial flotation kits include Fecalyzer (EVSCO Pharmaceuticals, Buena, NJ), Ovassay (Synbiotics, San Diego, CA), and Ovatector (BGS Medical Products, Venice, FL) (Figure 6-55). These kits are easy to use but expensive. Some practices reduce the expense by washing and reusing the vials and filters.

Figure 6-55
Three examples of commercial fecal flotation kits. From *left* to *right,* Fecalyzer (EVSCO Pharmaceuticals, Buena, NJ), Ovassay (Synbiotics, San Diego, CA), and Ovatector (BGS Medical Products, Venice, FL).

Figure 6-56
A, Vial filled with flotation solution, showing appearance of the meniscus. **B,** Test tube filled with flotation solution, showing appearance of the meniscus.

CENTRIFUGAL FLOTATION.   Centrifugal flotation for parasite eggs, oocysts, and other parasitic material is the most efficient method available. It requires less time to perform than the standard flotation method. The only drawback to this procedure is that it requires a centrifuge with a horizontal (nonfixed) rotor that can hold 15-ml centrifuge tubes (see Chapter 1). If such a centrifuge is available, centrifugal flotation is preferred because it is easy to perform and samples can be run individually or in batches.

If testing multiple samples, the veterinary technician may want to use a numbering system to keep the samples in order. A number is assigned to the patient and the corresponding centrifuge tube. This minimizes the chances of error (Procedure 6-5).

FECAL SEDIMENTATION.   Fecal sedimentation concentrates parasite eggs, oocysts, and other parasitic material by allowing them to settle to the bottom of a tube of liquid, usually water. A disadvantage of this technique is the amount of fecal debris that mixes with the parasitic material, which makes microscopic examination somewhat difficult.

This procedure is used to detect heavy eggs that would not float in flotation solution, or eggs that would become distorted by the flotation solution. Parasite eggs considered too heavy for flotation are trematode (fluke) eggs. Although some flotation solutions can be adjusted to a specific gravity of 1.300 to float these eggs, such solutions are not routinely used because distortion may occur (Procedure 6-6).

PROCEDURE **6-5**

Centrifugal flotation procedure

Materials

Same as for standard flotation, but omit the vials
15-ml centrifuge tube
Microscope slides and coverslips

Procedure

1. Prepare the fecal mixture as described in the standard flotation procedure.
2. Strain the mixture through cheesecloth into the 15-ml centrifuge tube. Fill the tube to the top. (If using a fixed-rotor centrifuge, the tube should be filled half way and a coverslip should not be used.) Apply a coverslip to the top of the tube. Always balance the centrifuge with a 15-ml tube filled with flotation solution and a coverslip placed on top. Be sure all tubes are marked for identification after centrifugation.
3. Centrifuge the tubes for 3 to 5 minutes at 1300 to 1500 rpm (400 to 650 gravities).
4. Remove the coverslip or use a wire loop or glass rod to remove the top part of fluid in the tube and place on a microscope slide. Microscopically examine the sample, using the 10× objective as previously described.

Quantitative Fecal Examination

Quantitative procedures are used to determine the number of eggs or oocysts present in each gram of feces. These procedures are used as a rough indication of the number of parasites present within a host. Their usefulness is limited, however, by the fact that the various parasite species produce different numbers of eggs. Also egg production by the parasites may be sporadic, and the number of eggs may not correlate with the number of parasites present. The last item is the most significant disadvantage because, in most cases, clinical signs of disease are caused by immature parasites that have not yet begun producing eggs or larvae.

Several quantitative procedures can be performed in veterinary hospitals. These include the Stoll egg count technique, the modified Wisconsin double centrifugation technique, and the McMaster technique. These procedures are fairly easy to perform; each requires its own equipment. Two quantitative techniques are described in Procedures 6-7 and 6-8. Other quantitative procedures may be found in the reference books listed at the end of this chapter.

PROCEDURE **6-6**

Fecal sedimentation procedure

Materials

Waxed paper cups
Cheesecloth cut in 6-inch × 6-inch squares
Wooden tongue depressors
Centrifuge and 15-ml tubes
Pasteur pipettes with bulbs
Microscope slides and coverslips

Procedure

1. Mix about 2 g of feces with tap water in a waxed paper cup. Strain the mixture through cheesecloth into a centrifuge tube (as described for the centrifugation procedure), filling the tube half full.
2. Balance the centrifuge with tubes filled with equal amounts of water. Centrifuge for 3 to 5 minutes at 1300 to 1500 rpm. If a centrifuge is unavailable, allow the tube to sit undisturbed for 20 to 30 minutes.
3. Slowly pour the liquid off the top without disturbing the sediment layer (including the fine, silty material) on the bottom.
4. Using a pipette, transfer a small amount of the fine sediment to a microscope slide. Also transfer a small amount of sediment to a different slide. Apply a coverslip to the drops of sediment and examine microscopically. Lugol's iodine may be mixed with the drop of sediment before a coverslip is applied; this facilitates identification of protozoal cysts or trophozoites.

PROCEDURE 6-7

Wisconsin double centrifugation technique

1. Weigh out a fecal sample (5 g for cattle, 2 g for horses or swine).
2. Place 12 ml of water in a small cup and add the feces to it.
3. Stir well with a wooden tongue depressor and mash the material until it is completely broken up.
4. Pour the mixture through an ordinary tea strainer into another cup, stirring the material while pouring.
5. Press the remaining material with the tongue depressor until nearly dry.
6. Squirt 2 to 3 ml of water into the small cup just emptied and rinse down the sides. Pour this rinsing fluid through the material in the strainer.
7. Press the material in the strainer until dry again and discard.
8. Stir the mixture in the second cup and immediately pour it into a 15-ml centrifuge tube.
9. Centrifuge the tube at 1500 rpm for 10 minutes.
10. Decant the fluid from the tube, being careful not to pour off the fine material on the surface of the sediment.
11. Fill the tube half full of sugar solution (specific gravity 1.27) and mix the sediment and sugar solution with a wooden applicator stick, being careful to scrape the sides and bottom of the tube while mixing.
12. Finish filling the tube with sugar solution and place in the centrifuge.
13. With a pipette, add sugar solution to the tube until it is full enough to place a coverslip on top. No air bubbles should be under the coverslip nor should the material overflow so that it runs down the sides of the tube.
14. Centrifuge at 1500 rpm for 10 minutes.
15. Remove the coverslip by lifting straight upward and place it on a microscope slide. If done properly, the material under the coverslip should be sufficiently thick.
16. Using the 10× objective, scan the entire slide, counting all parasite eggs.
    For cattle:
    Total number = eggs/5 g of feces; total number × 91 = eggs/g of feces
    For horses and swine:
    Total number = eggs/2 g of feces; total number × 227 = eggs/g of feces

PROCEDURE 6-8

Modified Wisconsin technique

1. Weigh 5 g of feces.
2. Mix the feces thoroughly with 45 ml of water in a small cup.
3. Withdraw 1 ml of suspended mixture and place into a 15-ml centrifuge cup.
4. Fill the tube with sugar solution (specific gravity 1.27) and place a coverslip on the tube.
5. Centrifuge the tube at 1200 rpm for 5 minutes.
6. Remove the coverslip and place on a microscope slide. Scan the slide, counting all parasite eggs or oocysts seen.
7. Multiply the number of eggs or oocysts counted by 10 to determine the eggs per gram (epg) of feces.

Examination of Feces for Protozoa and Coccidia

PROTOZOAL TROPHOZOITES. All of the previously described procedures may be used to detect protozoal cysts. However, some protozoans do not form cysts and pass out of the host in trophozoite form. Trophozoites are one-cell, motile organisms that lack the rigid wall of a cyst, making flotation without distortion or death of the trophozoite impossible. Therefore the direct smear technique, using saline and a stain, is the preferred procedure for examination of a fecal sample for protozoal organisms.

In a direct smear, trophozoites may be recognized by their movement. *Balantidium coli* is bean-shape and covered with cilia. It moves in a slow, tumbling fashion. *Giardia* species are pear shape and have five to eight flagella. They move with a jerky motion. Trichomonads are long, slender organisms with a single flagellum attached to the dorsal surface, forming a sail-like structure that ripples as the organism glides through debris. Amoebas move with a flowing motion, extending a part of the body (*pseudopod*) and moving the rest of the body after it.

Stains also may be used to recognize certain structural characteristics of trophozoites and cysts. Lugol's iodine and new methylene blue are common stains used with the direct smear procedure. These stains do not preserve the slide but do facilitate examination of the specimen, making identification easier (Procedure 6-9).

If a protozoal parasite cannot be identified on direct smears, fecal smears containing protozoal trophozoites can be dried, stained with Diff-Quik, Wright's, or Giemsa stain, and sent to a diagnostic laboratory. Many other procedures are used for staining and preserving protozoal trophozoites. Most of these procedures are used in diagnostic laboratories and are not explained here.

COCCIDIA. Several coccidian parasites require special staining techniques for identification. Two procedures are discussed in this chapter.

The acid-fast staining technique is used to identify *Cryptosporidium* species in the feces. *Cryptosporidium* is a parasite of the gastrointestinal tract of many animals,

---

PROCEDURE **6-9**

Preparation of Lugol's iodine

Before preparing this solution, the technician should remove all jewelry, as this solution permanently stains precious metals.
1. Dissolve 10 g of potassium iodide in 100 ml of distilled water in a glass beaker.
2. Add 5 g of powdered iodine crystals to the solution and stir until all of the iodine has dissolved. This produces a 5% Lugol's iodine solution (therapeutic strength). This solution should be stored in an amber bottle, away from light.
3. For staining, this 5% Lugol's solution must be diluted by adding 1 part 5% Lugol's solution to 5 parts distilled water. This staining solution must be remade every 3 weeks because it deteriorates.

including people. The oocysts are 2 to 8 μ in diameter and are almost undetectable in flotation solution to the inexperienced eye. Acid-fast staining can aid detection of the oocysts in a fecal smear (Procedure 6-10).

The second procedure uses Diff-Quik stain for identification of *Isospora* species. *Isospora* species are coccidia found in the gastrointestinal tract (especially the jejunum) of many animals, but they are of most concern in pigs. This parasite can cause the death of many piglets before any oocysts are found in the feces using conventional

PROCEDURE **6-10**

Acid-fast staining technique

Materials

Glass pipette
Microscope slide
Timer
Hot plate or Bunsen burner
Carbol fuchsin stain[a]
Acid alcohol[b]
New methylene blue stain[c]

Procedure

1. Make a thin (paper thin) smear of feces using a glass pipette and allow to air dry.
2. Fix the smear by heating on a hot plate at a setting of 1.5 for 2 to 3 minutes or by passing the slide through a Bunsen burner flame, specimen side up.
3. Flood the slide with carbol fuchsin stain and heat the slide until the stain steams.
4. Remove the slide from the heat and let it sit for 5 minutes. Rinse with tap water.
5. Decolorize by adding acid alcohol for 10 to 20 seconds, then rinse with tap water. Repeat this step until the film on the slide appears light pink.
6. Add new methylene blue stain for 20 to 30 seconds. Rinse with tap water.
7. Blot dry with a paper towel and examine microscopically using the oil-immersion objective.
8. Oocysts appear as bright fluorescent red objects, whereas bacteria and yeasts stain blue.

[a]*Carbol fuchsin stain:*	Basic fuchsin	0.3 g
	95% ethanol	10 ml
	Liquefied phenol	5 ml
	Distilled water	95 ml

Dissolve the basic fuchsin in ethanol. Mix the phenol with distilled water and then add this to the ethanol. Mix and let stand for several days. Filter before using.

[b]*Acid alcohol:*	95% ethanol	97 ml
	Concentrated hydrochloric acid	3 ml
[c]*Methylene blue stain:*	Methylene blue chloride	0.3 g
	Distilled water	100 ml

flotation methods. Therefore an intestinal mucosal scraping must be stained and examined for other diagnostic stages (schizonts, merozoites) of this parasite. This procedure involves scraping the mucosa of the jejunum and smearing the scrapings onto microscope slides. After the slides are air dried, they are stained with Diff-Quik and examined with the oil-immersion objective.

For accurate results with either of these procedures, several samples should be examined. If such examination is not possible, feces or intestines may be sent to a diagnostic laboratory. Collection and shipping of parasitic specimens are described later in this chapter.

Fecal Culture

Fecal cultures involve rearing infective larvae of strongyles, trichostrongyles, or hookworms for identification. Several techniques are available for this purpose.

The first procedure uses a covered glass jar rinsed with 0.1% sodium carbonate solution. Sodium carbonate solution is used to inhibit mold growth while allowing the parasite eggs to develop. Formed feces are placed in the jar, which is then stored at room temperature in a dark area for 7 to 10 days. The contents of the jar should be kept moist but not soggy. If no water droplets are seen condensing on the inside of the jar, a few drops of water or sodium carbonate are added. Vermiculite or sand should be added to bovine feces or feces that contain a lot of water.

Larvae may be found in the condensation droplets in the culture jar. The veterinary technician may collect the larvae by rinsing the jar with a small amount of water, collecting the rinsings, and concentrating the larvae by centrifugation. The larvae found in the sediment after centrifugation may be placed on a microscope slide and examined after coverslip application. The slide is then briefly heated with a match to "relax" or straighten the larvae and curtail their movement.

During examination for larvae, numbers of larvae do not necessarily correlate with numbers of eggs present in the feces. Development from egg to larva may take longer with some species than with others, and some parasite species may produce more eggs than others. For example, *Haemonchus contortus* and *Strongyloides papillosus* are found in greater numbers and their eggs develop faster than those of *Trichostrongylus* and *Cooperia* species.

Culture of canine feces for *Strongyloides stercoralis* filariform larvae uses the same technique described previously. Most filariform larvae appear within 24 to 48 hours. Rhabditiform larvae may be evident first. If this occurs, the sample should be allowed to stand for no less than 96 hours so that the larvae can mate and produce filariform larvae.

Another method uses a covered Petri dish and filter paper. Feces are placed in the middle of a piece of moistened filter paper, which is then placed in the Petri dish. The Petri dish is covered and placed in a dark area at room temperature for 7 to 10 days. The dish is rinsed and the rinsings are collected as previously described. Technicians who wish to do a fecal culture and identify larvae should refer to the chapters on larval identification in the reference by Bowman, listed at the end of this chapter.

◆ Sample Collection at Necropsy

Necropsy (postmortem examination) is an important method of diagnosing many diseases, including parasitism (see Chapter 10). The types of lesions produced by immature parasites, any adult parasites found in the body cavity and tissues, and histopathologic examination of infected tissues are used in diagnosis. Veterinary technicians are responsible for the samples collected, making sure they are contained, preserved, labeled, and shipped properly.

Two methods may be used to recover parasites from the digestive tract at necropsy: the *decanting method* and the *sieving method* (Procedures 6-11 and 6-12). With either method, the veterinary technician must separate the different parts of the digestive tract and work with the contents of each individually.

Parasites recovered from the digestive tract may be preserved in 70% alcohol or 10% neutral buffered formalin for later identification. Occasionally, bladder worms or cysticerci may be found attached to the viscera of domestic animals. A bladder worm is a fluid-filled, balloon-like structure that is actually a larval tapeworm. These should

---

PROCEDURE **6-11**

Decanting method

Materials

Buckets (large enough to hold the contents of each
  part of the digestive tract and an equal volume of water)
Knives   ·
Metal spatulas
Stirring spoons or paddles
Dissecting pans
Dissecting microscope or magnifying glass
Thumb forceps

Procedure

1. Open each section of the digestive tract and pour its contents into a bucket. Using a spatula, scrape the interior lining of the organ into the bucket or examine the scrapings separately.
2. Add an equal amount of water to the contents of each bucket and mix thoroughly.
3. Allow the contents to sit undisturbed for about 45 minutes.
4. Carefully pour off the liquid, leaving the sediment in the bottom of the bucket. Add an equal amount of water and repeat the above procedure until the water over the sediment becomes clear.
5. Pour off the clear water, then transfer the sediment to a dissecting pan.
6. Using a dissecting microscope or magnifying glass, examine a number of small samples of the sediment. Any parasites found should gently be removed with thumb forceps and preserved (discussed later in this chapter).

be handled with care because the fluid within the bladder can be allergenic and may also be zoonotic. To identify the parasites recovered, the veterinary technician should consult the references listed at the end of this chapter. If in-hospital diagnosis is not possible, the samples may be preserved as previously described and sent to a diagnostic laboratory for identification.

◆ Shipping Parasitologic Specimens

Any parasitologic specimen shipped to a diagnostic laboratory should be preserved with alcohol or formalin, unless otherwise directed by laboratory personnel. Specimens should be packaged in a leakproof container and sealed with Parafilm (American National Can, Greenwich, CT) or tape. If specimen containers are found leaking, the shipment will not be delivered. Feces can be sent fresh or mixed at a ratio of 1:3 with 10% formalin. Whole parasites or segments can be preserved in alcohol or formalin and placed in a leak-proof container (clean small jar, medicine vial, clot tube).

All specimen containers should be labeled as to the site from which the specimen was obtained, the owner's name, the animal's species, name, or identification number, and the referring veterinarian (including telephone number and address). The labeled specimen container should be placed in a shockproof shipping container to prevent breakage during shipping. Styrofoam containers filled with shredded newspaper work well for shipping parasitologic specimens.

A cover letter should be included with the specimen and should contain a brief history of the animal, findings upon necropsy, and the reason for submitting the samples to the laboratory (e.g., fecal examination, special staining, species identification). Without this background information, the diagnostic laboratory is unlikely to provide accurate results.

PROCEDURE 6-12

Sieving method

Materials

Same as for decanting method
Testing sieves (#18 and #45, Sargent-Welch Scientific)

Procedure

1. Place the contents of each section of digestive tract and the scrapings in a bucket and mix with water, as previously described.
2. Pour the mixture through the #18 sieve and then through the #45 sieve. Wash the sieves' contents with water.
3. Examine the solid material in the sieves, as described for the sediment in the decanting method.

Miscellaneous Procedures for Detection of Endoparasites

CELLOPHANE TAPE TECHNIQUE.   The cellophane tape technique is used to detect the equine pinworm, *Oxyuris equi* (Procedure 6-13). Pinworms are nematodes found in horses, rodents, and people. They live in the colon and, as adults, migrate out the rectum to lay eggs on the skin around the anus. The eggs are contained within a sticky substance and fall off as the substance hardens or as the animal scratches. For this reason, pinworm eggs usually are not seen in a routine fecal examination (see Figure 6-42).

BAERMANN TECHNIQUE.   The Baermann technique is used to recover nematode larvae from feces, tissues, or soil. This technique uses warm water to stimulate larvae to move about. As the larvae do so, they sink to the bottom of the funnel for collection and identification (Procedure 6-14).

This technique is performed with a Baermann apparatus (Figure 6-57). The apparatus consists of a ring stand and ring holder, a glass funnel with a piece of rubber tubing on the end, a clamp, and a wire net or cheesecloth. With the apparatus set up as shown in Figure 6-57, the sample is placed on the wire screen or cheesecloth, and warm water is added to barely cover the sample. All air bubbles are allowed to flow from the tube of the funnel by releasing the clamp. The apparatus is allowed to sit undisturbed for 12 to 24 hours.

A drop of fluid from the bottom of the funnel is removed (usually the first drop) and placed on a microscope slide. If any larvae are found swimming on the slide, the slide is heated with a match to render them immobile.

Larvae recovered from fresh large animal feces are almost always those of lungworms. Larvae from *Strongyloides stercoralis* can be found in *fresh* canine feces. If

---

PROCEDURE **6-13**

Cellophane tape technique

Materials

Transparent cellophane tape (e.g., Scotch tape)
Tongue depressor
Microscope slide

Procedure

1. Wrap the cellophane tape in a loop around the tongue depressor, with the sticky side out.
2. Press the tape to the skin around the horse's anus. Stand to the side of the horse and not directly behind it.
3. Place a drop of water on the slide. Remove the tape from the tongue depressor and place it, sticky side down, on top of the water.
4. Examine the slide for pinworm eggs (see Figure 6-42).

the feces are not fresh, all sorts of parasitic and nonparasitic larvae and adults may be seen. For more detailed information on the descriptions of larvae, consult the reference by Bowman.

PROCEDURE **6-14**

Baermann technique

Materials

Baermann apparatus
Cheesecloth or gauze square about twice the diameter of the funnel
Microscope slides and coverslips

Procedure

1. Spread the cheesecloth out on the support screen in the Baermann apparatus. Take 5 to 15 g of fecal, soil, or tissue sample and place it on the cheesecloth. Fold any excess cheesecloth over the top of the sample. Be sure the sample is covered by the warm water or saline; add more if necessary.
2. Allow the apparatus to remain undisturbed overnight.
3. Hold a microscope slide under the cut off pipette and open the pinch clamp only long enough to allow a large drop to fall on the slide. Apply a coverslip to the slide and examine it microscopically for larvae. Repeat by examining several slides before concluding the sample is negative.

Figure 6-57
Baermann apparatus.

DIAGNOSIS OF BLOOD PARASITISM

Dirofilaria immitis, the canine heartworm, is the most important parasite of the vascular system in domestic animals in the United States. For this reason, in-hospital blood examinations are commonly performed to detect heartworms.

The following procedures can be performed by veterinary technicians to identify *D. immitis.* As mentioned earlier, a clean environment and proper handling of samples are vital to quality control in any laboratory. Any sample handled improperly may result in inaccurate results.

◆ Collection of Blood Samples

Sterile equipment and alcohol are required for collecting a blood sample from an animal. Blood may be collected using a syringe and needle or a Vacutainer (Becton-Dickinson, Rutherford, NJ). If blood is collected with a syringe and needle, the inside of the syringe should be coated with an anticoagulant, such as heparin. If a Vacutainer is used, an EDTA (lavender top) tube is used. Unless serum is required, as with some of the immunodiagnostic test kits, a clot tube (red top) should be used. All samples should be labeled with the owner's name, animal's name, and date of collection.

Microfilariae are more numerous in the blood stream at certain times of the day. To increase the probability of collecting microfilariae, blood should be collected in the afternoon because the microfilariae of *D. immitis* are most numerous in the circulating blood at this time.

◆ Examination of the Blood

General observations of the blood should be noted. For example, a blood sample that appears watery may be due to anemia. Clinical pathology tests on the blood also may aid in diagnosis of parasitism. Heartworm microfilariae may be seen during the differential white blood cell (WBC) count. A high eosinophil count may also indicate parasitism (Procedure 6-15).

Direct Examination

Direct examination of the blood for microfilariae is the simplest procedure to perform. This procedure detects movement of microfilariae and other parasites among the RBCs. As with direct examination of feces, direct examination of blood requires only a small sample. However, unless parasites are present in large numbers, they may be missed. For this reason, the direct smear is *not* a good diagnostic technique for diagnosing microfilariae.

Microfilariae of primary interest are those of *D. immitis,* the canine heartworm, and *Dipetalonema reconditum,* a subcutaneous parasite of dogs. Differentiation between the two is extremely important, as treatment for heartworms is expensive, somewhat stressful, and involves use of arsenical compounds.

In a direct blood smear, microfilariae of *Dirofilaria* species coil and uncoil, whereas those of *Dipetalonema* species may glide smoothly across the slide. How-

PROCEDURE 6-15

Direct examination of blood

Materials

Blood collection equipment
Microscope slides and coverslips

Procedure

1. Immediately after collecting the blood sample, place a single drop of blood onto the microscope slide and add a coverslip.
2. Examine the slide using the 10× microscope objective. Watch for localized areas of movement among the red blood cells, which may indicate the presence of parasites.

ever, this is not always the case. Also, the number of *Dirofilaria* species microfilariae in a sample is greater than that of *Dipetalonema* species. Again, this is not always the case. Direct examination of the blood is only used to determine the presence of microfilariae, not the type. For this, a concentration technique, which "relaxes" and stains microfilariae, is used. These procedures are discussed later in this chapter.

Trypanosomes are another type of parasite found in the blood. These protozoa occur in tropical areas and occasionally in the United States. Trypanosomes can be seen swimming among the cells of a diluted blood smear (single-cell thickness) but are more easily identified in stained smears.

Microfilariae can also be found in large animals. *Setaria* is a long, white nematode found in the serous membranes of cattle and horses. Adults are most often seen during abdominal surgery, and microfilariae are found during differential WBC count.

Thin Blood Smear

The thin blood smear is prepared and stained in exactly the same way as a blood smear for a differential WBC count (Procedure 6-16). When doing a differential WBC count on an animal, the veterinary technician should note any parasitic organisms seen. Occasionally, microfilariae may be found. Because of their size, microfilariae usually are found along the feathered edge. Because differentiation of the microfilariae is not possible in a thin blood smear, other procedures must be performed for identification. Trypanosomes, protozoans, and rickettsiae also may be found among or within cells. As with the direct smear procedure, a small blood sample is used and mild parasitic infections may be missed.

Thick Blood Smear

A thick blood smear examines a slightly greater volume of blood than does a thin blood smear. Again, microfilariae may be seen, but they cannot be easily differentiated using this method (Procedure 6-17).

PROCEDURE **6-16**

Thin blood smear

Materials

Microscope slides
Blood smear stain (Diff-Quik, Wright's, Giemsa)

Procedure

1. Place a glass slide on a flat surface. Add a drop of blood near one end of the slide.
2. Place the end of a second slide near the middle of the first slide at a 45-degree angle (Figure 6-58). Holding the second slide at that angle, gently pull the slide backward, into the drop of blood. Allow the blood to spread across the edge of the second slide.
3. Holding the first slide firmly, smoothly push the second slide across and off the end of the first slide. This should form a thin smear on the first slide, with a nice feathered edge.
4. Allow the slide to air dry, and stain. After staining, the slide can be examined using the oil-immersion objective.

Figure 6-58
As viewed from the side, the correct angle and direction of movement for preparation of a thin blood smear.

Buffy Coat Method

The buffy coat method is a concentration technique used on a small volume of blood. When blood is placed in a microhematocrit tube and centrifuged for determining the packed cell volume (PCV), it separates into three layers: plasma, WBC layer (buffy coat) and RBC layer (Figure 6-59). Microfilariae can be found on the surface of the buffy coat layer (Figure 6-60). This technique is quick and may be performed in conjunction with a PCV and total protein evaluation. However, differentiation of microfilariae is not possible (Procedure 6-18).

PROCEDURE 6-17

Thick blood smear

Materials

Microscope slides
Distilled water
Methyl alcohol
Giemsa stain, diluted 1:20 with distilled water
Wooden applicator stick

Procedure

1. Place 3 drops of blood on the slide and spread them with a wooden applicator stick to make a 2-cm circle.
2. Allow the slide to air dry.
3. Place the slide in a slanted position, smear side down, in a beaker filled with distilled water. Allow the slide to remain in the water until the smear loses its red color.
4. Remove the slide and allow it to air dry. Immerse the slide in methyl alcohol for 10 minutes. Stain the slide with Giemsa stain for 30 minutes. Rinse off excess stain.

Figure 6-59
Buffy coat in a hematocrit tube.

Figure 6-60
Microfilaria in a buffy coat smear from canine blood.

PROCEDURE **6-18**

Buffy coat method

Materials

Microhematocrit tubes and sealer
Microhematocrit centrifuge
Small file or glass cutter
Microscope slides and coverslips
Saline
Methylene blue stain (diluted 1:1000 with distilled water)

Procedure

1. Fill the microhematocrit tube with blood, and seal.
2. Centrifuge for 3 minutes.
3. Read the PCV, if desired, then find the buffy coat layer between the red blood cells and plasma (Figure 6-59).
4. Using a file, scratch the tube at the level of the buffy coat. Carefully snap the tube and save the part of the tube containing the buffy coat and plasma. Gently tap the tube onto a slide, ejecting the buffy coat layer with a small amount of plasma. Save the rest of the plasma for a total protein determination, if desired.
5. Add a drop of saline and a drop of stain to the buffy coat. Apply a coverslip and examine for microfilariae (Figure 6-60).

PROCEDURE **6-19**

Modified Knott's technique

Materials

15-ml centrifuge tube
Centrifuge
2% formalin (2 ml of 40% formalin diluted with 98 ml of distilled water)
Methylene blue stain (diluted 1:1000 with distilled water)
Pasteur pipettes and bulbs

Procedure

1. Mix 1 ml of blood with 9 ml of 2% formalin in a centrifuge tube.
2. Centrifuge the tube at 1300 to 1500 rpm for 5 minutes.
3. Pour off the liquid supernatant, leaving the sediment at the bottom of the tube.
4. Add 2 to 3 drops of stain to the sediment. Using a pipette, mix the sediment with the stain.
5. Place a drop of this mixture onto a glass slide. Apply a coverslip and examine for microfilariae using the 10× objective.

The following concentration techniques may be used for differentiating *D. immitis* from *D. reconditum.*

MODIFIED KNOTT'S TECHNIQUE. The modified Knott's technique is a simple procedure that allows differentiation of microfilariae (Procedure 6-19). This technique concentrates, "relaxes," and stains microfilariae, while lysing red blood cells to make the microfilariae more visible.

Figures 6-61 and 6-62 and Table 6-1 show the characteristics that may be used when identifying microfilariae. The veterinary technician should always examine as many microfilariae as possible because mixed infections can occur. The most accurate method for differentiation is measuring the length and width of the body. However, with some practice, general characteristics of the microfilariae may be used for identification if a means of measuring microfilariae is not available.

FILTER TECHNIQUE. Filter techniques are the most common method used in veterinary practices for detection of microfilariae in the blood. Several diagnostic kits are available for this procedure, including Di-Fil Test Kit (EVSCO, Buena, NJ) and

Figure 6-61
Microfilaria of *Dirofilaria immitis,* found using the modified Knott's technique. Note the straight tail and tapering cranial end of the microfilaria.

Figure 6-62
Cranial **(A)** and caudal **(B)** ends of a *Dipetalonema reconditum* microfilaria.

TABLE 6-1		
Differentiation of microfilariae using the modified Knott's technique		
	Dirofilaria immitis	*Dipetalonema reconditum*
Body length	>310 μ	<290 μ
Mid-body width	>6 μ	<6 μ
Head	Tapered	Blunt
Tail	Straight	Hooked

Filarassay*F Heartworm Diagnostic Test Kit (Pitman-Moore, Mundelein, IL). These kits come complete with filters, lysing solution, stain, and directions for use.

Most kits require 1 ml of whole blood to test for heartworms. The blood is mixed with nine parts of lysing solution and passed through a filter. The filter is rinsed, removed, and placed on a slide. A drop of stain is added, a coverslip is applied, then the filter is microscopically examined for microfilariae (Figure 6-63). Differentiation of microfilariae is possible but difficult using the filter technique. If microfilariae are present, it is best to perform other diagnostic procedures for identification purposes.

ENZYME-LINKED IMMUNOSORBENT ASSAY. Enzyme-linked immunosorbent assay (ELISA) kits do not directly detect microfilariae but instead test the host's response to the parasites. These types of tests can be used for differentiating *Dirofilaria immitis* from *Dipetalonema,* and they can be used to identify an occult heartworm infection. An occult infection is one in which only one sex of adult worms is present, and no microfilariae are produced. Also, when an animal is treated with drugs that kill circulating microfilariae or render the adults unable to reproduce, again no circulating microfilariae exist.

Some ELISA kits detect the host's antibody response to the adult heartworms, whereas others detect the host's antibody response to the microfilariae (see Chapter 9). The most reliable ELISA kits test for the presence of *Dirofilaria* species antigen in the host's blood. Dirochek (Synbiotics, San Diego, CA) and CITE Heartworm Test Kit (IDEXX, Portland, ME) are two such diagnostic kits. These two procedures rely on a color change to indicate a positive response. As with any procedure, ELISA immunodiagnostic tests should be performed exactly according to the manufacturer's directions and in a clean environment to avoid contamination.

MISCELLANEOUS TESTS. Another type of heartworm diagnostic test kit (Heartworm Identification Test: ImmunoVet, Tampa, FL) works on the same principle as the Knott's and filter techniques, except the microfilariae remain alive. This test relies on the movement of the microfilariae, which can be unreliable at times.

Other tests use special stains to bring out certain characteristics of the microfilariae. These procedures are too cumbersome to be useful in private practice and usually are performed in diagnostic laboratories.

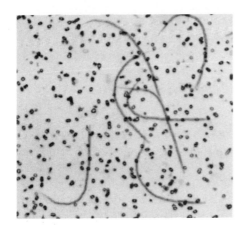

Figure 6-63
Microfilariae in canine blood on a filter. The small, irregular structures are the pores in the filter paper, and the small circular objects are RBCs.

Recommended Reading

Bowman DD, Lynn RC, Georgi JR: *Georgi's parasitology for veterinarians,* ed 7, Philadelphia, 1999, WB Saunders.

Hendrix CM: *Diagnostic veterinary parasitology,* ed 2, St Louis, 1998, Mosby.

Sloss MW, et al: *Veterinary clinical parasitology,* ed 6, Ames, Iowa, 1994, Iowa State University Press.

CHAPTER 7

External Parasites

CHARLES M. HENDRIX

If a parasite resides on the surface of its host, it is termed an *ectoparasite*. The majority of ectoparasites are either insects (e.g., fleas, lice, flies) or arachnids (e.g., ticks, mites). A few nematodes have immature stages that occur in the skin or subcutaneous tissues.

This chapter is designed to aid the veterinary technician in diagnosis of ectoparasitism in dogs, cats, cattle, sheep, goats, horses, and swine. To diagnose an ectoparasitic infestation, the technician must be able to collect the ectoparasite and then identify the organism involved. This chapter explains procedures commonly used to collect ectoparasites from the host and describes those parasites so that a correct diagnosis can be made.

Although a complete review of the biology of ectoparasites is beyond the scope of this chapter, a brief review of the life cycles of the major groups of ectoparasites is included.

COLLECTION OF SAMPLES

◆ Skin Scrapings

Skin scraping is one of the most common diagnostic procedures used in evaluating animals with dermatologic problems. Equipment needed includes an electric clipper with #40 blade, a scalpel or spatula, mineral oil in a small dropper bottle, and a compound microscope. Typical lesions or sites likely to harbor the particular parasite should be scraped (e.g., ear margins for *Sarcoptes scabiei* variety *canis*).

The scraping is performed with a #10 scalpel blade, used with or without a handle. A 165-mm stainless-steel spatula (Sargent-Welsh Scientific, Detroit, MI) is preferred by some clinicians. The scalpel blade should be held between the thumb and forefinger (Figure 7-1). Before the skin is scraped, the blade is dipped in a drop of mineral oil on the slide, or a drop of mineral oil may be placed on the skin.

Figure 7-1
A scalpel blade may be held safely between the thumb and forefinger for skin scrapings.

During the scraping process, the blade must be held perpendicular to the skin. Holding it at another angle may result in an accidental incision. The average area scraped should be about 6 to 8 cm².

The depth of the scraping varies with the typical location of the parasite in question. When scraping for mites that live in tunnels (e.g., *Sarcoptes* species) or in hair follicles (e.g., *Demodex* species), the veterinary technician should scrape the skin until a small amount of capillary blood oozes from the scraped area. Clipping the area with a #40 blade before scraping enables better visualization of the lesion and removes excess hair that impedes proper scraping and interferes with collection of epidermal debris. For surface-dwelling mites (e.g., *Cheyletiella* or *Chorioptes* species), the skin is scraped superficially to collect loose scales and crusts. Clipping before scraping is not necessary when infestation with surface dwellers is suspected.

All scraped debris on the forward surface of the blade is then spread in a drop of mineral oil on the slide. A glass coverslip is placed on the material, and the slide is ready for microscopic examination using the 4× (scanning) objective. The slide should be examined systematically in rows so that the entire area under the coverslip is evaluated. Low light intensity and high contrast increase visualization of translucent mites and eggs. If necessary, the slide may be evaluated using the 10× (low-power) objective.

Demonstration of the characteristic mite or egg is frequently diagnostic for most diseases. In certain circumstances, however, more than just identification of the parasite is necessary. For example, determination of live:dead ratios and observation of immature larval and nymphal stages of demodectic mites are important in determining a patient's prognosis. A decrease in the number of live mites and eggs during treatment is an excellent prognostic indicator.

◆ Cellophane Tape Preparation

When attempting to demonstrate lice or mites that live primarily on the surface of the skin (e.g., *Cheyletiella* species), the veterinary technician may use a cellophane tape preparation instead of a skin scraping. Clear cellophane tape (Scotch Transparent Tape, 3M, Minneapolis, MN) is applied to the skin to pick up epidermal debris. A ribbon of mineral oil is placed on a glass slide, and the adhesive surface of the tape is then placed on the mineral oil. Additional mineral oil and a coverslip may be placed on the tape to prevent the tape from wrinkling, but this is not necessary. The slide is then examined microscopically for parasites.

◆ Parasite Identification

When arthropods or helminths cannot be grossly identified, the intact specimen should be collected in a sealed container containing 10% formalin or ethyl alcohol and submitted to an arthropodologist/parasitologist for identification. A complete history should accompany the specimen. The specimen should not be fragmented or squashed, which could distort morphologic features necessary for proper identification. Forensic identification of parasites is difficult.

TERMINOLOGY

Ectoparasites usually live on or in skin surfaces or feed on them. Ectoparasites infest the skin or external surfaces of animals and produce an infestation on the animal. By contrast, internal parasites, or endoparasites, infect the internal organs of domestic animals and produce an infection within that animal. In diagnostic parasitology, these terms always should be used in the proper context.

Life cycle describes the development of a parasite through its various life stages. Every parasite's life cycle has a definitive host and may have one or more intermediate hosts. The definitive host harbors the adult, sexual, or mature stages of a parasite. *The intermediate host* harbors the juvenile, asexual, or immature stages of a parasite.

Many of the ectoparasites in this chapter belong to the phylum Arthropoda or, more simply, are considered arthropods. All adult arthropods have jointed legs. Later in this chapter is a discussion of ectoparasites that reside within the skin; these ectoparasites are not arthropods but rather belong to the phylum Nematoda, or more simply, the roundworms.

CLASSIFICATION SYSTEM

In beginning biology, students must learn the classification scheme perfected by Linnaeus, an early biologist. Every living organism on this planet may be classified using the following classification scheme: kingdom, phylum, class, order, family, genus, and species. Students often remember this scheme with this simple mnemonic device, "King Philip came over for good spaghetti," in which each letter in the sentence corresponds to the first letter in the Linnaean classification scheme.

Every living thing is known by a scientific name that is made up of two components: the *genus* and the *specific epithet*. The dog's scientific name is *Canis familiaris: Canis* is the genus and *familiaris* is the specific epithet or species.

Similar species are grouped together into the same genus. Similar genera (plural of genus) are grouped together into the same family. Similar families are grouped together into the same order. Similar orders are grouped together into the same class. Similar classes are grouped together into the same phylum. Similar phyla are grouped together into the same kingdom. Therefore the dog's classification scheme is as follows:

Kingdom: Animalia
      Phylum: Chordata
            Subphylum: Vertebrata
                Class: Mammalia
                    Order: Carnivora
                        Family: Canidae
                            Genus: *Canis*
                              Species: *familiaris*

Every living thing on earth has a distinct classification scheme.

PHYLUM: ARTHROPODA

◆ Class: Insecta

The first part of this chapter discusses the orders belonging to the class Insecta and the families belonging to the class Acarina and how these ectoparasites are relevant to veterinary practice.

Order: Hymenoptera

Hymenoptera includes ants, bees, and wasps. Fire ants are indigenous to the southeastern United States and can bite and sting almost any domestic animal. "Downer cows" and young newborn animals are particularly at risk to the perils of fire ants.

Bees, wasps, and hornets can sting domestic animals, particularly curious dogs and cats. When stung, the animals may show an extremely swollen nose or face.

Africanized honeybees, or "killer bees," have now crossed the Mexico/United States border. Almost any domestic animal (and people) could stumble on a hive of these bees, angering the inhabitants. Death often results from thousands of killer bee stings.

DIAGNOSIS.   If ants, bees, wasps, or hornets are suspected to be causing problems, the intact hymenopteran should be collected in a sealed container containing 10% formalin or ethyl alcohol and submitted to an entomologist for identification.

Order: Hemiptera

Members of Hemiptera are true bugs. Two groups of hemipterans are of veterinary importance: Reduviid bugs (kissing bugs) and bed bugs. Reduviid bugs (kissing bugs) are periodic parasites, making frequent visits to the host to obtain a blood meal. Kissing bugs serve as intermediate hosts for *Trypanosoma cruzi,* a protozoan parasite that can produce a rare disease in people and dogs called *Chagas' disease.* This disease also is called *South American trypanosomiasis* and rarely occurs in the United States. Kissing bugs take blood meals from an infected host and transmit the parasite as they defecate.

Bed bugs are dorsoventrally flattened, wingless hemipterans that often infest homes. They are periodic parasites, making frequent visits to the host to obtain a blood meal. Although bed bugs are human parasites, they also may be found in rabbit colonies, poultry houses, and pigeon colonies.

DIAGNOSIS. If Reduviid bugs or bed bugs are suspected to be causing problems, the intact hemipteran should be collected in 10% formalin or ethyl alcohol and submitted to an entomologist for identification.

Orders: Mallophaga and Anoplura

Lice are some of the most prolific ectoparasites of domestic animals. Two orders of lice exist: the Mallophaga (chewing or biting lice) and Anoplura (sucking lice). Lice are dorsoventrally flattened, wingless insects. They have three body divisions: the head, with its mouthparts and antennae; the thorax, with its three pairs of legs and no wings; and the abdomen, the portion that bears the reproductive organs. These body divisions and their relationship to each other are important in diagnostic veterinary parasitology.

Members of the order Mallophaga, or chewing/biting lice, are smaller than sucking lice. They are usually yellow and have a large, round head. The mouthparts are mandibulate and are adapted for chewing or biting. Characteristically, the head of every chewing louse is wider than the widest portion of the thorax. On the thorax are three pairs of legs, which may be adapted for clasping or for moving rapidly among feathers or hairs. Chewing/biting lice may parasitize birds, dogs, cats, cattle, sheep, goats, and horses (Figure 7-2).

Members of the order Anoplura (sucking lice) are larger than members of the order Mallophaga (chewing lice). These lice are red to gray; their color usually depends on the amount of blood ingested from the host. In contrast to the big head of the Mallophagans, Anoplurans' heads are narrower than the widest part of the thorax. Their mouthparts are piercing and are adapted for sucking. Their pincerlike claws are adapted for clinging to the host's hairs. Although they are found on many species of domestic animals, sucking lice do not parasitize birds or cats (Figure 7-3).

Anoplurans and Mallophagans have the same type of life cycle. This life cycle has only three developmental stages: the egg, nymphal, and adult stages.

The egg stage is also called a "nit." The nit is tiny, approximately 0.5 to 1.0 mm in length. It is oval, white, and usually found cemented to the hair or feather shaft. Figure 7-4 shows a gravid female sucking louse and an associated nit collected from a dog. Nits hatch about 5 to 14 days after being laid by the adult female louse.

Figure 7-2
Damalinia caprae, Goniodes dissimilis, and *Goniodes gallinae,* assorted chewing lice of goats and fowl.

Figure 7-3
Solenopotes capillatus, Pedicinus obtusus, and *Linognathus setosus,* assorted sucking lice of sheep, monkeys, and dogs.

Figure 7-4
Linognathus setosus, a gravid female sucking louse and associated nit collected from a dog.

The nymphal stage is similar in appearance to the adult. However, it is smaller and lacks functioning reproductive organs and genital openings. The three nymphal stages are each progressively larger than its predecessor. The nymphal stage lasts from 2 to 3 weeks.

The adult stage is similar in appearance to the nymphal stage but larger. It has functional reproductive organs. Male and female lice copulate, the female lays eggs, and the life cycle begins again. It takes 3 to 4 weeks to complete the cycle. Nymphal and adult stages live no longer than 7 days if removed from the host. Eggs hatch within 2 to 3 weeks during warm weather but seldom hatch off the host.

Lice usually are transmitted by direct contact, but all life stages may be transmitted by fomites (inanimate objects such as blankets, brushes, and other grooming equipment). Lice are easily transmitted among young, old, and malnourished animals. Veterinarians often cannot understand why certain animals in a flock or herd are heavily infested, whereas others have only a few lice.

Infestation by lice (whether Mallophagan or Anopluran) is referred to as *pediculosis.* Sucking lice can ingest blood to such a degree that they produce severe anemia; fatalities can occur, especially in young animals. The packed cell volume can drop as much as 10% to 20%. Severely infested animals may have as many as a million lice. Infested animals become more susceptible to other diseases and parasites and may succumb to stresses not ordinarily pathologic to uninfested animals. When animals are poorly fed and kept in overcrowded conditions, they often become severely infested with lice and quickly become anemic and unthrifty.

DIAGNOSIS. Careful examination of the haircoat or feathers of infested animals easily reveals lice and their accompanying nits. Hair clippings also serve as a good source for lice. Infestation of animals with a thick haircoat may be easily overlooked. A hand-held magnifying lens or a binocular headband magnifier may aid observation of adult/nymphal lice crawling through or clinging to hair or feathers, or tiny nits cemented to individual hairs.

Any lice and/or their nits observed may be collected with thumb forceps and placed in a drop of mineral oil on a glass microscope slide. A coverslip should be placed over the specimen and the slide examined using the 4× or 10× objective.

Identification of louse to genus and specific epithet is difficult. A better method is to identify the specimen as being Anopluran (sucking) or Mallophagan (chewing or biting) by visual examination of head size.

Order: Diptera

Diptera is a large, complex order of insects. As adults, most members have one pair of wings, which is the origin of the ordinal name: *di-,* meaning two, and *-ptera,* meaning wing. Its members vary in size, food source preference, and developmental stage that parasitizes the animal or produces lesions.

Dipterans produce two contrasting pathologic scenarios. As adults, they may feed intermittently on vertebrate blood, saliva, tears, and mucus. As larvae, they may develop in the subcutaneous tissues. Dipterans that make frequent visits to the vertebrate host to intermittently feed on blood are referred to as *periodic parasites.* When Dipteran larvae develop in the tissue or organs of vertebrate hosts, they produce a condition known as *myiasis.*

As periodic parasites, blood-feeding Dipterans may be classified as to which sex feeds on vertebrate blood and as to food preference. In certain Dipteran groups only the females feed on vertebrate blood; these female flies require vertebrate blood for laying their eggs. In this group are the biting gnats (e.g., *Simulium, Lutzomyia,* and *Culicoides* species), the mosquitoes (e.g., *Anopheles, Aedes,* and *Culex* species), the horse flies (e.g., *Tabanus* species), and the deer flies (e.g., *Chrysops* species).

In the second group of blood-feeding Dipterans, both male and female flies require a vertebrate blood meal. These species include the stable fly *Stomoxys calcitrans,* the horn fly *Haematobia irritans,* and the sheep ked *Melophagus ovinus. Musca autumnalis* (face fly) feeds on mucus, tears, and saliva of large animals, particularly cattle.

In the first Dipteran group of periodic parasites, only the female Dipterans feed on vertebrate blood. The tiniest members of this group are the biting gnats, *Simulium, Lutzomyia,* and *Culicoides* species.

SIMULIUM (BLACK FLY).   Members of the genus *Simulium* are commonly called "black flies," although their coloration may vary from gray to yellow. They also are called "buffalo gnats" because their thorax is humped over the head, giving the appearance of a buffalo's hump (Figure 7-5). These are tiny flies, ranging from 1 to 6 mm in length. They have broad, unspotted wings with very prominent veins along the cranial margins of the wings. These tiny flies have serrated, scissor-like mouthparts that inflict painful bites.

Because the females lay their eggs in well-aerated water, these flies often are found in the vicinity of swiftly flowing streams. They move in great swarms, inflicting painful bites and sucking the host's blood. These flies may keep cattle from grazing or cause them to stampede. The animal's ears, neck, head, and abdomen are favorite feeding sites. These flies also feed on poultry and can serve as an intermediate host for the protozoan parasite *Leukocytozoon.*

Figure 7-5
Simulium species, black flies. These tiny flies range in size from 1 to 6 mm in length.

Diagnosis. Black flies are most often collected in the field and are not found on animals presented to a veterinary clinic. They are identified by their small size, humped back, and strong venation in the cranial region of the wings. Identification of black flies is probably best left to an entomologist.

LUTZOMYIA (NEW WORLD SAND FLY). Members of the genus *Lutzomyia* are commonly referred to as "New World sand flies." They are tiny, mothlike flies, rarely more than 5 mm long. A key feature for identification is that their bodies are covered with fine hairs. They tend to be active only at night and are weak fliers. These tiny flies transmit the protozoan parasite *Leishmania* species.

Diagnosis. Like black flies, sand flies most often are collected in the field and are not found on animals presented to a veterinary clinic. They are identified by their small size and hairy wings and body. Identification of sand flies is probably best left to an entomologist.

CULICOIDES SPECIES. *Culicoides* gnats are also commonly known as "no-see-ums," "punkies," or "sand flies." They are tiny gnats (1 to 3 mm in length), similar in appearance to black flies. They inflict painful bites, suck the blood of their hosts, and are active at dusk and dawn, especially during the winter months. These gnats tend to feed on the dorsal or ventral areas of the host; the feeding site depends on the species of biting gnat.

Horses often become allergic to the bites of *Culicoides* gnats, scratching and rubbing bitten areas, causing alopecia, excoriations, and thickening of the skin. This condition has several names, including "Queensland itch," "sweat itch," "sweet itch," and "summer dermatitis" (the latter name because it is often seen during the warmer months of the year). These flies also serve as the intermediate host for *Onchocerca cervicalis*, a nematode whose microfilariae are found in the skin of horses. These flies also transmit the bluetongue virus of sheep.

Diagnosis. In contrast to the clear, heavily veined wings of black flies, the wings of *Culicoides* species are mottled. Identification of *Culicoides* species is probably best left to an entomologist.

Anopheles, Aedes, and *Culex* Species (Mosquitoes)

Although they are tiny, fragile Dipterans, mosquitoes are some of the most voracious blood feeders on domestic animals and people (Figure 7-6). Mosquitoes can plague livestock and in swarms have been known to keep cattle from grazing or to cause them to stampede. The feeding of large numbers of swarming mosquitoes may cause significant anemia in domestic animals. Large numbers of mosquitoes may be produced from eggs laid in relatively small bodies of water. Although they are known for spreading malaria (*Plasmodium* species), yellow fever, and elephantiasis among people, mosquitoes are probably best known in veterinary medicine as the intermediate host for the canine heartworm, *Dirofilaria immitis.*

DIAGNOSIS.   Adult mosquitoes have wings and body parts covered by tiny, leaf-shape scales. Identification of adult and larval *Anopheles, Aedes*, and *Culex* species is probably best left to an entomologist.

Chrysops and *Tabanus* Species (Deer Fly, Horse Fly)

Chrysops species (deer flies) and *Tabanus* species (horse flies) are large (up to 3.5 cm long), heavy-body, robust Dipterans with powerful wings and large eyes. Horse flies and deer flies are the largest flies in the Dipteran group, in which only the females feed on vertebrate blood. Figure 7-7 shows Tabanus species, the largest blood-feeding Dipterans. Horse flies are larger than deer flies. Deer flies have a dark band passing from the cranial to the caudal margin of the wings.

Adult flies lay eggs in the vicinity of open water. Larval stages of these flies are found in aquatic to semiaquatic environments, often buried deep in mud at the bottom of lakes and ponds. Adults are seen in summer and are fond of sunlight. Female flies feed in the vicinity of open water and have reciprocating, scissorlike mouthparts. They use these sharp, bladelike mouthparts to lacerate tissues and lap up the oozing vertebrate blood. These flies feed primarily on large animals, such as cattle and horses. Preferred feeding sites include the underside of the abdomen around the navel, the legs, or the neck and withers.

Horse flies and deer flies feed a number of times at multiple feeding sites before they stop feeding. When disturbed by the animal's swatting tail or by the panniculus reflex (skin twitching), the flies leave the host, but the blood continues to ooze from the open wound. These fly bites are painful. Affected cattle and horses become restless. These flies may act as mechanical transmitters of anthrax, anaplasmosis, and the virus of equine infectious anemia.

DIAGNOSIS.   These flies are most easily recognized by their large, robust size and lacerating, scissorlike mouthparts. Species identification of intact adult and larval horse and deer flies is probably best left to an entomologist.

In the second group of blood-feeding Dipterans, both male and female adult flies require a vertebrate blood meal. These species include the stable fly *Stomoxys calcitrans,* the horn fly *Haematobia irritans,* and the wingless ked *Melophagus ovinus.*

Figure 7-6
Culex species, one genus among several genera of mosquitoes.

Figure 7-7
Tabanus species, the largest blood-feeding Dipteran. This tabanid is approximately 2.5 cm in length.

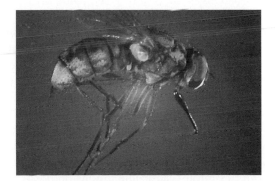

Figure 7-8
Stomoxys calcitrans, the stable fly. Note the bayonet-like proboscis that protrudes forward from the head. The stable fly is approximately the same size as a housefly.

Stomoxys calcitrans (Stable Fly)

The stable fly, *Stomoxys calcitrans,* is often called the "biting housefly." It is approximately the size of *Musca domestica,* the housefly. Rather than a sponging type of mouthpart, the stable fly has a bayonet-like proboscis that protrudes forward from the head (Figure 7-8). These flies are found worldwide. In the United States, they are found in the central and southeastern states, where cattle are raised. Both male and female flies are avid blood feeders, feeding on any domestic animal. They usually attack the legs and ventral abdomen and may also bite the ears. These flies also feed on the tips of the ears of dogs with pointed ears, especially the German Shepherd.

This fly feeds on both horses and cattle, with horses the preferred host. The fly usually lands on the host with its head pointed upward. It is a sedentary fly, not moving on the host. The flies inflict painful bites that puncture the skin and bleed freely. Stable flies stay on the host for short periods, during which they obtain the blood meals. This is an outdoor fly; however, in the late fall and during rainy weather, it may enter barns.

Stable flies are mechanical vectors of anthrax in cattle and equine infectious anemia. They are the intermediate host for *Habronema muscae,* a nematode found in the stomach of horses. When large numbers of stable flies attack dairy cattle, milk production can fall. Beef cattle may refuse to graze in the daytime when they are attacked by large numbers of flies; as a result, these cattle do not gain the usual amount of weight.

DIAGNOSIS. The veterinary technician can easily identify the stable fly by its size (approximately the same size as a housefly) and its bayonet-like proboscis that protrudes forward from the head.

Haematobia irritans (Horn Fly)

Haematobia irritans is often called the *horn fly.* This dark-colored fly is approximately 3 to 6 mm in length, half the size of *Stomoxys calcitrans,* the biting housefly. Like the stable fly, the horn fly has a bayonet-like proboscis that protrudes forward from the head. These flies are found almost exclusively on cattle throughout North America.

When the air temperature is below 70° F, horn flies cluster around the base of the horns; this is the origin of the name *horn fly.* In warmer climates, thousands of flies often cluster on the hosts' shoulders, backs, and side; these areas are least disturbed by tail switching. On hot, sunny days, horn flies congregate on the ventral abdomen.

Adult horn flies spend most of their life on cattle and leave the host only to deposit their eggs in fresh cow manure. Using their tiny bayonet mouthparts, they feed frequently, sucking blood and other fluids, and cause considerable irritation. Female flies are more aggressive than males. Harassment by the flies and loss of blood often reduces weight gains and milk production in cattle. Horn flies probably cause greater losses in cattle in the United States than any other blood-sucking fly. Adult horn flies also cause focal midline dermatitis on the ventral abdomen of horses. These flies also serve as the intermediate host for *Stephanofilaria stilesi,* a filarial parasite that produces ventral, plaque-like lesions on the ventral abdomen of cattle.

DIAGNOSIS. The veterinary technician can easily identify the horn fly by its dark color and its size (approximately half the size of a stable fly). Like the stable fly, the horn fly's bayonet-like proboscis protrudes forward from the head.

Melophagus ovinus (Sheep Ked)

Melophagus ovinus is often called the *sheep ked.* Members of the order Diptera usually have one pair of wings (two wings). Keds are an exception to that rule; they are *wingless Dipterans.* Keds are hairy, leathery, and 4 to 7 mm in length. The head is short and broad, the thorax brown, and the abdomen broad and grayish-brown. The legs are strong and armed with stout claws (Figure 7-9). Some say that keds have a "louse-like" appearance.

Keds are permanent ectoparasites of sheep and goats. Their pupal stages are often found attached to the wool or hair of the host. Keds are avid blood feeders. Heavy infestations can reduce the condition of the host considerably and even cause anemia. Their bites cause pruritus over much of the host's body; infested sheep often bite, scratch, and rub themselves, damaging the wool. Ked feces often stain the wool and do not wash out readily. Keds are most numerous in the cold temperatures of the fall and winter months. Their numbers decline as temperatures warm in the spring and summer months.

DIAGNOSIS. Close inspection of the wool and underlying skin reveals infestation by these wingless Dipterans, with their unique appearance.

Musca autumnalis (Face Fly)

The final periodic parasite among the Dipteran flies is one that is not a blood feeder but instead feeds on mucus, tears, and saliva of large animals, particularly cattle. Face flies, *Musca autumnalis,* are so named because they gather around the eyes and muzzle of livestock, particularly cattle. They also may be found on the withers, neck, brisket, and sides. Face flies feed mostly on saliva, tears, and mucus. They usually are not considered blood feeders because their mouthparts are not piercing or bayonet-like. Instead, their mouthparts are adapted for sponging up saliva, tears, and mucus (Figure 7-10). They follow blood-feeding flies, disturb them during their feeding process, and then lap up the blood and body fluids that accumulate on the host's skin. Face flies are found on animals outdoors; they usually do not follow animals into barns.

Face flies produce considerable annoyance to the host. The irritation around the host's eyes stimulates the flow of tears, which attracts even more flies. This harassment ultimately interferes with the host's productivity. Face flies may be involved in the transmission of *Moraxella bovis,* a bacterium associated with infectious kerato-conjunctivitis or pinkeye in cattle.

Figure 7-9
Melophagus ovinus, the sheep ked. Keds are hairy, leathery, and 4 to 7 mm in length. The head is short and broad. The thorax is brown, and the abdomen broad and grayish-brown. The legs are strong and armed with stout claws.

Figure 7-10
Musca autumnalis, *the face fly. Its mouth-parts are adapted for sponging saliva, tears, and mucus.*

DIAGNOSIS. Face flies are morphologically similar to the housefly, *Musca domestica.* These two species may be differentiated through minor differences in eye position and color of the abdomen. The veterinary technician probably should not attempt to speciate this fly; speciation requires the skills of a trained entomologist. If the fly is found around the face of cattle or horses, it is probably a face fly.

Myiasis-Producing Flies

With regard to their roles as ectoparasites, larval Dipterans may develop in the subcutaneous tissues of many domestic animals. When Dipteran larvae develop in the tissue or organs of vertebrate hosts, they produce a condition known as *myiasis.* Based on the degree of host dependence, myiases are divided into two types. In *facultative myiasis,* the fly larvae are usually free-living. Under certain circumstances, these "normally free-living" larvae can adapt to a parasitic dependence on a host. In *obligatory myiasis,* the fly larvae are completely parasitic; that is, they are completely dependent on the host to develop through the life cycle. In other words, without the host, the obligatory parasites die.

Facultative Myiasis-Producing Flies

This group of flies includes *Musca domestica (housefly)* and *Calliphora, Phaenicia, Lucilia, Phormia* (blowfly, bottle fly), and *Sarcophaga (flesh fly)* species.

Dipteran larvae that produce facultative myiasis include the housefly *M. domestica,* the blowflies or bottle flies *Calliphora, Phaenicia, Lucilia,* and *Phormia* species, and the flesh fly *Sarcophaga* species. Larval stages of these flies usually are associated with skin wounds contaminated with bacteria or with a matted haircoat contaminated with feces.

Under normal conditions, adult flies of these genera lay their eggs in decaying animal carcasses or in feces. In facultative myiasis, the adult flies are attracted to an animal's moist wound, skin lesion, or soiled haircoat. These sites provide the adult fly with a moist medium on which it feeds. As adult female flies feed in these sites, they lay eggs. These eggs hatch, producing larvae (maggots) that move independently about the wound surface, ingesting dead cells, exudate, secretions, and debris, but not live tissue. This condition is known as "fly strike" or "strike." These larvae irritate, injure, and kill successive layers of skin and produce exudates.

Maggots can tunnel through the thinned epidermis into the subcutis. This process produces tissue cavities in the skin that measure up to several centimeters in diameter. Unless the process is halted by appropriate therapy, the infested animal may die from shock, intoxication, histolysis, or infection. A peculiar, distinct, pungent odor permeates the infested tissue and the affected animal. Advanced lesions may contain thousands of maggots. As adults, these flies can be pestiferous flies in a veterinary clinical setting. These flies are "vomit drop" feeders and fly from feces to food, spreading bacteria on their feet and their disgorged stomach contents.

DIAGNOSIS. A tentative diagnosis of maggot infestation in any domestic animal can easily be made by a veterinary technician, as maggots can be observed in an existing wound or among the soiled, matted haircoat. When facultative myiasis has been diagnosed, the veterinarian must rule out the possibility of obligatory myiasis caused by *Cochliomyia hominivorax.*

Obligatory Myiasis-Producing Flies

COCHLIOMYIA HOMINIVORAX (PRIMARY SCREWWORM).
In obligatory myiasis, the Dipteran larvae lead a parasitic existence. Only one fly in North America, *Cochliomyia hominivorax,* is a primary invader of fresh, uncontaminated skin wounds of domestic animals. These larvae must not be confused with the larvae of the facultative myiasis-producing flies described previously. *C. hominivorax* is often referred to as the "screwworm fly." Economically it is the most important fly that attacks livestock in the southwestern and southern United States.

Adult female flies are attracted to fresh skin wounds on any warm-blooded animal, where they lay batches of 15 to 500 eggs in a shinglelike pattern at the edge of wounds. The female lays several thousand cream-color, elongated eggs during her lifetime. They hatch within 24 hours. Larvae enter the wound, where they feed for 4 to 7 days before developing into third-stage (fully-grown) larvae. They may be as long as 1.5 cm in length. At this stage they resemble a wood screw; this is the origin of the name "screwworm." When fully grown, the larvae drop to the ground and pupate for about a week, after which the adult flies emerge. The adult male and female fly breed only once during their lifetime, a fact that is used to control these flies biologically.

Diagnosis. Adult flies are shiny and greenish-blue, with a reddish orange head and eyes, and are 8 to 15 mm long. Larvae often are identified by their wood screw shape and by the deeply pigmented tracheal tubes on the dorsal aspect of the caudal ends. Because of the obligatory nature of the screwworm with regard to breeding in the fresh wounds of any warm-blooded animal, the veterinarian must report any screwworm infestations to both state and federal authorities. *C. hominivorax* has been eradicated from the United States but occasionally surreptitiously enters the country in imported animals.

Cuterebra Species (Wolf, Warble)

Larvae of the genus *Cuterebra* infest the skin of rabbits, squirrels, mice, rats, chipmunks, and occasionally dogs and cats. A large discrepancy exists concerning the descriptions of larval *Cuterebra*. Most of the specimens recovered in a veterinary setting are second- or third-stage larvae. Second-stage larvae are grublike, 5 to 10 mm long, and cream to grayish white. They are often sparsely covered with tiny, black, toothlike spines. Third-stage larvae are large, robust, coal-black, and heavily spined. Larval stages usually are found in swollen, cystlike subcutaneous sites, with a fistula or pore communicating to the outside environment. The larval *Cuterebra* species breathes through this pore.

Adult flies lay eggs near the entrance to rodent burrows. Pets usually contract this parasite while investigating or hunting rodent prey. As a result, the most commonly affected sites in dogs and cats are the subcutaneous tissues of the neck and face. Most cases occur during the late summer and early fall. Among the myiasis-producing flies, this Dipteran larva is known for its aberrant or erratic migrations, having been found in a variety of extracutaneous sites, the cranial vault, the eye, and the pharyngeal regions. Clinical signs vary with the site of infection or infestation. Larvae often are discovered in subcutaneous sites during physical examination. They usually are removed surgically by enlarging the breathing pore and removing the larva with thumb forceps. Great care must be taken not to crush the larva during extraction because anaphylaxis might result.

DIAGNOSIS.   Cuterebrosis is diagnosed by observing the characteristic swollen, cystlike subcutaneous lesion, with a fistula or central pore communicating to the outside environment. Second- or third-stage larvae usually are removed from this lesion.

Hypoderma Species (Ox Warble, Cattle Grub)

Two larval stages of *Hypoderma* flies infect cattle: *Hypoderma lineatum* and *Hypoderma bovis. H. lineatum* is found in southern United States; both species are found in northern United States and in Canada. The adult flies are heavy and resemble honeybees; the adults often are called "heel flies."

The life cycle is almost a year. Adult flies are bothersome to cattle because they approach cattle to lay eggs. Animals often become apprehensive and disturbed and attempt to escape the fly by running away, an action that is called *gadding*. The eggs are about 1 mm long and attached to hairs on the legs of cattle. *H. lineatum* deposits a row of six or more eggs on an individual hair shaft, whereas *H. bovis* lays its eggs singly. The larvae hatch in about 4 days and crawl down the hair shaft to the skin, through which they penetrate. They wander through the subcutaneous connective tissue in the leg, migrating to the esophagus (*H. lineatum*) or the region of the spinal canal and epidural fat (*H. bovis*), until they reach the subcutaneous tissues of the back. Here the larvae create breathing holes in the skin of the dorsum, through which they later exit and fall to the ground to pupate. The adult flies emerge from the pupae.

DIAGNOSIS. Adults are beelike and covered with yellow to orange hairs. Mature larvae are 25 to 30 mm long, cream to dark brown, and covered with small spines. Lesions consist of large, cyst-like swellings on the back, with a central breathing pore. As with *Cuterebra* species, great care must be taken not to crush the larva during extraction because anaphylaxis might result.

◆ Order: Siphonaptera (Fleas)

Of all the ectoparasites discussed thus far, the flea is perhaps the most economically important insect to the veterinarian; treating flea infestations can be a veterinary practice builder. Because of the extreme popularity of dogs and cats and the prolific nature of the flea (it is able to return after populations are exterminated on the animal and in the animal's environment), special attention should be paid to detecting the various life cycle stages of fleas both on the pet and in the pet's environment.

Fleas are Siphonapterans, small (4 to 5 mm in length), laterally compressed, wingless insects with powerful hind legs that are used for jumping. Figure 7-11 shows the life stages of *Ctenocephalides felis,* the cat flea. Adult fleas have piercing-sucking (siphon-like) mouthparts that are used to suck the blood of their host. Figure 7-12 shows the morphologic details of the adult female and male *C. felis,* the cat flea. More than 2000 species of fleas have been identified throughout the world. Adult fleas are always parasitic, feeding on both mammals and birds. Dogs and cats are host to comparatively few species of fleas.

C. felis, the cat flea, is the most common flea found on dogs and cats. The dog flea, *C. canis,* is uncommon and occurs far less frequently on dogs than does the cat flea.

Echidnophaga gallinacea is also known as the "stick-tight flea" of poultry (Figure 7-13). A common flea of chickens and guinea fowl, it also feeds on dogs and cats. This flea has unique feeding habits. The female flea inserts its mouthparts into the skin of the host and remains attached at that site. These specimens resemble attached ticks; however, they are indeed fleas.

Figure 7-11
Life stages of *Ctenocephalides felis,* the cat flea. *Left* to *right,* pupae, larvae, eggs, adult male and female.

Figure 7-12
Morphologic details of the adult female and male *Ctenocephalides felis,* the cat flea.

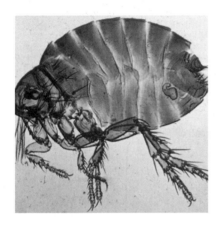

Figure 7-13
Adult *Echidnophaga gallinacea,* the stick-tight flea of poultry.

Fleas are not commonly found on horses or ruminants. In barns where feral cats abound and where excessive bedding is used, fleas have been found on calves in large numbers and can produce significant anemia. *Pulex irritans,* the human flea, has been recovered from dogs and cats, especially in the southeastern United States.

Although the adult flea is the stage most commonly encountered, the veterinary technician also may be presented with flea eggs, larval fleas, or flea droppings from the pet's environment. Flea eggs and larvae are commonly found in the owner's bedclothes, the pet's bedding, travel carriers, doghouses, or clinic cages. Flea eggs resemble tiny pearls; they are non-sticky, 0.5 mm long, white, oval, and rounded at both ends (Figure 7-14). Flea larvae resemble tiny fly maggots. They are 2 to 5 mm long, white (after feeding they become brown), and sparsely covered with hairs (Figure 7-15). Flea larvae spin a sticky, silky cocoon that often becomes covered with environmental debris. This is the pupal stage (Figure 7-16).

DIAGNOSIS.   Because adult fleas spend most of their time on the host, flea infestation is usually obvious. However, in animals with flea-allergy dermatitis, fleas may be so few on the pet as to make diagnosis of flea infestation difficult.

Figure 7-14
Eggs of *Ctenocephalides felis,* the cat flea.

Figure 7-15
Larva of *Ctenocephalides felis,* the cat flea.

Figure 7-16
Sand-covered pupae of *Ctenocephalides felis,* the cat flea.

Definitive diagnosis of flea infestation requires demonstration of the adult fleas and/or their droppings (flea dirt, flea feces, flea frass) (Figure 7-17). Adult fleas defecate large quantities of partially digested blood, commonly called "flea dirt." These feces are reddish-black and can appear as fine pepperlike specks, comma-shape columns, or long coils.

Figure 7-17
Flea dirt, flea feces, or flea frass of *Ctenocephalides felis,* the cat flea.

Adult fleas usually are encountered on the animal but also may be collected in the pet's environment. When recovered from the pet, the larger fleas with an orange to light brown abdomen are females; the smaller, darker specimens are males.

Flea collection is facilitated by spraying the pet with an insecticide. In a few minutes, dead fleas drop off the animals. Alternatively, fleas may be collected using a fine-tooth flea comb, available at any veterinary supply store or pet store.

"Flea dirt" may be used to diagnose current or recent flea infestation. To collect a sample of flea dirt, the pet should be combed with a flea comb and the collected samples placed on a white paper towel moistened with water. Rubbing the flea dirt with a fingertip causes the flea dirt to dissolve, producing a characteristic blood red or rust-red color.

CONTROL.   Flea control is important because fleas cause discomfort and irritation to the pet and serve as intermediate hosts to certain helminth parasites. Fleas serve as intermediate host for *Dipylidium caninum,* the double-pore tapeworm of dogs and cats, and as intermediate host for *Dipetalonema reconditum,* a filarial parasite that resides in the subcutaneous tissues of dogs. Some types of fleas also may transmit disease, such as bubonic plague and endemic typhus, to people.

◆ Class: Acarina (Mites and Ticks)

Mites and ticks of veterinary importance are members of the class Acarina.

Mites of Veterinary Importance

The first group of parasitic mites may be classified together as "sarcoptiform" mites. Sarcoptiform mites have several key characteristics or features in common. These mites may produce severe dermatologic problems in a variety of domestic animals. This dermatitis usually is accompanied by a severe pruritus. Sarcoptiform mites are small, barely visible to the naked eye, and approximately the size of a grain of salt. Their bodies have a round to oval shape. Sarcoptiform mites have legs with pedicels or stalks at the tip. The pedicels may be long or short. If the pedicel is long, it may be straight (unjointed) or jointed. At the tip of each pedicel, there may be a tiny sucker. Veterinarians and veterinary technicians should use the description of the pedicel (long or short, jointed or unjointed) to identify these sarcoptiform mites.

Sarcoptiform mites may be divided into two basic families: Sarcoptidae, which burrow or tunnel within the epidermis, and Psoroptidae, which reside on the surface of the skin or within the external ear canal. The Sarcoptidae includes *Sarcoptes, Notoedres,* and *Cnemidocoptes* species, whereas the Psoroptidae includes *Psoroptes, Chorioptes,* and *Otodectes* species.

FAMILY: SARCOPTIDAE. Sarcoptic mites burrow or tunnel within the epidermis of the infested definitive host. The entire four-stage life cycle is spent on the host. Male and female mites breed on the skin surface. Female mites penetrate the keratinized layers of the skin and burrow or tunnel through the epidermis. Over a 10- to 15-day period, the female deposits 40 to 50 eggs within the tunnel. After egg deposition, the female dies. Larvae emerge from the eggs in 3 to 10 days and exit the tunnel to wander on the skin surface. These larvae molt to the nymphal stage within minute pockets in the epidermis. Nymphs become sexually active adults in 12 to 17 days and the life cycle begins again.

SARCOPTES SCABIEI (SCABIES MITES). The disease caused by *Sarcoptes scabiei* is called *scabies* or *sarcoptic acariasis.* This condition is considered extremely pruritic.

Certain varieties of mites infest specific hosts. For example, *S. scabiei* variety *canis* infests only dogs, and *S. scabiei* variety *suis* infests only pigs. Almost every domestic species has its own distinct variety of this mite.

Scabies in dogs is caused by *S. scabiei* variety *canis,* which produces an erythematous, papular rash. Scaling, crusting, and excoriation are common. The ears, lateral elbows, and ventral abdomen are most likely to harbor mites. The host's entire body, however, may be infested. These mites are spread by direct contact and can affect all dogs in a household or kennel. Scabies is extremely contagious. Also, the dog owner can become infested with this mite, but the infestation in people is self-limiting. The mites burrow into human skin, producing a papulelike lesion, but they do not establish a full-blown infestation in people. This mite is considered to cause a *zoonosis,* that is, a disease that can be transmitted from animals to people. Some dogs may be asymptomatic carriers of this mite. *Sarcoptes scabiei* variety *felis,* which causes scabies in cats, is an extremely rare mite.

Among large animals, pigs most commonly are affected by scabies. Lesions caused by *Sarcoptes scabiei* variety *suis* include small, red papules, alopecia, and crusts, most commonly on the trunk and ears. Scabies in cattle (*Sarcoptes scabiei* variety *bovis*) is rare. The main infested areas are the head, neck, and shoulders. Scabies in horses (*Sarcoptes scabiei* variety *equi*) is even more rare. The main infested area is the neck. *Sarcoptes scabiei* variety *ovis* does not infest the fleece of sheep and goats; rather, the face is the main area affected.

Diagnosis.   Areas with an erythematous, papular rash and crust should be scraped, especially the areas most associated with sarcoptic infestation (ears, lateral elbows, and ventral abdomen of dogs). Repeated scrapings may be necessary to detect mites. Adult sarcoptic mites are oval and 200 to 400 μ in diameter, and have eight legs. The key morphologic feature used to identify this species is the long, unjointed pedicel with sucker on the end of some of the legs (Figure 7-18). The anus is located on the caudal end of the body. The eggs of *Sarcoptes* mites are oval (Figure 7-19).

***NOTOEDRES CATI* (FELINE SCABIES MITE).**   *Notoedres cati* infests mainly cats; but on occasion it can parasitize rabbits. This sarcoptiform mite is found chiefly on the ears, back of the neck, face, feet, and in extreme cases on the entire body. The life cycle is like that of *S. scabiei,* with the mite burrowing or tunneling in the superficial layers of the epidermis. The characteristic lesion of notoedric acariasis is a yellowing crust in the region of the ears, face, or neck.

Diagnosis.   Notoedric mites are easier to demonstrate in cats than sarcoptic mites in dogs. Likely infestation sites should be scraped. Like *Sarcoptes* species, *Notoedres* mites have a long, unjointed pedicel with sucker on the end of some of the

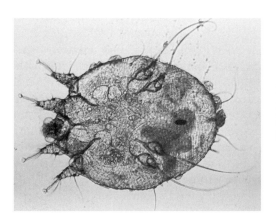

Figure 7-18
Adult *Sarcoptes scabiei* mite. Note the long, unjointed pedicels (stalks), with suckers on the ends.

Figure 7-19
Oval eggs of *Sarcoptes scabiei.* Note the emergence of a six-legged larval mite.

legs. Adult notoedric mites are similar to sarcoptic mites but are smaller, with a dorsal anus. The eggs of notoedric mites are oval.

CNEMIDOCOPTES PILAE (SCALY LEG MITE OF BUDGERIGARS). *Cnemidocoptes pilae* causes scaly leg in budgerigars or parakeets. This mite tunnels in the superficial layers of the epidermis of the pads and shanks of the feet. In severe cases the beak and cere also may be affected. The mite characteristically produces a yellow to gray-white mass that resembles a honeycomb. This condition may be disfiguring to the parakeet. The parasites pierce the skin underlying the scales, causing an inflammation with exudate that hardens on the surface and displaces the scales superficially. This process causes the thickened, scaly nature of the skin. A related species, *Cnemidocoptes mutans*, produces "scaly leg" in chickens and turkeys.

Diagnosis. Infested sites should be scraped. Great care should be taken in handling infested birds because parakeets are fragile. The eight-legged, globular mites are about 500 μ in diameter. Adult female mites have very short legs and no suckers on the end of their legs (Figure 7-20). Adult males have longer legs and a long, unjointed pedicel with suckers on the end of some of the legs.

Family: Psoroptidae

Members of the family Psoroptidae reside on the surface of the skin or within the external ear canal. The entire five-stage life cycle (egg, larva, protonymph, deutonymph or pubescent female, adult ovigerous female) is spent on the host. Adult male and female mites breed on the skin surface. The female produces 14 to 24 elliptic, opaque, shiny white eggs that hatch within 1 to 3 days. The six-legged nymphs are small, oval, soft, and grayish-brown. The eight-legged nymphs are slightly larger than larvae. Larval and nymphal stages may last 7 to 10 days. The life cycle is completed in 10 to 18 days. Under favorable conditions, psoroptic mites can live off the host for 2 to 3 weeks or longer. Under optimum conditions, mite eggs may remain viable for 2 to 4 weeks.

Figure 7-20
Adult female *Cnemidocoptes pilae* mite. The adult male has longer legs and a long, unjointed pedicel with suckers on the end of some of the legs.

PSOROPTES CUNICULI (EAR CANKER MITE OF RABBITS).   *Psoroptes cuniculi* occurs most commonly in the external ear canal of rabbits but also has been found in horses, goats, and sheep. These mites live on the surface of the skin and feed on the rabbit host by puncturing the epidermis to obtain tissue fluids. Within the external ear canal of the infested host are the characteristic dried crusts of coagulated serum. The rabbit's ears appear to be packed with dried corn flakes. Affected animals shake their head and scratch their ears. Lesions sometimes occur on the head and legs. Severely infested animals may become debilitated. Loss of equilibrium may occur, with head tilt.

   Diagnosis.   The mites within the crusty debris inside the ear can be easily isolated. The brownish-white female is large, up to 750 μ long. The mites exhibit characteristic long, jointed pedicels with suckers on the ends of some of the legs (Figures 7-21 and 7-22). The anus is in a terminal slit.

PSOROPTES SPECIES (SCAB MITE OF LARGE ANIMALS).   *Psoroptes ovis, Psoroptes bovis,* and *Psoroptes equi* are the scab mites of large animals, residing on sheep, cattle, and horses, respectively. These mites are host-specific and reside within the thick-hair or long-wool areas of the animal. They are surface dwellers and feed by puncturing the epidermis to feed on lymphatic fluid. Serum exudes through the puncture site. After the serum coagulates and forms a crust, wool is lost. The feeding site is ex-

Figure 7-21
Adult *Psoroptes cuniculi* mites.

Figure 7-22
Detail of the long, jointed pedicel on the leg of *Psoroptes cuniculi.*

tremely pruritic and the animal excoriates itself, producing further wool loss. The mites then migrate to adjacent undamaged skin. As the mites proliferate, tags of wool are pulled out and the fleece becomes matted. Finally, patches of skin are exposed and the skin becomes parchment-like, thickened, and cracked. The skin may bleed easily. Infested sheep constantly rub against fences, posts, farm equipment, and anything else that might serve as a scratching post. The disease is spread by direct contact or infested premises.

P. bovis in cattle produces lesions on the withers, neck, and rump. These consist of papules, crusts, and wrinkled, thickened skin. *P. equi* in horses is rare and affects the base of the mane and the tail.

Because of the intense pruritus and the highly contagious nature of the infestation, the occurrence of *Psoroptes* species in large animals should be reported to state and federal authorities and the United States Department of Agriculture.

Diagnosis.   These mites are host-specific. Adults are up to 600 µ long. Psoroptic mites exhibit characteristic long, jointed pedicels with suckers on the ends of some of the legs.

***CHORIOPTES* SPECIES (FOOT AND TAIL MITE, ITCHY LEG MITE).**   *C. equi, C. bovis, Chorioptes caprae,* and *Chorioptes ovis* are the foot and tail mites of large animals, residing on horses, cattle, goats, and sheep, respectively. These mites are found on the skin surface on the distal (lower) part of the hind legs but may spread to the flank and shoulder area. On cattle, they are frequently found in the tail region, especially in the area of the escutcheon. These mites do not spread rapidly or extensively. They puncture the skin, causing serum to exude. Thin crusts of coagulated serum form on the skin surface. The skin eventually wrinkles and thickens although pruritus is not severe.

Infested horses stamp, bite, and kick, especially at night. Mites typically infest the pasterns, especially those of the hind legs.

Diagnosis.   The characteristic mites can be identified from skin scrapings of infested areas. Chorioptic mites have short, unjointed pedicels, with suckers on the ends of some of the legs (Figure 7-23). The female mites are about 400 µ long.

Figure 7-23
Female and male *Chorioptes* species. Note this mite's short, unjointed pedicels.

***OTODECTES CYNOTIS* (EAR MITE).**   Ear mites, *Otodectes cynotis,* are a common cause of otitis externa in dogs and cats. Although they occur primarily in the external ear canal, ear mites may be found on any area of the body. A common infestation site is the tail and head region. As dogs and cats curl up to sleep, their head (and ears) are often in close proximity to the base of the tail. These mites are spread by direct contact and are highly transmissible both among and between the canine and feline species.

Ear mites are found within the external ear canal, where they feed on epidermal debris and produce intense irritation. Infection is usually bilateral. The host responds to the mite infestation by shaking its head and scratching its ears. Severe infestations may cause otitis media, with head tilt, circling, and convulsions. Auricular hematomas may develop.

Diagnosis.   Mites usually are identified by using an otoscope; through an otoscope the mites appear as white, motile objects. The brown exudate collected by swabbing the ear may be placed in mineral oil on a glass slide and the mites observed with a low-power microscopic objective. These mites are fairly large, approximately 400 μ; they also may be easily seen with a magnifying glass or even the unaided eye. The mites exhibit characteristic short, unjointed pedicels, with suckers on the ends of some of the legs (Figures 7-24 and 7-25). The anus is terminal.

Figure 7-24
Adult female *Otodectes cynotis* mite.

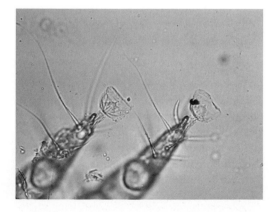

Figure 7-25
Detail of the leg of *Otodectes,* with a short, unjointed pedicel.

Miscellaneous Mites

This group of parasitic mites may be grouped together because they are not sarcoptiform mites. They can, however, produce severe dermatologic problems in a variety of domestic animals. These mites lack pedicels or stalks on their legs that are so important in identifying sarcoptiform mites.

DEMODEX SPECIES. Mites of the genus *Demodex* reside in the hair follicles and sebaceous glands of people and most domestic animals. In many species, they are considered normal, nonpathogenic fauna of the skin. These mites are host-specific and are not transmissible from one host species to another. The clinical disease, caused by an increased number of these mites, is called *demodicosis*.

Demodex mites resemble "eight-legged alligators." They are elongated mites with short, stubby legs. Adult and nymphal stages have eight legs, whereas the larvae have six. Adult *Demodex* mites are approximately 250 µ long (Figure 7-26). The eggs are spindle-shape or tapered at each end (Figure 7-27).

The life cycle of *Demodex* species has five stages: egg, larva, protonymph, deutonymph, and adult. The developmental periods of these various life cycle stages are not well known.

Figure 7-26
Adult *Demodex canis* mite.

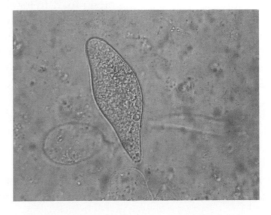

Figure 7-27
Egg of *Demodex canis*.

Of all the domestic animals infested with *Demodex* species, the dog is the most commonly and most seriously infested. Small numbers of these mites are considered part of the normal skin flora of all dogs. In dogs with immunodeficiencies, however, these mites proliferate and cause skin disease.

Demodicosis occurs in two forms in dogs: localized demodicosis and generalized demodicosis. The predominant clinical sign of the localized form is patchy alopecia, especially of the muzzle, face, and forelimbs. The mites presumably are acquired during intimate contact when the puppy nurses the dam. As a result of that close contact, localized demodicosis often develops in the region of the face. Generalized demodicosis is characterized by diffuse alopecia, erythema, and secondary bacterial contamination over the entire body surface of the dog. An inherited defect in the dog's immune system is thought to be an important factor in development of generalized demodicosis.

Cats are infested by two species of demodectic mites: *Demodex cati* and an unnamed species. *D. cati* is an elongated mite, similar to *D. canis*. The unnamed species has a broad, blunted abdomen, as compared with the elongated one of *D. cati*. The presence of either species on the skin of cats is rare. In localized feline demodicosis are patchy areas of alopecia, erythema, and occasionally crusting on the head (especially around the eyes), ears, and neck. In generalized feline demodicosis, the alopecia, erythema, and crusting usually involve the entire body. Demodicosis also has been associated with ceruminous otitis externa.

Demodectic mites reside in the hair follicles of other species of domestic animals but rarely produce clinical disease. Cattle and goats are most commonly infested but then only rarely.

In cattle, *Demodex bovis* causes large nodules (abscesses) on the shoulders, trunk, and lateral aspects of the neck. In goats, *Demodex caprae* occurs in small papular or nodular lesions on the shoulders, trunk, and lateral aspect of the neck. In sheep, *Demodex ovis* rarely causes pustules and crusting around the coronet, nose, ear tips, and periorbital areas. In pigs, *Demodex phylloides* rarely produces pustules and nodules on the face, abdomen, and ventral neck. In horses, *Demodex equi* occurs around the face and eyes and rarely produces clinical disease.

Diagnosis. Skin areas with altered pigmentation, obstructed hair follicles, erythema, or alopecia should always be scraped. In localized demodicosis, the areas most commonly affected are the forelegs, perioral region, and periorbital regions. In generalized demodicosis, the entire body may be affected; however, the face and feet usually are the most severely involved. In dogs, areas of apparently normal skin also should be scraped to determine if the disease is generalized. The areas should be clipped and a fold of skin gently squeezed to express any mites from the hair follicles. Scraping should be continued until capillary blood oozing is observed because these mites live deep in the hair follicles and sebaceous glands (Figure 7-28).

Nodular lesions in large animals should be incised with a scalpel and the caseous material within smeared on a slide with mineral oil, covered with a coverslip, and examined microscopically for mites.

The mites on the slide should be counted and the live:dead ratio determined. The presence of any larval or nymphal stages or eggs should be noted. During therapy for

Demodex species, a decrease in the number of eggs and live mites is a good prognostic indicator.

CHEYLETIELLA SPECIES (WALKING DANDRUFF). Mites of the genus *Cheyletiella* are surface dwelling (nonburrowing), residing in the keratin layer of the skin and in the haircoat of the definitive host, which may be a dog, cat, or rabbit. These mites ingest keratin debris and tissue fluids. *Cheyletiella* mites are sometimes referred to as "walking dandruff" because the mites resemble large, mobile flakes of dandruff. Cheylettid mites have distinct key morphologic features. They are large (386 by 266 μ) and visible to the naked eye. With the compound microscope, their most characteristic key morphologic feature may easily be seen: their enormous hooklike accessory mouthparts (palpi). These palpi assist the mite in attaching to the host as it feeds on tissue fluids. The mite also has comblike structures at the tip of each leg. Members of the genus also are known for their characteristic body shape resembling a shield, a bell pepper, an oak acorn, or a western horse saddle when viewed from above (Figure 7-29). Eggs are 235 to 245 μ long and 115 to 135 μ wide (smaller than louse nits) and supported by cocoonlike structures bound to the host's hair shaft by strands of fibers. Two or three eggs may be bound together on one hair shaft.

Figure 7-28
A deep skin scraping produces numerous mites of *Demodex canis.*

Figure 7-29
Adult *Cheyletiella* mite.

Diagnosis.   The key feature of *Cheyletiella* species infestation is often the moving white "dandruff" flakes along the dorsal midline and head of the host. A hand-held magnifying lens or Optivisor (binocular headband magnifier) often are used to view questionable flakes or hairs; these are perhaps the quickest methods of diagnosing cheyletiellosis. A fine-tooth flea comb may be used to collect mites; combing dandruff-like debris onto black paper often facilitates visualization of these highly mobile mites. Using clear cellophane tape to entrap mites collected from the haircoat often simplifies viewing with the compound microscope.

***LYNXACARUS RADOVSKYI* (FELINE FUR MITE).**   *Lynxacarus radovskyi,* the feline fur mite, is found attached to the shafts of individual hairs on the back, neck, thorax, and hind limbs of cats residing in tropical or warm areas of the United States, such as Florida, Puerto Rico, and Hawaii. These fur mites are laterally compressed. The adults are approximately 500 μ long (Figure 7-30). Pruritus is not always associated with infestations of L. *radovskyi* in cats. This mite also may affect humans who handle infested cats, producing a papular dermatitis.

Diagnosis.   These mites are diagnosed by observation of the mites attached to individual hair shafts and by examination of the dander and other debris after combing.

***TROMBICULA* SPECIES (CHIGGER).**   The chigger (*Trombicula* species) is yellow to red, has six legs, and is 200 to 400 μ in diameter. The larval stage is the only developmental stage that parasitizes people, domestic animals, and wild animals. The larvae are most common in the late summer and early fall and are transmitted by direct contact with the ground or with foliage in fields or heavy underbrush. Nymphal and adult chiggers are nonparasitic and are free living in nature.

Chigger larvae do not burrow into the skin as commonly believed nor do they feed primarily on host blood. Their food consists of the serous components of tissues. Chiggers attach firmly to the host and inject a digestive fluid that liquefies host cells. The host's skin becomes hardened and a tube called a *stylostome* forms at the chigger's attachment site. Chiggers suck the liquefied host tissues. When the mite has finished feeding, it loosens its grip and falls to the ground. The injected digestive fluid causes the attachment site to itch intensely. Cutaneous lesions tend to be restricted

Figure 7-30
Adult *Lynxacarus radovskyi,* the feline fur mite, attaches to the hair shafts on the back, neck, thorax, and hind limbs of cats.

to areas of the body that come in contact with the ground, such as the limbs, inter-digital areas, and ventrum, in addition to the head and ears.

The most common chigger mite affecting animals and people is *Trombicula alfreddugesi* (the North American chigger). Lesions consist of an erythematous, often pruritic papular rash on the ventrum, face, feet, and legs.

Diagnosis. Chigger infestation (trombiculosis) is diagnosed by an orange, crusting dermatosis, a history of exposure (roaming the outdoors), and identification or the typical six-legged larvae in skin scrapings or on collection from the host. The larvae remain attached to the skin only for several hours. Consequently, trombiculosis may be difficult to diagnose because the pruritus persists after the larvae have dropped.

PNEUMONYSSOIDES (PNEUMONYSSUS) CANINUM (NASAL MITE OF DOGS).

Pneumonyssoides (Pneumonyssus) caninum is a rare mite that lives in the nasal passages and associated sinuses of dogs. Nasal mites are generally considered to be nonpathogenic; however, reddening of the nasal mucosa, sneezing, head shaking and rubbing the nose often accompany infestation. Fainting, labored breathing, asthma-like attacks, and orbital disease have been associated with this mite. Sinusitis caused by these mites may lead to disorders of the central nervous system. Owners may observe these mites exiting the animal's nostrils.

The life cycle is unknown, but it apparently takes place entirely within the host. Adult males, adult females, and larvae have been identified, but no nymphal stages have been observed. Transmission probably occurs via direct contact with an infested animal.

Diagnosis. The mites are oval and pale yellow. They measure 1 to 1.5 mm by 0.6 to 0.9 mm. They have a smooth cuticle, with few hairs. The larvae have six legs and the adults have eight legs. All legs are located on the cranial half of the body.

ORNITHONYSSUS SYLVIARUM (NORTHERN MITE OF POULTRY) AND DERMANYSSUS GALLINAE (RED MITE OF POULTRY).

These two mites parasitize poultry, but they differ in the sites they tend to infest. *Ornithonyssus sylviarum* is a 1-mm, elongated to oval mite usually found on birds but also may be found in their nests or houses. They feed intermittently on the birds, producing irritation, weight loss, decreased egg production, anemia, and even death. These mites have been known to bite people.

Dermanyssus gallinae is another 1-mm, elongated to oval, whitish, grayish or black mite that feeds on birds. This mite has a distinct red color when it has recently fed on its host's blood. *D. gallinae* lays its eggs in cracks and crevices in the walls of poultry houses. Nymphs and adults are periodic parasites, hiding in the crevices of the poultry houses and making frequent visits to the host to feed. Because of their blood-feeding activity, they may produce significant anemia and much irritation to the host. Infested birds are listless and egg production may drop. Loss of blood may result in death. These mites also occur in birds' nests in the eaves of houses or in air conditioners. The mites can migrate into homes and infest people.

Diagnosis.   *O. sylviarum* usually is found on the avian host, whereas *D. gallinae* is a periodic parasite, usually found in the host's environment. Specimens should be cleared in lactophenol and the anal plates examined with a compound microscope. The anus of *O. sylviarum* is on the cranial half of the anal plate, whereas the anus of *D. gallinae* is on the caudal half.

Ticks of Veterinary Importance

Ticks are small- to medium-size acarines with dorsoventrally compressed, leathery bodies. The tick's head, the capitulum, has cutting organs called *chelicerae,* a penetrating, anchorlike sucking organ, the hypostome, and four accessory appendages, two chelicerae and two pedipalps, which act as sensors and supports when the tick fastens to the host's body. The tick's body may be partially or entirely covered by a hard, chitinous plate, the scutum. Mouthparts may be concealed under the tick's body or may extend from the cranial border. Most ticks are inornate; that is, they are reddish or mahogany, without markings. Some species are ornate; that is, they have distinctive white patterns on the dark scutum background. Adult ticks have eight legs, with claws on the ends of the legs.

Ticks are important parasites because of their voracious blood feeding activity. They are important also because they can transmit many parasitic, bacterial, viral, and other diseases, such as borreliosis (Lyme disease), among animals and from animals to people. These pathogenic organisms may be transmitted passively or the tick may serve as an obligatory intermediate host.

The salivary secretions of some female ticks are toxic and can produce a syndrome known as "tick paralysis" in people and animals. Tick species commonly associated with tick paralysis are *Dermacentor andersoni* (the Rocky Mountain spotted fever tick), *Dermacentor occidentalis* (the Pacific Coast tick), *Ixodes holocyclis* (the paralysis tick of Australia), and *Dermacentor variabilis* (the wood tick).

Ticks of veterinary importance may be divided into two families: the Argasid, or soft, ticks and the Ixodid, or hard, ticks. Argasid ticks lack a scutum, or hard, chitinous plate. The mouthparts of the adults cannot be seen when viewed from the dorsal aspect. Ixodid ticks have a hard, chitinous scutum that covers all of the male tick's dorsum and about a third or less of the female's dorsum. Depending on the degree of engorgement, male ticks are much smaller than female ticks.

Two species of Argasid ticks are important: *Otobius megnini* (the spinose ear tick) and *Argas persicus* (the fowl tick). Thirteen economically important tick species are in the Ixodid family. These include *Rhipicephalus sanguineus, Ixodes scapularis, Dermacentor* species, and *Amblyomma* species. Of these species, only *R. sanguineus* infests buildings; the remaining ticks attack their hosts outdoors.

Specific identification of ticks is difficult and should be performed by a veterinary parasitologist or a trained arthropodologist. Ticks usually are identified by the shape and length of the capitulum, the shape and color of the body, and the shape and markings on the scutum. Male and unengorged female ticks are easier to identify than engorged females. Determining the species of larval or nymphal ticks is most difficult.

Common species may be identified by their size, shape, color, body markings, host, and location on the host.

Four major stages exist in the life cycle of ticks: egg, larva, nymph, and adult. After engorgement on the host, female ticks drop off the host and seek protected places, such as within cracks and crevices or under leaves and branches to lay their eggs (Figure 7-31). The six-legged larvae, or *seed ticks,* hatch from the eggs and feed on a host (Figure 7-32). The larva molts to the eight-legged nymphal stage, which resembles the adult stage but lacks the functioning reproductive organs of the adult stage. After one or two blood meals, the nymph matures and molts to the adult stage. During the larval, nymphal, and adult stages, ticks may infest one to three or even many different host species. This ability to feed on several hosts during the life cycle plays an important role in the transmission of disease pathogens among hosts. Any infestation of domestic animals by mites or ticks is referred to as *acariasis.*

Most ticks do not tolerate direct sunlight, dryness, or excessive rainfall. They can survive as long as 2 to 3 years without a blood meal, but females require blood before egg fertilization and deposition. Tick activity is restricted during the cold winter months.

Figure 7-31
Adult female *Dermacentor variabilis* tick laying hundreds of eggs.

Figure 7-32
Six-legged larval *Rhipicephalus sanguineus.*

ARGASID (SOFT) TICKS

Otobius megnini (spinose ear tick). *Otobius megnini,* the spinose ear tick, is an unusual soft tick in that only the larval and nymphal stages are parasitic. The adult stages are not parasitic but are free living, found in the environment of the definitive host, usually in dry, protected places, in cracks and crevices, under logs, and on fence posts. The larval and nymphal stages feed on horses, cattle, sheep, goats, and dogs. These ticks usually are associated with the semiarid or arid areas of the southwestern United States. With widespread interstate movement of animals, this soft tick may occur throughout North America. As with most soft ticks, the mouthparts may not be visible when viewed from the dorsal aspect (Figure 7-33). The nymphal stage is widest in the middle, almost violin shape. It is covered with tiny, backward-projecting spines, which is the origin of the name *spinose.* Larvae and nymphs usually are found within the ears of the definitive host, which is the origin of the name ear tick.

Spinose ear ticks are extremely irritating to the definitive host. They often occur in large numbers, deep within the external ear canal. These ticks imbibe large amounts of host blood; however, because they are soft ticks, they do not enlarge with feeding. Large numbers may produce ulceration deep within the ear. The ears become highly sensitive and the animals may shake their head. The pinnae may become excoriated by the animal's shaking and rubbing its head.

Diagnosis. The ticks may be visualized in the ear with an otoscope. Any waxy exudate should be examined for larval and nymphal spinose ear ticks.

Argas persicus (fowl tick). *Argas persicus,* the fowl tick, is a soft tick of chickens, turkeys, and wild birds. These ticks are periodic parasites, hiding in cracks and crevices during the day and becoming active during the night, when they feed intermittently on the avian host. The adults are 7 mm long and 5 mm wide. In the unengorged state, they are reddish brown. After engorgement, they are slate blue. These ticks are flat and leathery, and the tegument is covered with tiny bumps. As soft ticks, they lack a scutum. The mouthparts are not visible when the adult tick is viewed from the dorsal aspect.

Heavily infested birds may develop anemia. These ticks are worrisome to birds, particularly at night. Egg production by hens may decrease or cease.

Figure 7-33
Otobius megnini, *the spinose ear tick, is an unusual soft tick in that only the larval and nymphal stages are parasitic. These mouthparts may not be visible when viewed from the dorsal aspect.*

Diagnosis. All stages of this tick may be collected from birds, but they usually are found in cracks, crevices, and contaminated bedding in poultry houses.

IXODID (HARD) TICKS

Rhipicephalus sanguineus (brown dog tick). *Rhipicephalus sanguineus,* the brown dog tick, is an unusual hard tick; it may invade both kennel and household environments. This tick is distributed throughout North America. It has an inornate, uniformly reddish-brown scutum, and it feeds almost exclusively on dogs. *R. sanguineus* also has a distinguishing morphologic feature. Its basis capitulum has prominent lateral extensions that give this structure a decidedly hexagonal appearance (Figure 7-34). The engorged female is often slate gray. In southern climates, the tick is found outdoors, but in northern climates it becomes a serious household pest, breeding indoors.

The bites of this tick can irritate dogs. Severe infestations may cause heavy blood loss. This tick is also an intermediate host for *Babesia canis,* the agent that causes piroplasmosis in dogs.

Diagnosis. This tick may be identified by its inornate brown color and characteristic lateral projections of the basis capitulum. These ticks are unique; they may be found in indoor or kennel environments.

Dermacentor variabilis (American dog tick, wood tick). *Dermacentor variabilis,* the American dog tick or wood tick, is found primarily in the eastern two thirds of the United States; however, with increased mobility of American households, the tick may occur throughout the country. Unlike *R. sanguineus,* this tick only inhabits grassy, scrub brush areas, especially roadsides and pathways. This three-host tick initially feeds on small mammals and rodents; however, dogs (and people) can serve as hosts for this ubiquitous tick. This tick is a seasonal annoyance to people and domestic animals. It can serve as a vector of Rocky Mountain spotted fever, tularemia, and other diseases, and

Figure 7-34
Lateral expansion of the basis capitulum (base of the head) (*arrows*) of an adult *Rhipicephalus sanguineus.* This key morphologic feature is used to identify this parasite, which can breed in the host's environment.

may also produce tick paralysis in animals and people. This tick has a dark brown, ornate scutum, with white striping. Unfed adults are approximately 6 mm long, whereas adult engorged females are about 12 mm long and blue-gray (Figure 7-35).

Diagnosis.   This tick may be identified by its morphologic features. It has a rectangular base of the capitulum and characteristic white markings on the dorsal shield.

Amblyomma americanum (lone star tick).   *Amblyomma americanum,* the Lone Star tick, gets its common name from a characteristic white spot on the apex of its scutum. The spot is more conspicuous on male ticks than on female ticks. This tick is distributed throughout the southern United States but is found also in the Midwest and on the Atlantic coast.

This three-host tick is found most often in the spring and summer months, parasitizing the head, belly, and flanks of wild and domestic animal hosts. It also feeds on people and is said to have a painful bite. It can produce anemia and has been incriminated as a vector of tularemia and Rocky Mountain spotted fever.

Diagnosis.   *A. americanum* is easily identified by a characteristic white spot on the apex of the scutum.

Amblyomma maculatum (Gulf Coast tick).   *Amblyomma maculatum,* the Gulf Coast tick, is a three-host tick found in the ears of cattle, horses, sheep, dogs, and people. It occurs in areas of high humidity on the Atlantic and Gulf coasts. It produces severe bites and painful swellings and also is associated with tick paralysis. This tick has silvery markings on its scutum. Larval and nymphal stages occur on ground birds throughout the year. The number of adult ticks on cattle decreases during the winter and spring and increases in the summer and fall. When the ear canals of cattle and horses are infested, the pinna may droop and become deformed.

Diagnosis.   *A. maculatum* is easily identified by the silvery markings on its scutum (Figure 7-36).

Boophilus annulatus (Texas cattle fever tick).   *Boophilus annulatus* is often called the *Texas cattle fever tick* or the *North American tick.* This one-host tick has historical significance in that it is the first arthropod shown to serve as an intermediate host for a protozoan parasite, *Babesia bigemina* of cattle, a milestone in veterinary parasitology. This tick has been completely eradicated from the United States; however, any *Boophilus* species infestation should be reported to the proper regulatory agencies. The tick should be identified by a specialist and control methods applied. *B. annulatus* frequently enters the United States from Mexico.

The engorged female is 10 to 12 mm long and the male 3 to 4 mm. The mouthparts are short and no festoons are on the caudal aspect of the abdomen.

Because this is a one-host tick, larvae, nymphs, and adult ticks may be found on the same animal. They do not have to leave the host to complete the life cycle. Animals with heavy infestations are restless and irritated. In an attempt to rid themselves of

Figure 7-35
Adult female *Dermacentor variabilis.* Unfed adults are approximately 6 mm long, while engorged adult females are about 12 mm long and a blue-gray color.

Figure 7-36
Ornate adult male *Amblyomma maculatum.*

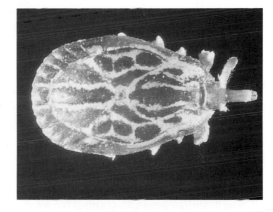

ticks, they rub, lick, bite, and scratch themselves. Irritated areas may become raw and secondarily infected. Heavily infested cattle may become anemic.

Diagnosis. Suspect ticks from an enzootic area or from animals originating from the Texas-Mexico border should be submitted to a laboratory recommended by regulatory agencies.

PHYLUM: NEMATODA (ROUNDWORMS)

◆ Class: Secernentea

The next part of this chapter discusses the superfamilies belonging to the class Secernentea and how these skin-dwelling parasites are relevant to veterinary practice.

Superfamily: Rhabditoidea

PELODERA STRONGYLOIDES (FREE-LIVING SAPROPHYTIC NEMATODE). *Pelodera strongyloides* is a free-living saprophytic nematode that normally lives in moist soil. These are facultative parasites. They are normally free living; however, under certain circumstances, they can invade mammalian skin and develop to a parasitic existence. Male and female adult *P. strongyloides* nematodes are found in soil mixed with moist organic debris, such as straw. The females produce eggs that hatch into first-stage larvae. These larvae invade the superficial layers of damaged or scarified skin, producing mild dermatitis. The skin may become reddened, denuded, and covered with a crusty material. Occasionally a pustular dermatitis develops. Because dogs become infested by lying on contaminated soil, these lesions usually are observed on the ventrum or medial (inner) surface of the limbs. Larvae of *P. strongyloides* also may be recovered from the skin of cattle recumbent on soil containing these larvae.

Diagnosis.   These larvae (and possibly adults) can be identified in superficial skin scrapings. Larvae of *P. strongyloides* are 596 to 600 μ long. These larvae must be differentiated from the microfilariae of the canine heartworm, *D. immitis*, the microfilariae of *D. reconditum*, and the first-stage larvae of *Dracunculus insignis*.

Superfamily: Spiruroidea (Spirurid Nematodes)

HABRONEMA AND DRASCHIA SPECIES.   Adult *Habronema* nematodes are found on the stomach mucosa of horses, under a thick layer of mucus. Adult *Draschia* species produce large, fibrous nodules in the equine stomach wall; the nematodes reside within the nodules. The adults do not parasitize the skin; however, their larval stages can be deposited by flies (*Musca domestica, Stomoxys calcitrans*) into skin wounds on horses. Here the larvae produce a condition known as "cutaneous habronemiasis," "cutaneous draschiasis," or "summer sores."

The lesions vary in size and have an uneven surface consisting of a soft, reddish-brown material covering a mass of firmer granulations. These lesions are seen on body parts most susceptible to trauma, such as the legs, withers, male genitalia, and medial canthus of the eye. Infested wounds tend to increase in size and do not respond to ordinary treatment until the following winter, when they spontaneously heal.

Diagnosis.   Diagnosis of cutaneous habronemiasis is based on clinical signs and skin biopsies, which may reveal cross or longitudinal sections of these aberrant *Habronema* or *Draschia* larvae.

Superfamily: Filarioidea (Filarial Nematodes)

ONCHOCERCA CERVICALIS.   Microfilariae of *Onchocerca cervicalis*, the filarial parasite of horses, produce recurrent dermatitis and periodic ophthalmia. The adults live in the ligamentum nuchae. Females produce microfilariae that migrate to the dermis via connective tissue. This parasite is spread by the biting midge, *Culicoides* species. The midge feeds on a horse's blood and ingests the microfilariae, which develop to the infective third stage within the fly. When the fly bites another horse, larvae are injected into the connective tissue and develop to adults during migration to the ligamentum nuchae.

The characteristic signs of cutaneous onchocerciasis include patchy alopecia, scaling on the head, neck, shoulders, and ventral midline, and sometimes intense pruritus.

Many infected horses are asymptomatic. Microfilariae of *Onchocerca* species concentrate in certain areas, with the ventral midline the most common area of concentration. Because more than 90% of normal hosts are probably infected with *O. cervicalis*, detection of microfilariae in the skin of the ventral midline is not diagnostic for cutaneous onchocerciasis. However, the presence of microfilariae in diseased skin is highly indicative, though not diagnostic, of cutaneous onchocerciasis.

Diagnosis. *Onchocerca* microfilariae may be demonstrated by the following procedure. After clipping the skin site and performing a surgical scrub, a 6-mm punch biopsy is used to obtain a skin sample (see Skin Biopsy, Chapter 12). With a single-edge razor blade or scalpel blade, half of the tissue is minced in a small amount of preservative-free physiologic saline on a glass slide and allowed to stand for 5 to 10 minutes. Drying of the specimen is prevented by placing the slide in a covered chamber with a small amount of saline. The slide is then examined with a low-power (10×) objective. Because the translucent microfilariae are difficult to observe, low-intensity light and high contrast (achieved by lowering the condenser) are essential. Live microfilariae are identified by their vigorous swimming activity at the edge of the tissue. *O. cervicalis* microfilariae are slender and 207 to 140 μ long. The other half of the biopsy should be submitted for routine histopathologic examination.

STEPHANOFILARIA STILESI. *Stephanofilaria stilesi* is a small nematode found in the skin of ruminants, such as cattle, goats, and buffalo, and of wild mammals. It commonly causes dermatitis along the ventral midline of cattle in the United States. The infective larvae are transmitted by the bites of horn flies, *Haematobia irritans*. The skin lesions are thought to be caused by both adult and microfilarial stages.

The lesions caused by *S. stilesi* are located near the umbilicus and consist of small, red papules initially. Later, the lesions develop into large pruritic areas (up to 25 cm) of alopecia, with thick, moist crusts.

Diagnosis. The adults (less than 6 mm long) and microfilariae may be found in deep skin scrapings after the crusts have been removed from the lesions.

DIPETALONEMA RECONDITUM (SUBCUTANEOUS FILARIAL PARASITE OF DOGS). Adult *Dipetalonema reconditum* is a nonpathogenic parasite that resides in the subcutaneous tissues of the dog. It also may be found within a body cavity. Occasional subcutaneous abscesses and ulcerated areas have been associated with this parasite. The intermediate host for this parasite is the flea, *C. felis*. Because this parasite is found in enzootic areas where *D. immitis* is present, it is necessary to differentiate the microfilariae of these two filarial parasites (see Chapter 6).

Diagnosis. Adults of *D. reconditum* rarely are recovered from their subcutaneous sites. Microfilariae may be recovered rarely in deep skin scrapings that draw blood. When subjected to the modified Knott's procedure, the microfilariae of *D. reconditum*

Figure 7-37
Aberrant adult *Dirofilaria immitis* heartworm in a subcutaneous interdigital cyst in a dog.

average about 285 μ long, with a button-hook tail and a blunt (broom handle–shape) cranial end. They must be differentiated from microfilariae of *D. immitis,* first-stage larvae of *Pelodera strongyloides,* and first-stage larvae of *Dracunculus insignis.*

***DIROFILARIA IMMITIS* (CANINE HEARTWORM).** *Dirofilaria immitis,* the canine heartworm, normally resides in the right ventricle and pulmonary arteries of its definitive host, the dog. Adult heartworms also may occur aberrantly and may be found in a variety of extravascular sites, including cystic spaces in the subcutaneous sites (Figure 7-37). When adult heartworms are found aberrantly, they are usually single, immature, isolated worms. Any female heartworms found within the cyst have not been fertilized by a male heartworm. Therefore such females are not gravid and do not produce microfilariae.

Adult female heartworms in the right ventricle and pulmonary arteries may produce microfilariae after mating with adult males. These microfilariae may be recovered occasionally in deep skin scrapings that draw blood.

Diagnosis. Aberrant adult *D. immitis* heartworms within cystic spaces in the skin can be removed surgically. When subjected to the modified Knott's procedure, the microfilariae of *D. immitis* are 310 to 320 μ long, with a straight tail and tapering cranial end. They must be differentiated from the microfilariae of *D. reconditum,* first-stage larvae of *Pelodera strongyloides,* and first-stage larvae of *Dracunculus insignis.*

Superfamily: Dracunculoidea

***DRACUNCULUS INSIGNIS* (GUINEA WORM).** *Dracunculus insignis,* the Guinea worm, is a nematode found in the skin of dogs. The adult female nematode resides subcutaneously and produces a draining, ulcerous lesion in the skin,

Figure 7-38
Unique first-stage larva of *Dracunculus insignis*. These larvae are 500 μ to 750 μ long and have a characteristic long tail.

usually on the dog's limb. The cranial end of the female worm extends from this ulcer. When the female worm within the lesion comes in contact with water, its uterus prolapses through the worm's cranial end and ruptures, releasing a mass of first-stage larvae into the water. These larvae are 500 to 750 μ long and have a unique, long tail (Figure 7-38). The larvae are ingested by tiny crustaceans in the water; within the crustaceans, the larvae develop to the infective third stage. Dogs become infected with D. insignis by drinking water containing the infected crustaceans.

Diagnosis. If *D. insignis* infection is suspected, the ulcer with its associated worm should be dipped in cool water. The cool water is a stimulus for the female worm to expel her larvae. The water containing expelled larvae should be centrifuged and the sediment examined for the characteristic first-stage larvae. Larvae of *D. insignis* must be differentiated from the microfilariae of *D. immitis*, microfilariae of *D. reconditum*, and first-stage larvae of *P. strongyloides*. Once identified, the adult female worm may be removed surgically.

PHYLUM: ANNELIDA (SEGMENTED WORMS)

◆ Class: Hirudinea (Leeches)

Order: Gnathobdellida

HIRUDO MEDICINALIS **(MEDICINAL LEECH).** Leeches are annelids; they are not considered to be true helminths but are often described as *parasitic worms*. As ectoparasites of people, domestic animals, and wild animals, leeches are members of the phylum Annelida and the class Hirudinea. Leeches may have a pathologic or beneficial role in veterinary medicine.

The term *hirudiniasis* is derived from the classic Linnaean nomenclature and is defined as invasion of the nose, mouth, pharynx, or larynx by leeches, or the attachment of leeches to the skin. Leeches are voracious blood feeders; depending on the number that attach to the host, the host may become anemic and may die from blood loss. Leeches have recently gained favor as postsurgical tools in reconstructive and microvascular surgery. *H. medicinalis,* the medicinal leech, has been used in reconstructive and microvascular surgery in people; such use in veterinary medicine is forthcoming.

Diagnosis.   Leeches are segmented worms with slender, leaf-shape bodies devoid of bristles. A typical leech has two suckers, a large and adhesive caudal sucker and a smaller cranial one that surrounds the mouth. Most leeches are found in fresh water and a few in salt water; some are terrestrial varieties.

Recommended Reading

Bowman DD, Lynn RC, Georgi JR: *Georgi's parasitology for veterinarians,* ed 7, Philadelphia, 1999, WB Saunders.

Hendrix CM: *Diagnostic veterinary parasitology,* ed 2, St Louis, 1998, Mosby.

Sloss MW et al: *Veterinary clinical parasitology,* ed 6, Ames, Iowa, 1994, Iowa State University Press.

Function Tests

RAFAEL RUIZ DE GOPEGUI
BERNARD FELDMAN

Function tests are challenges: they provoke organs to demonstrate their operational integrity. Because they probe function, these tests may discover abnormalities that are latent or even disguised in other clinical data. A single test may be employed to examine different links in this chain. The veterinary technician must be familiar with these links to identify which links have failed when a test result is abnormal.

Most function tests involve direct observation of a traceable substance in the body. Prerequisite to interpretation of alterations are an understanding of the normal path of this substance and the values deemed normal by the reference laboratory. If normal values are unavailable, normal control samples should accompany each test procedure; otherwise the data obtained may be misleading and/or useless.

Four main types of function tests exist: gastrointestinal, hepatic, renal, and endocrine. Pulmonary function tests are also important but are performed in specialized hospitals only.

TESTS OF GASTROINTESTINAL FUNCTION

The principal functions of the gastrointestinal (GI) tract are the assimilation of nutrients (digestion and/or absorption) and excretion of waste products. Most nutrients are ingested in a form either too complex or insoluble for absorption. Within the GI tract these substances are solubilized and degraded enzymatically to simple molecules that may be absorbed across the mucosal epithelium.

Gastrointestinal diseases are common in veterinary practice. Specific diagnosis is essential, especially when the disease is chronic. In cases of malabsorption, intestinal biopsy tends to be required to obtain a definitive diagnosis. However, function tests are performed previously to rule out other diseases and confirm the need of more invasive diagnostic procedures. Therefore function tests are useful in guiding treatment.

Malassimilation may be classified by pathophysiologic process into maldigestive or malabsorptive forms. *Maldigestion* results from altered gastric secretion and lack of

365

or decreased amounts of digestive enzymes, usually secreted by the pancreas and, less often, the intestinal mucosa. *Malabsorption* most often is caused by an acquired disease of the small intestinal wall or by bacterial overgrowth syndromes. Before clinical signs of maldigestion are seen, about 90% of the pancreas must be either nonfunctional or destroyed. The small intestine of a dog can function well with up to 85% loss, but greater than 50% loss may result in "short bowel syndrome" that cannot be compensated for by adaptive mechanisms.

Laboratory tests may evaluate gastric hydrochloric acid secretion, but most of them are directed to detect malassimilation and its origin. Gastric acid secretion also may be indirectly estimated by determining gastric juice pH; normal dogs have a fasting gastric pH from 0.9 to 2.5. Gastric juice pH may be continuously monitored by radiotelemetric technique.[1]

Malassimilation tests are based on examination of feces for fecal dietary nutrients, fecal enzyme activities, and serum for concentrations of orally administered substrates or metabolites and specific tests for endogenous substances.

◆ Gastrin Secretion

The diagnosis of Zollinger-Ellison syndrome (gastrinoma) may be required after identification of gastrointestinal ulceration and amine precursor uptake and decarboxylation (APUD), neoplasia (prevalently located in the pancreas), and the assessment of high serum gastrin concentrations. However, some cases may require provocative tests to document the excessive gastrin secretion. Stimulation of gastrin secretion may be accomplished by test meal, intravenous calcium infusion, or intravenous secretin infusion. Serum samples for gastrin determination must be obtained before, 2, 5, 15, and 30 minutes after intravenous administration of 2 to 4 IU/kg of secretin. A positive test is considered if twofold increase gastrin concentration occurs 2 and/or 5 minutes after administration.[2]

◆ Fecal Examination

The senses of sight and smell must not be ignored. First insights into GI function come from simple fecal examinations. In this case, the functional challenge is provided by the patient's diet; no clinical intervention is needed. Grossly, stools may reveal excess fat (*steatorrhea*). They may be bulky, pale, and malodorous, especially with severe pancreatic insufficiency.

◆ Microscopic Examination

Microscopic examination explores these abnormalities or reveals them when the stool appears normal. Procedure 8-1 shows a protocol for microscopic examination. Performance of these tests on a normal animal eating the same diet as the patient is useful for comparison. These tests are qualitative and they point the veterinarian in the right direction. Fecal fat, starch, and muscle tests vary with diet content and intestinal motility. It is wise to repeat them.

PROCEDURE **8-1**

Protocol for microscopic examination of feces

Fecal Neutral Fat

1. Add 2 drops of water to a stool sample on a glass slide and mix.
2. Add 2 drops of 95% ethanol with several drops of saturated Sudan III or IV stain in 95% ethanol.
3. Mix, apply coverslip, and examine for more than a few red-orange droplets.

Fecal Free Fatty Acids

1. Add several drops of glacial acetic acid to a stool sample on a glass slide and mix.
2. Add several drops of Sudan III or IV stain, mix, apply coverslip, and heat gently over a Bunsen burner until it just bubbles.
3. Air cool and repeat two to three times.
4. Examine for more than a few red-orange droplets.

Fecal Starch and Muscle Fiber

1. Mix a stool sample with several drops of Lugol's iodine on a glass slide.
2. Apply a coverslip.
3. Examine for blunt, striated muscle fibers or blue-black starch granules. Muscle fiber also may be seen in unstained smears.

Of the nutrients, absorption of fat is the least physiologically efficient; the entire small intestine is required. Steatorrhea, then, is a forerunner and accompaniment of nearly all malabsorption syndromes. Steatorrhea of neutral fats (undigested/nonsplit) is revealed by treating the stool with Sudan III or IV stains. Large oil globules stain red-orange. Up to two or three such globules normally are found per high-power field (HPF, 40× objective). Larger numbers suggest pancreatic lipase deficiency.

Digested fats (free fatty acids/split fats) do not color with Sudan stains unless acidification (acetic acid 36%) and heat melt them into neutral droplets that stain as above. Again, more than two or three droplets per high-power field indicate malfunction, particularly intestinal malassimilation. Fecal protease activity should be present in such cases (see Fecal Protease Test).

Lugol's iodine 2% demonstrates starch granules in feces (amylorrhea); these stain blue-black, with a turquoise fringe. Persistent amylorrhea indicates pancreatic amylase deficiency, but it is a relatively insensitive test for pancreatic malfunction.

Also seek creatorrhea (fecal muscle fibers) in a patient eating a meat-based diet. A fresh fecal smear is stained with Lugol's, methylene blue, or Wright's stain and examined under high power. Undigested fibers have blunt ends and prominent cross striations. The presence of two or three striated muscle fibers per high-power field is supportive of maldigestion. They are products of deficient protein digestion (usually pancreatic). However, the results tend to be excessively variable and insensitive because most carnivorous pets usually eat cooked meat.

◆ Fecal Protease Test

Observing the effect of a fecal suspension on gelatin (Procedure 8-2) makes a quick, inexpensive estimate of pancreatic protease function. The substrate is provided in a test tube of gelatin (tube test). Digestion of the gelatin implies fecal (and presumably intestinal) protease activity. The test's convenience is offset by inaccuracy.

A negative test (i.e., a test with no protease activity) may mean true pancreatic insufficiency, but normal animals often have negative tests because of the normal daily flux in fecal protease concentrations. False negatives also may arise from trypsin inhibitors or exhaustion of proteases during digestion. The x-ray film digestion test is simply inaccurate. The technician should always run simultaneous controls. Negative tests should be repeated at least three times before they are given credence.

For correct interpretation of these results, fresh feces must be used. If not quickly analyzed, the sample should be frozen.

The credibility of positive results should also be doubted. The protease activity revealed may be only bacterial. This is pronounced when the client is tardy in submitting feces collected 1 to 2 days earlier. Serial fecal dilutions exceeding 1:100 in the tube test reduce the influence of these bacterial proteases.

◆ Fecal Occult Blood

Blood loss into the gut is another cause of protein-losing gastroenteropathy. Dramatic bleeding is evident as black feces (melena) or frank fecal blood (hematochezia). Less obvious, subtle bleeding is a significant sign of GI ulcers, neoplasia or parasitism. Chronic, low-level bleeding may lead to iron-deficiency anemia.

Useful reagents to detect insidious bleeding include orthotoluidine (Occultest: Ames, IA) and benzidine (Hemoccult: Beckman Coulter Inc., Fullerton CA). Impreg-

---

PROCEDURE **8-2**

Protocol for the fecal protease test

Tube Test

1. Dilute 1 part feces with 9 parts 5% sodium bicarbonate.
2. Add 1 ml of the above mixture to 2 ml of melted 7.5% gelatin at 37° C.
3. Incubate at 37° C for 1 hour or at room temperature for 2.5 hours.
4. Refrigerate for 20 minutes.
5. If the mixture fails to form a gel, the test is positive. Confirm positive tests by diluting feces up to 1:100. Negative results at these dilutions indicate fecal protease deficiency.

Run Two Control Samples

1. Diluent only (negative control)
2. Normal feces (positive control)

nated strips or tablets are oxidized to a colored product by hemoglobin peroxidase activity in the feces. Both reagents are so sensitive that they respond to dietary hemoglobin and myoglobin; therefore the patient's diet must be meat free for 3 days before the test. It is recommended that the patient consume a cottage cheese and rice diet, 50% of each, before the test is performed. This precaution is less pertinent to herbivores, but the technician must check that the diet has not been supplemented with meat or bone meal.

Guaiac Test

The guaiac test is the preferred test because it is less affected by diet (Procedure 8-3). It is less sensitive but still detects fecal blood volumes as small as 5 to 20 ml. Dietary restriction is still advised. Guaiac also may be used to test for blood in urine and gastric juice. Many gum guaiac preparations vary in sensitivity. Alcohol solutions of guaiac and solutions of 3% hydrogen peroxide are unstable. These solutions should be checked with known positive controls. False negatives also are caused by excess reducing compounds in the medium (as with vitamin C supplementation). This situation may be a problem when trying to demonstrate blood in canine urine. Dogs overproduce vitamin C; the excess vitamin C is found in the urine.

Fecal Proteolytic Activity

The assay for fecal proteolytic activity was found to be effective for the evaluation of exocrine pancreatic insufficiency in cats and other species. Fecal proteolytic activity can be determined colorimetrically using an azocasein or azoalbumin substrate, or radial enzyme diffusion (RED) method.[3] Dogs with EPI may seldom have normal fecal proteolytic activity. A reliable RED requires fecal samples of 3 different days. Normal values of diameter of digestion halo are 10.7 ± 2.7 mm in dogs and 9.6 ± 3.4 mm in cats.[4,5]

PROCEDURE 8-3

Protocol for the guaiac fecal occult blood test

1. Smear feces sparingly on a piece of filter paper. Also smear a positive control sample (0.05 ml of venous blood in 50 ml of water) on another paper.
2. Add two drops each of glacial acetic acid, gum guaiac solution (20 g in 100 ml 95% ethanol), and 3% hydrogen peroxide (fresh) to each sample.
3. Observe for color change and rapidity of color change.
   Trace: faint green-blue in 1 minute
   1+: light blue appearing slowly
   2+: clear blue appearing fairly fast
   3+: deep blue almost immediately
   4+: deep blue immediately
4. The control should give a 1+ reaction.

Fecal α_1-Protease Inhibitor (α-1-Antitrypsin)

This plasma protease resists intraluminal proteolytic degradation. Detection of alpha$_1$-protease inhibitor may be accomplished by radial immunodiffussion or ELISA in dogs.[6] The assay is species specific. Documentation of protein-losing enteropathy or gastrointestinal hemorrhage is appropriate.

The best method for diagnosing protein-losing enteropathy is quantitative loss of ^{52}Cr-labeled albumin. The test is based on intravenous administration of radioactive chromium, which links to circulating plasma albumin; albumin loss is proportional to radioisotope quantity (radioactivity) in feces.[7]

◆ Serum Tests

Fat, or Lipid, Absorption

Lipid absorption relies on bile, pancreatic lipase and a healthy intestinal mucosa. Associated lesions cause steatorrhea and prevent the normal hyperlipemia that follows a fatty meal. Lipemia, as judged by plasma turbidity, is then a gauge of GI function.

The patient must be fasted for 12 hours and a baseline blood sample must be drawn and centrifuged. If fasting lipemia is encountered (e.g., in diabetes mellitus, starvation, feline steatitis, hypothyroidism, hyperadrenocorticism, liver/biliary disease, familial hyperlipemia of Schnauzers, white muscle disease of sheep or hyperlipemia of ponies, among others), the test must be abandoned. If the plasma is clear, either corn oil (3 ml/kg) or peanut oil (2 ml/kg) is administered *per os.* Blood samples are drawn at hourly intervals for 4 hours. This plasma should be cloudy. Clear follow-up samples indicate disturbed absorptive function, but its site of disturbance may not be known. Some argue that this test reveals nothing more than the simple discovery of steatorrhea.

A variation of this method may better define the lesion. The test is repeated on another day; however, the oil is preincubated at room temperature for 20 minutes with pancreatic enzymes. A cloudy postchallenge plasma implies a pancreatic enzyme deficiency. If it is clear, inadequate bile production or intestinal malassimilation must be considered. The fat absorption test may yield false negatives (no fat absorption) with delayed gastric emptying (fat induces this), gastric inactivation of added pancreatic enzymes, or enteritis.

Slight lipemia before oil administration indicates increased levels of low lipoproteins (mainly triglycerides and cholesterol). The enzyme, lipoprotein lipase, usually clears plasma of triglycerides; the activity of this enzyme is enhanced by insulin, thyroid hormones, glucagon and heparin. Determination of triglyceride concentrations of slightly lipemic plasma may reveal increased triglyceride concentration, which could be attributed to disease of hepatic, pancreatic, renal, or endocrine origin. Slight postprandial lipemia also may be seen in some canine patients with malabsorptive syndromes.

Monosaccharide Absorption Tests

These tests more specifically probe intestinal function. Again, the agent is given *per os;* blood concentrations are the measure of absorption.

D-XYLOSE ABSORPTION. D-xylose is a five-carbon sugar absorbed passively in the jejunum and excreted rapidly by the kidneys. Because xylose absorption is simple and the agent is not metabolized, its fate is readily traced. Xylose absorption is inefficient and often affected by some intestinal diseases. Nonetheless, the test is relatively insensitive because control values are variable.

The test is performed in dogs and horses as described in Procedure 8-4. Interference from rumen flora precludes use of the oral test in cattle and sheep; the alternative injection of monosaccharides into the abomasum is difficult enough to make its use rare.

PROCEDURE **8-4**

Protocol for the monosaccharide absorption test in dogs and horses

Oral Xylose Absorption in Dogs

1. Fast the patient for 16 hours.
2. Collect a heparinized blood sample for baseline xylose measurement.
3. Give 5% xylose solution at 500 mg/kg via stomach tube.
4. Draw heparinized blood samples at 30, 60, 90, 120, 180, and 240 minutes after xylose administration and submit for xylose determination.[23]
5. Plot a blood xylose concentration vs. time curve. A peak of less than 45 mg/dl between 30 and 90 minutes is abnormal. Peak values of 45 to 50 mg/dl are possibly abnormal. A peak above 50 mg/dl is probably normal.

Glucose and Xylose Absorption in Horses

1. Fast the patient for 12 to 18 hours.
2. Withhold water for the first 2 hours of the test.
3. Collect baseline blood samples (heparinized for xylose, sodium fluoride for glucose).
4. Give xylose at 0.5 g/kg as a 10% aqueous solution or anhydrous glucose at 1 g/kg as a 20% aqueous solution via stomach tube.
5. Collect blood at 30-minute intervals for 4 to 5 hours. Centrifuge and keep plasma at 0° C (32° F) until analyzed.
6. Maximum blood xylose level of 20.6 ± 4.8 mg/dl is expected at 60 minutes. The preadministration blood glucose concentration should be doubled by 120 minutes.
7. Do not run tests simultaneously because they cause mutual interference.

Abnormal xylose absorption indicates intestinal malassimilation, specifically malabsorption. However, only slight differences separate normal and abnormal ranges; diseased animals may have normal results. Animals with lymphangiectasia still may have normal results because the lymphatics do not participate in xylose absorption. The rate of xylose absorption depends only on the amount given, the size of the absorptive area, intestinal blood circulation, and gastric emptying. The latter may be delayed by cold or hypertonic solutions, pain, apprehension, or feeding. Fasting or radiographs to confirm an empty stomach are required. Vomiting, however, falsely lowers blood values, as does ascites (xylose enters pooled fluids). Bacteria have the ability to metabolize xylose; therefore bacterial overgrowth may be monitored by this test. If bacterial overgrowth is suspected (in cases of intestinal stasis or pancreatic enzyme deficiency), the test should be repeated after 24 hours' use of oral tetracycline. Finally, renal disease falsely elevates blood xylose concentrations.

The fate of D-xylose also has been followed in dogs by collecting a 5-hour urine sample after a 25-g oral dose and determining the total xylose excreted. This method is more laborious but requires only one xylose assay.

Cats were thought to have plasma concentrations and kinetics similar to dogs.[8] Other studies found xylose uptake to be variable in cats; plasma concentration did not increase to the levels found in dogs.[9,10] Peak plasma concentration of xylose in normal cats ranged between 12 and 42 mg/dl when a dosage of 500-mg/kg body weight was used.[11]

False-negative results may be caused by delayed gastric emptying, abnormal intestinal motility, reduced intestinal blood flow, bacterial overgrowth, and sequestration of xylose in ascitic fluid. False-positive results may be caused by decreased glomerular filtration rate, therefore ensuring the patient is fully hydrated and not azotemic at the time of testing is important.

Of the oral dose of xylose, 18% is excreted through the kidneys within 5 hours. This test has been improved performing D-xylose and 3-O-Methyl-D-Glucose (3MG) absorption test comparing the differential absorption of two sugars to eliminate the nonmucosal effects of D-xylose absorption.[12]

Serum Folate and Cobalamin

Serum concentrations of folate and cobalamin may be assessed by radioimmunoassay (RIA). Both concentrations tend to be decreased in malabsorption. Folate is absorbed in the proximal intestine, whereas cobalamin is absorbed in the ileum. Bacterial overgrowth also may alter these concentrations; folate synthesis is increased in bacterial overgrowth, whereas some bacteria may decrease the cobalamin availability. Reference intervals in dogs are 3.7 to 8.8 µg/L of folate and 200 to 490 ng/L of cobalamin in serum.[13]

Trypsin-Like Immunoreactivity

Trypsin-like immunoreactiviy is the most convenient and accurate test of pancreatic digestive function. Most of the pancreatic secretions enter the pancreatic duct, but small amounts leak from the basolateral aspect of the acinar cells into the blood. The serum content of the enzyme trypsinogen is derived only from the pancreas. This unique characteristic of trypsinogen prompted development of a radioimmunoassay technique for detecting the minute amount of serum trypsinogen or trypsin-like immunoreactivity (TLI) using antibodies to trypsin. These antibodies are species specific. TLI provides a sensitive and specific test for diagnosis of exocrine pancreatic insufficiency in dogs.[14] Assays for TLI also have been developed for feline species.[15]

Dogs with exocrine pancreatic insufficiency have a serum TLI of less than 2.5 µg/L. Normal dogs have a range of 5 to 35 µg/L. Dogs with other causes of malassimilation may have normal serum TLI. Dogs with chronic pancreatitis may have normal TLI values or between 2.5 and 5 µg/L. Normal cats have 14 to 82 µg/L TLI, whereas cats with EPI have less than 8.5 µg/L.

Serum TLI decreases in parallel with functional pancreatic mass. The inflammation associated with acute and probably chronic pancreatitis may enhance leakage of trypsinogen and trypsin from the pancreas and increase TLI. Also decreased glomerular filtration rate increases TLI (trypsinogen is a small molecule that easily passes into the glomerular filter). Serum TLI is an important indicator of functional pancreatic mass. It is most informative if coupled with BT-PABA and fecal fat results to characterize and diagnose malassimilation.

Serum TLI increases after eating (especially proteins), but values remain within reference intervals. In addition, pancreatic enzyme (exogenous) supplementation does not alter TLI. Therefore food should be withheld for at least 3 hours and preferably 12 hours before taking a blood sample. The blood is coagulated at room temperature and the serum stored at $-20°$ C until assay.

Breath Hydrogen Test

Enterocytes do not release hydrogen in carbohydrate catabolism as many bacteria do. Part of hydrogen is absorbed to the bloodstream and then excreted in the breath. Expired hydrogen is minimal in healthy animals, but when bacterial overgrowth and subsequent bacterial carbohydrate metabolism occur, breath hydrogen increases. Breath hydrogen in fasting healthy dogs is 0.9 ± 0.1 ppm, peak concentration 8 hours after feeding is 1.4 ± 0.2 ppm.[16] The test is performed using an anesthesia induction mask, a valve, and 1 L latex bag to recover the expired gas, hourly up to 8 hours after eating a carbohydrate-rich diet. Hydrogen concentration of gas samples may be measured by thermal conductivity gas chromatography or hydrogen-sensitive electrochemical cells. Higher than normal hydrogen concentrations, in expired air, are observed in dogs with carbohydrate malabsorption, and highest concentrations result from bacterial overgrowth.

TESTS OF LIVER FUNCTION

The liver's metabolic and transport functions are numerous. The liver plays a key role in conjugation and excretion of exogenous compounds, such as bilirubin and bile acids, in addition to numerous exogenous drugs. Production of various proteins, metabolism of carbohydrates and lipids, and conversion of ammonia to urea are also important metabolic functions, making the liver an essential organ for maintenance of life. Malfunctions in these pathways result in predictable clinical signs of jaundice, hypoalbuminemia, problems with hemostasis, hypoglycemia, hyperlipoproteinemia, and hepatoencephalopathy.

◆ Dye Excretion

Among the liver's many functions is excretion of certain wastes and foreign substances. This function may be utilized to test the liver's health.

BSP Clearance

Sulfobromophthalein (BSP) is an organic dye. Although an excellent test, its usefulness is limited by the availability of the dye. Injected intravenously, BSP is retrieved by the liver, conjugated and excreted in the bile by a pathway shared by bilirubin. Its disappearance from the plasma then depends on hepatic blood flow, bile flow, and hepatocellular integrity. This disappearance is assayed as a half-life or percent dye retention (Procedure 8-5).

This test has not been used any more in human beings because of hypersensitivity reaction reported in late 1960s. BSP was discontinued as a commercially available drug in 1984; as a result the application in veterinary medicine was restricted to research institutions. However, two new references have been published about BSP test application in canine medicine.[17,18]

BSP clearance is a sensitive hepatic function test, especially useful for detecting chronic lesions or portosystemic shunts with no leakage of liver enzymes. Coagulation defects and mysterious anemias sometimes may be explained by BSP test results. In horses, the test is handy to differentiate the jaundice of hepatic disease from that of simple anorexia, and hepatoencephalopathy from the wobbler syndrome. Specific indications in ruminants include fascioliasis, liver abscesses, ketosis, and photosensitization. BSP clearance may aid in diagnosis of aflatoxicosis in swine.

Hepatic lesions delay BSP excretion. Delays due to hepatocellular injury indicate a loss of at least 55% of the liver's functional mass. The magnitude of delay is poorly correlated to both the extent of hepatic lesions, when mild, and the clinical signs of liver dysfunction.

Delayed BSP clearance can be erroneous. Slowed BSP excretion results from perivascular dye injection (which can be painful), poor hepatic perfusion (shock, heart failure, dehydration) and fever. Ascites also interferes with BSP clearance because the dye lingers in pooled fluids. Certain inborn defects of BSP metabolism occur without liver disease, notably in some Southdown and Corriedale sheep. Obesity prolongs BSP retention because the amount of BSP per unit of body mass is relatively increased. In conclusion, bilirubin competes with BSP for excretion by the liver. For this reason, the BSP test should not be performed in animals with hyperbilirubinemia of 3 mg/dl or more. The results reveal nothing more than the already apparent jaundice.

PROCEDURE **8-5**

Protocol for BSP clearance

Dogs and Cats

1. Fast the patient for 12 hours. Also withdraw all medication for this period.
2. Inject BSP IV at 5 mg/kg. (*Caution:* Perivascular BSP causes major sloughing! Also, old solutions of BSP can crystallize and cause anaphylaxis.)
3. Collect a 5-ml blood sample from the opposite cephalic vein 30 minutes after BSP injection. Centrifuge and avoid hemolysis.
4. Submit plasma for BSP determination and calculate the percentage of retention at 30 minutes.
5. Normal is less than 5% retention at 30 minutes.

Cattle and Horses (1000 lb or More)

1. Collect an initial blood sample.
2. Inject 20 ml of 0.5% BSP (or 1 g of BSP) IV.
3. Collect blood samples from the opposite jugular vein at 2- to 3-minute intervals between 5 and 15 minutes postinjection (record the times).
4. Centrifuge the samples, avoid hemolysis, and submit for BSP analysis.
5. Plot the clearance curve and calculate the half-life.
6. Normal half-life is 2.5 to 4 minutes.

Sheep and Goats

1. Half-life or percent retention may be determined.
2. For percent retention, inject BSP IV at 5 mg/kg and collect blood samples from the opposite jugular vein 10 minutes later. Centrifuge the sample and submit plasma for BSP analysis. Calculate percent retention at 10 minutes.
3. For half-life determination, collect an initial blood sample, inject BSP IV at 5 mg/kg, and collect two to three blood samples from the opposite jugular vein within 7 minutes of injection (record the times). Submit plasma for BSP analysis and half-life determination.
4. Normal percent retention (sheep) is 6% ± 2% at 10 minutes. Normal half-life for sheep and goats is about 2 ± 0.3 minutes.

Swine

1. Determine percent retention as for sheep and goats. Give BSP IV at 6 mg/kg.
2. Normal percent retention at 10 minutes is 3% to 4% for a 100-kg pig, and 1.4% ± 0.9% for a 30-kg pig.

Two conditions may disguise liver disease by speeding BSP clearance. Because albumin carries BSP in the plasma, hypoalbuminemia (nephrotic syndrome, protein-losing gastroenteropathies, extreme liver disease) speeds clearance by increasing hepatic access to the free dye. Phenobarbital use also hastens BSP clearance. BSP clearance has no correlation with the extent of fatty infiltration of the liver.

Indocyanine Green Clearance

Indocyanine green (ICG) is a similar organic dye. Introduced to human medicine because of occasional reactions to BSP, it is used to estimate hepatic blood flow. ICG clearance is now being used by veterinarians instead of BSP because BSP is no longer available for clinical use.

Preinjection plasma is required to prepare a blank and a standard solution. This test can be used in both fed and fasted animals, but the latter are preferred. An IV dosage of 0.8 to 1.1 mg/kg body weight is recommended for horses, whereas 1 mg/kg body weight is recommended for dogs and 1.5 mg/kg body weight is recommended for cats. Usually five to six plasma samples are taken between 0, 5, 10, 15 and 30 minutes postinjection. ICG concentration is measured photometrically at 805 nm, and the half-life is determined. Normal ICG clearances are as follows: dogs, 8.4 ± 2.3 minutes; horses (fed), 3.5 ± 0.67 minutes; horses (fasted), 1.6 ± 0.57 minutes. Normal 30-minute retention is < 14.7% ± 5% percent in dogs and <7.3% ± 2.9% in cats.[19] Delayed ICG clearance has been reported in a variety of disorders, such as hyperbilirubinemia, hypoproteinemia, decreased hepatic blood flow, hepatic necrosis, and extrahepatic bile duct obstruction.[20]

◆ Ammonia Tolerance

The liver's enzyme constituents include those involved in the urea cycle. Liver disease may impair ammonia detoxification, leading to hepatoencephalopathy. Random blood ammonia measurements may be normal in these patients, but challenge with overwhelming exogenous ammonia loads may reveal liver dysfunction. Rectal administration is more reliable because some dogs regurgitate ammonium chloride solution when it is given orally. However, oral administration of ammonium chloride may be accomplished with dry powder in gelatin capsules (Procedure 8-6).

The ammonia tolerance test is used to detect urea cycle enzyme deficiencies (argino-succinate synthetase) and abnormal portal blood flow, particularly congenital portovascular anomalies.[21] In affected animals, plasma liver enzyme levels are often normal. The test's chief limitation is in the handling of blood samples. The clinic's reference laboratory must be consulted for sample handling recommendations. In general, the blood must be centrifuged immediately and the serum placed on ice and analyzed within 1 to 3 hours of collection or frozen at −20° C. Whole blood cannot be tested because its ammonia content increases with storage. Although the test can dramatically elevate the blood ammonia level, it does not cause or worsen neurologic signs. Occasional vomiting is the only problem.

◆ Bile Acid Concentrations

Bile acids are synthesized by hepatocytes from cholesterol and are conjugated with glycine or taurine. Conjugated bile acids are secreted across the canalicular membrane and reach the duodenum via the biliary system. When bile acids reach the ileum, they are transported to the portal circulation and travel back to the liver. Spillover bile acids that escape from enterohepatic circulation may be detected in normal animals; serum

PROCEDURE 8-6

Protocol for the ammonia tolerance test

1. Consult your regional diagnostic laboratory about blood specimen handling.
2. Fast the patient for 12 hours and give enemas to clear the lower bowel of feces. Obtain a baseline blood sample.
3. For rectal administration, give ammonium chloride at 0.1 g/kg as a 5% solution infused 20 to 30 cm into the rectum. For oral administration, give 0.1 mg/kg (maximum of 3 g) dissolved in 20 to 50 ml of water via stomach tube.
4. Collect a second blood sample 30 minutes after administration and another at 60 minutes postadministration. The blood should be kept on ice until it is analyzed (within 3 hours).
5. Blood ammonia levels:

	Before ammonia loading	After ammonia loading
Normal	80 ± 36 μg/dl	156 ± 71 μg/dl
Abnormal	236 ± 116 μg/dl	1049 ± 256 μg/dl

6. Rectal ammonia tolerance results increase only minimally in normal blood (less than 2.5 times the baseline). Increases greater than 2.5 times the baseline value indicate hepatic failure or portosystemic shunting.

Note: Always consult your diagnostic laboratory for their reference intervals ("normal values").

concentrations of bile acids correlate portal concentrations. As a result, postprandial serum bile acid concentrations are higher than fasting concentrations. Any process that impairs the hepatocellular, biliary, or portal enterohepatic circulation of bile acids results in elevated serum bile acid (SBA) levels. The great advantage of SBA determinations as a liver function test is that they evaluate the major anatomic component of the hepatobiliary system, and they are stable *in vitro* (Procedure 8-7).

Bile acids may be determined by several methods; the most commonly used is an enzymatic method. The 3-hydroxy bile acids react with 3-hydroxisteroid dehydrogenase and then with diformazan. Color generation is measured by end-point spectrophotometry. Lipemic postprandial samples must be cleared by centrifugation to avoid interference with spectrophotometry.

Increased fasting SBA levels were observed in patients with extrahepatic biliary obstruction, cholangiohepatitis, portosystemic shunt, biliary cirrhosis, and hepatic lipidosis. Postprandial values are more valuable in portosystemic vascular abnormalities or acquired shunts. Fasting bile acid levels may be greater than postprandial levels in spontaneous gallbladder contraction, slow intestinal transit, altered response to cholecystokinin, and altered gastrointestinal flora. Low bile acid levels may appear in hepatobiliary disease if diarrhea and steatorrhea are present. Additional comparative studies are needed to evaluate this test in comparison with other established tests in determination or diagnosis of hepatopathy in each animal species.

PROCEDURE 8-7

Protocol for determination of serum bile acid concentrations

1. Obtain blood samples from dogs after fasting for 12 hours and again 2 hours after eating (see fat/lipid absorption).
2. Separate serum from blood cells within 1 hour and store at –20° C.
3. Determine bile acid concentration by radioimmunoassay or an enzymatic colorimetric procedure. The latter also has been validated for equine serum.

Enzymatic Method

This measures all nonsulfated conjugated and unconjugated 3-alphahydroxy bile acids.

1. To each of two test tubes, add 0.2 ml of serum and 0.2 ml of 200-mM sodium pyruvate.
2. To one tube add 0.5 ml of the 3-alpha-hydroxysteroid dehydrogenase reaction mixture (prepared as described in step 6, or from the kit, Enzabil [Nyegaard & Co., Oslo, Norway]).
3. To the other tube add 0.5 ml of the reference reaction mixture (prepared or from the kit). This mixture has the same constituents as the reaction mixture described above, except it has no 3-alpha-hydroxysteroid dehydrogenase.
4. Incubate the tubes at 37° C (water bath) for 10 minutes. Add 0.1 ml of 1.33-M phosphoric acid solution to each tube after incubation and mix thoroughly.
5. The final volume in each tube is 1 ml. Read the light absorbance at 540 nm to determine the difference between the reaction tube and the reference tube.
6. A standard solution is prepared from sodium taurocholate (400 μmol/L), pooled serum (species specific), and various buffers.[7]
7. Bile acid concentration equals:

Sample concentration × Standard concentration/Standard concentration

Radioimmunoassay Method

The conjugated bile acid, solid-phase radioimmunoassay kit (Conjugated Bile Acids Solid-Phase Radioimmunoassay Kit: Becton-Dickinson Immunodiagnostics, Orangeburg, NJ) consists of assay tubes coated with rabbit antiserum against conjugated bile acids, a bile acid tracer that contains iodoglycocholic acid dissolved in buffers, and sodium taurocholate standards (0, 0.4, 2.0, 6.0, 15, and 50 μmol/L) in buffer solutions.

1. Mix 25 μl of serum or standard with 1 ml of bile acid tracer solution in the assay tube and incubate the tubes for 1 hour in a 37° C water bath to allow antigen-antibody interaction.
2. Aspirate the solution from each tube and rinse the tubes with 1 ml of sterile distilled water. Determine the radioactivity remaining in the tubes with an automatic gamma scintillation counter calibrated for[125]I measurement.
3. Calculate the conjugated bile acid concentration (μmol/L) of each sample from the standard curve.[29]

PROCEDURE 8-7

Protocol for determination of serum bile acid concentrations—cont'd

Results

Normal fasting concentrations:

Dogs   ≤ 5.0 µmol/L
Cats   ≤ 2.0 µmol/L
Horses   5.9 ± 2.7 µmol/L

Normal values 2 hours after feeding:

Dogs   ≤ 15.5 µmol/L
Cats   ≤ 10.0 µmol/L
Horses   5.9 ± 2.7 µmol/L

Equine bile acid concentrations do not change after feeding; only an insignificant increase is observed.

Notes: In horses, an increase of 17 times greater than the baseline value is expected in cholestasis. An increase greater than ten-fold above the baseline value was observed in hepatocellular necrosis.

Fasting concentrations in dogs and cats >15 µmol/L are suggestive of disease.

Postprandial levels >25 µmol/L in dogs and >20 µmol/L in cats are suggestive of disease.

◆ Caffeine Clearance

This is a specific assay of hepatic microsomal function. Demethylation of caffeine is dependent only upon the specific P448 microsomal system of healthy hepatocytes; therefore it accurately reflects aberrations in hepatocellular function. This test is now used in human medicine; few experimental studies have been performed in canine species.[22]

Caffeine sodium benzoate is dissolved in 2 ml of sterile water (50:50 wt/wt) and 7 mg of caffeine/kg body weight are then injected IV. Plasma samples are collected from 15 to 480 minutes, and the caffeine concentration (µg/ml) is measured by automated enzyme immunoassay. Plasma caffeine clearance and half-life are calculated.

Normal half-life values in dogs are 6 ± 0.6 hours and clearance is 1.7 ± 0.1 ml/min/kg. Elimination of caffeine is prolonged in hepatic insufficiency, with a clearance of 0.8 ± 0.1 ml/min/kg.

◆ Delta Bilirubin Concentration

Delta bilirubin has been identified as a fourth, firmly bound bilirubin fraction of total bilirubin. It comprises a portion covalently bound to albumin and a portion that is nonenzymatically derived from albumin and monoconjugated bilirubin.

The Kodak Ektachem multilayer dry film method measures total bilirubin by the classic diazo reaction and unconjugated and conjugated bilirubin by the difference in their spectral properties. Delta bilirubin is then calculated by the following equation:

Delta bilirubin = Total bilirubin − (Unconjugated bilirubin + Conjugated bilirubin)

The total bilirubin, unconjugated bilirubin, and conjugated bilirubin values are determined with the Kodak Ektachem unit. The Kodak method is sensitive and superior for determination of bilirubin fractions. The observed delta bilirubin concentration range in one study in healthy horses was 3 to 6 μmol/L, and the concentration range in sick horses was 0 to 36 μmol/L.[23]

TESTS OF KIDNEY FUNCTION

The kidney must not be compared with a filter. Blood coursing through the kidney is not just cleansed, it is changed. Ion concentrations are regulated, and influential messengers, such as renin, erythropoietin, and activated vitamin D, are added. Therefore monitoring kidney function may be critical.

◆ Tests of Glomerular Function (Glomerular Filtration Rate)

Plasma decay techniques may be used to estimate glomerular filtration rate (GFR) if nonmetabolizable substances exclusively excreted by the kidneys are monitored. Clearance is the volume of plasma cleared of a marker substance per unit time. Plasma clearance method may be based on measures on plasma and urine (previously described) or only plasma. The second group of methods avoids the repeated or continued bladder catheterization and subsequent urinary tract infection risks. The rate of disappearance of sodium sulfanilate, inulin, phenosulfonphtalein, iohexol, and radioactive isotopes such as ^{125}I-iothalamate, ^{131}I-iodohippurate, ^{14}C-inulin, ^{3}H-tetraethylammonium, and ^{99M}Tc-diethylenetriaminepentaacetic acid is related with renal (glomerular) function. The complexity of the latter methods, need of isotope disposal, and scintigraphy facilities, have limited their usefulness. As a result, they rarely are used outside research institutions.[24]

Single-Injection Inulin Clearance

Inulin is excreted entirely by glomerular filtration, without tubular secretion, reabsorption or catabolism. As a result, inulin clearance using a constant infusion rate and quantitative urine sampling may be considered the best method to evaluate GFR. Single-injection inulin clearance is a simpler method that alternatively may be used. After 12-hour fast (free access to water is permitted during the test), inulin is injected intravenously at a dosage of 100 mg/kg or 3 g/m² (body surface calculation gives more accurate results); then, serum samples are obtained at 20, 40, 80, and 120 minutes. Total inulin clearance is calculated from the decrease of serum inulin concentration using a two-compartment model. Normal dogs present a GFR of 83.5 to 144.3 ml/min/m^2.[25]

Sodium Sulfanilate

Kidney filtration is evaluated by injecting inert traceable substances excreted in the urine. Sodium sulfanilate is removed only by glomerular filtration in dogs (Procedure 8-8); its disappearance from the plasma is an index of glomerular filtration. The test can detect unilateral nephrectomy and diminished renal function in dogs before azotemia develops. The half-life of sodium sulfanilate is prolonged up to five times in horses with glomerulonephritis. Although the test also is performed in cats, the mode of sodium sulfanilate excretion is not confirmed in this species.

PSP Clearance

Phenolsulfonphthalein (PSP) is an organic dye excreted by the renal tubules. Nonetheless, its clearance is accepted as a measure of renal blood flow because this

---

PROCEDURE 8-8

Protocol for sodium sulfanilate and PSP clearance

Sodium Sulfanilate Clearance in Dogs, Cats, and Horses

1. Inject sodium sulfanilate IV at 20 mg/kg (10 mg/kg for horses).
2. Obtain heparinized blood samples at 30, 60, and 90 minutes postinjection. Submit for sodium sulfanilate analysis.
3. Plot the disappearance curve and determine half-life.
4. Dogs: normal half-life is 66 ± 11 minutes; cats: normal half-life is 45.1 ± 7 minutes; horses: normal half-life is 39.5 ± 4 minutes.

PSP Urinary Test

1. Empty the bladder.
2. Give 6 mg of PSP IV, regardless of patient size.
3. Insert a urinary catheter 10 minutes later.
4. Empty the bladder 15 minutes after PSP injection and rinse with sterile saline until 20 minutes after PSP injection. Save the urine sample and the rinse.
5. Submit an aliquot of the bladder rinse for PSP analysis and determine the percent of total PSP dose excreted.
6. Normal PSP clearance is 43.8 ± 11.1%. Any value less than 30% is abnormal.

PSP Plasma Test in Dogs and Cats

1. Give PSP IV at 5 mg/kg.
2. Obtain 3.0-ml blood samples in EDTA at 15, 25, and 35 minutes after PSP injection. Submit for PSP determination.
3. Plot the disappearance curve and determine half-life.
4. Normal half-life is 18 to 24 minutes.

PROCEDURE 8-9

Protocol for endogenous creatinine clearance

1. Obtain a blood sample for creatinine analysis.
2. Catheterize the bladder and rinse the bladder several times with sterile saline. Discard the rinse. Empty the bladder.
3. Begin timing immediately and collect all urine for a 20-minute or 24-hour period (the latter is more precise).
4. At the end of this period (20 minutes or 24 hours), empty the bladder. Measure the total urine volume collected. Rinse the bladder thoroughly with sterile saline. Empty the bladder and save the rinses. Submit an aliquot of urine rinse saline for creatinine analysis:
5. Calculate creatinine clearance with the following equation:

Creatinine clearance = Uv × Uc/Pc

Uv, urine volume; Uc, urine creatinine concentration; Pc, plasma creatine concentration
6. Normal clearance in dogs is 2.8 ± 0.96 ml/min/kg.

---

usually limits its efflux more than tubular secretion rates. PSP clearance (Procedure 8-9) is decreased only when more than two thirds of the nephrons are nonfunctional or when renal perfusion is compromised.

These two tests have been used, with success, in the past. Because they are no longer commonly used, many veterinarians have not heard of them. They are useful and easily performed and have been included here for completeness. Both of the above tests have been abandoned in favor of the other GFR tests.

◆ Endogenous Creatinine Clearance

Creatinine is derived from degraded muscle or dietary creatinine. It is always present in the blood. Because creatinine appears in the glomerular filtrate with negligible tubular secretion, it is a natural tracer of glomerular filtration. Fortunately, its short-term blood concentrations are stable enough to satisfy the clearance formula used for steady infusion studies of inulin and p-aminohippuric acid, the renal function standards.

The test is relatively simple (Procedure 8-10). A measure of blood creatinine and an accurate, timed urine collection are required for this test. Precision is of the utmost importance. Sloppy bladder catheterization and sampling ruin the results, especially with the briefer methods. The bladder must be rinsed before and after the test, saving the after-rinses with the urine for creatinine analysis. Clearance is calculated by dividing urinary creatinine excretion (urine creatinine concentration times urine volume) by plasma creatinine concentration. The estimate, if imprecise, is practical.

To avoid errors, plasma creatinine should be determined by the combination creatinine PAP test instead of the Jaffe method. The combination creatinine PAP test is an

PROCEDURE 8-10

Protocol for the exogenous creatinine clearance determination

1. Creatinine is administered subcutaneously at 100 mg/kg (dogs of more than 20 kg) or 75 mg/kg (smaller dogs).
2. Administer, via stomach tube, an amount of water equivalent to 3% of the dog's body weight.
3. Catheterize and rinse the urinary bladder and obtain a serum sample for creatinine determination 40 minutes after SC creatinine administration.
4. Collect urine during 20 minutes and obtain a second serum sample.
5. Repeat step 4 to increase reliability.
6. Calculate creatinine clearance using the mean values of both periods (steps 4 and 5).
7. Normal values in the dog are 4.09 ± 0.52 ml/kg/min.

enzymatic chromogenic method to determine creatinine concentration. The Jaffe method also determines noncreatinine chromogens in plasma, which do not appear in urine.

◆ Exogenous Creatinine Clearance

Exogenous creatinine clearance is an accurate method to measure GFR in small animals. Plasma creatinine concentration increases, making plasma noncreatinine chromogens concentration negligible. This allows the application of the Jaffe method to determine creatinine concentrations (Procedure 8-11). Avoiding dehydration in the animal is critical in the performance of this test; free access to water must be ensured before any glomerular filtration tests.

◆ Modified Water-Deprivation Test, Vasopressin Response

Polyuria or polydipsia may lead to suspicions about the kidney, which may be an erroneous assumption. Diuresis and subsequent polydipsia may mean failing nephrons, or kidney function disrupted by hyperadrenocorticism (Cushing's disease), diabetes mellitus, or nephrogenic diabetes insipidus. The kidneys may be normal but not receiving the signal to concentrate urine, as in neurogenic diabetes insipidus. Finally, the diuresis may be a totally appropriate renal compensation for pathologic water intake (psychogenic polydipsia).

Some background on the control of urine concentration is essential. Vasopressin or antidiuretic hormone (ADH), from the neurohypophysis, signals the kidneys to retain water. Targeted on the renal collecting duct, it increases the duct's permeability to water. Water in the urine passes out of the collecting duct and into the hypertonic renal medulla, concentrating the urine that remains behind in the collecting duct. If the system fails (e.g., inappropriate diuresis), either the neuroendocrine pathway that releases ADH in response to hypovolemia/plasma hyperosmolarity has been interrupted or the nephrons are unable to respond.

PROCEDURE 8-11

Protocol for the modified water-deprivation test in dogs

Preparation

1. 72 hours before the test, limit water intake to 120 ml/kg/day in small portions.
2. 48 hours before the test, limit water intake to 90 ml/kg/day.
3. 24 hours before the test, limit water intake to 60 to 80 ml/kg/day.

Water Deprivation

Before the test:
1. Withdraw food and all water.
2. Empty the bladder completely.
3. Determine the exact body weight.
4. Check the urine osmolality/specific gravity.
5. Obtain a BUN determination to check for azotemia.
6. Check hydration and CNS status.

During the test:
1. Completely empty the bladder and determine the exact body weight every 30 to 60 minutes.
2. Check the urine specific gravity and osmolality at each interval.
3. Check hydration and CNS status at each interval.
4. Recheck the BUN and serum osmolality values.
5. Weigh the patient at each interval.

After the test:
If the dog is clinically dehydrated, appears ill, or has lost about 5% of its body weight:
1. Obtain a blood sample for determination of the vasopressin concentration.
2. Empty the bladder.
3. Collect a final urine sample and check specific gravity and osmolality.

Vasopressin Response

1. Give 2 to 5 pressor units of aqueous vasopressin IM.
2. Continue withholding food and water.
3. Monitor the patient as follows:
   a. Empty the bladder every 30 minutes for 1 to 2 hours maximum.
   b. Check urine osmolality ± specific gravity.
   c. Check BUN.
   d. Check hydration and CNS status.
   e. Weigh patient.

After Testing

1. Introduce small amounts of water (10 to 20 ml/kg) every 30 minutes for 2 hours.
2. Monitor the patient for vomiting, hydration, and CNS status.
3. If the patient is well 2 hours after the test, provide water *ad lib.*

PROCEDURE 8-11

Protocol for the modified water-deprivation test in dogs—cont'd

Test Results

Normal:
1. Urine specific gravity ≥1.048
2. Urine osmolality ≥1700 mOsm/kg
3. Exogenous ADH does not further concentrate the urine after water deprivation.

Psychogenic polydipsia:
1. Urine osmolality is below normal. It can be similar to or above that of serum.
2. Urine specific gravity is 1.015 to 1.020.
3. Exogenous ADH does not further concentrate urine.

Nephrogenic diabetes insipidus:
1. Urine osmolarity does not exceed that of plasma (290 to 310 mOsm).
2. Urine specific gravity is 1.010 to 1.012.
3. Exogenous ADH does not further concentrate urine.
4. The animal dehydrates rapidly.

Neurogenic diabetes insipidus:
1. Urine osmolarity does not exceed 300 mOsm.
2. Urine specific gravity is 1.010 to 1.012.
3. Exogenous ADH causes a 50% to 500% increase in urine concentration (specific gravity 1.020 to 1.030).
4. The animal dehydrates rapidly.

Partial diabetes insipidus:
1. Urine osmolarity is 300 to 1000 mOsm.
2. Exogenous ADH does not further concentrate urine.
3. The animal dehydrates slowly.

Hyperadrenocorticism (Cushing's disease):
1. Urine osmolarity is 300 to 1000 mOsm.
2. Exogenous ADH concentrates urine slightly.
3. The animal dehydrates slowly.

◆ Water-Deprivation Test

This test is performed by observation of the response to endogenous or exogenous ADH. The basis for this test is to safely dehydrate the patient until a definite stimulus exists for endogenous ADH release (usually at about 5% body weight loss). That endpoint may vary. When denied water, patients dehydrate at different rates and must be monitored for weight loss, clinical signs of dehydration, and increased urine osmolarity or specific gravity. At the endpoint, the kidney should be under strictest endocrine orders to concentrate urine. Continued diuresis and dilute urine indicate lack of endogenous ADH or unresponsive nephrons. In dogs with kidney failure, this unresponsiveness precedes azotemia.

Contraindications to this test include dehydration and azotemia. Dehydrated patients risk hypovolemia and shock. They already should have maximal ADH release; if they could concentrate urine, they would. The test then is useless and dangerous, especially in animals with diabetes insipidus or neurogenic diabetes insipidus. Azotemia already attests to kidney dysfunction. Again, the test reveals nothing new and adds a prerenal component to the azotemia.

Vasopressin Response

When patients demonstrate the above-mentioned signs or a previous water-deprivation test has failed, a vasopressin response test is indicated. The vasopressin response test is simply a challenge with exogenous ADH; it focuses on the kidneys' abilities to respond. Urine osmolarity or specific gravity is the index of function. Normal kidneys should concentrate urine with this technique, despite the patient's free access to water. Vasopressin must be handled carefully because it is a labile drug and settles out in oil suspensions. Test failures may result from use of old or poorly mixed solutions. Also, IM vasopressin injection causes pain. Because of vasopressin's vasomotor activity, its use is theoretically contraindicated in pregnancy. However, the authors have observed no ill effects from its use.

In both tests, even normal kidneys may be unable to concentrate urine to normal extremes. Diuresis quickly washes solutes from the renal medulla, weakening the osmotic gradient that draws water from the collecting ducts. Gradual water deprivation over 3 to 5 days before use of the water deprivation test is recommended to renew renal solutes and to allow an evaluation of the impact of dehydration on the animal. Some may argue, though, that this technique is not superior but simply increases the costs of hospitalization. A more rapid test is preferred, at least initially.

Modified Water-Deprivation Test

Both of these tests may be combined in a single protocol that may differentiate several causes of polyuria/polydipsia (see Procedure 8-11). The modified water-deprivation test is specifically contraindicated in patients with known renal disease, uremia resulting from prerenal or primary renal disorder, or suspected or obvious dehydration.

Urine Protein/Creatinine Ratio

Quantitative assessment of renal proteinuria is of diagnostic significance in renal disease. In the absence of inflammatory cells in the urine, proteinuria indicates glomerular disease. For accurate determination of proteinuria, a 24-hour urinary protein value should be determined. This is a tedious task and errors are common. A mathematical method that compares the urine protein level to the urine creatinine levels in a single urine sample is more accurate and comprehensive. This urine protein to creatinine (P/C) ratio is based on the concept that the tubular concentration of urine increases both the urinary protein and creatinine concentrations equally.

This method has been validated for the canine species. Usually 5 to 10 ml of urine are collected between 10 AM and 2 PM, preferably by cystocentesis. The urine sample should be kept at 4° C or stored at −20° C. The sample is centrifuged and the supernatant is used. The protein concentration for each sample can be determined by the trichloroacetic acid-ponceau S method (mg/dl), or by using commercial kits for microprotein determination (Microprotein Rapid Stat Diagnostic Kit: Lancer Division of Sherwood Medical, St. Louis, MO). The creatinine concentration may be determined in mg/dl by the alkaline picric method or the semiautomated chemistry method (CKDA: American Monitor Corp, Indianapolis, IN).

The urine P/C ratio for healthy dogs should be less than 1. The urine P/C ratio between 1 and 5 may have prerenal (hyperglobulinemia, hemoglobinemia, myoglobinemia) or functional origin (exercise, fever, hypertension), whereas the urine P/C ratio greater than 5 is caused by renal disease.[27]

◆ Fractional Clearance of Electrolytes

The fractional clearance (FC) of sodium, potassium, phosphorus, and chloride is increased with renal parenchymal damage. Those tests allow differentiation between prerenal and renal failure because in prerenal failure, normal results may be expected. Normal results are as follows[26]:

- Dogs: sodium <1; potassium <20; chloride <1; phosphorous <39
- Cats: sodium <1; potassium <24; chloride <1.3; phosphorous <73

$$\mathbf{FC_{electrolyte}} = \frac{[(\mathbf{U_{electrolyte}} \times \mathbf{P_{creatinine}})}{(\mathbf{U_{creatinine}} \times \mathbf{P_{electrolyte}})] \times 100}$$

U = concentration in urine
P = concentration in plasma

◆ Urethral Pressure Profilometry

Urinary incontinence is a common complaint in canine medicine. Most cases are caused by sphincter mechanism incompetence. The specific functional test to explore the urethral sphincter mechanism is the urethral pressure profilometry.[27]

This test requires appropriate equipment and is restricted to referral institutions. A double sensor microtip pressure transducer catheter is used. The catheter is inserted through the urethra into the urinary bladder. The tip sensor measures intravesical pressure at the same time as the other sensor records urethral resistance to perform a continuous comparison.

TESTS OF ADRENOCORTICAL FUNCTION

◆ The Adrenal Axis

Adrenocortical function tests are relatively common. Adrenal dysfunction is increasingly common, too often because of misuse of corticosteroids.

The adrenal axis starts with the hypothalamus. Stimuli originating in the brain, such as from stress, cause the hypothalamus to secrete corticotropin-releasing factor

(CRF). Under the influence of CRF, the adenohypophysis secretes adrenocorticotrophic hormone (ACTH), the hormone that stimulates adrenocortical growth and secretion, particularly of glucocorticoid-synthesizing tissue. Cortisol is the major hormone released in domestic mammals. It, in turn, feeds back to inhibit both CRF and ACTH release, completing a balanced system.

True or mimicked hyperfunction of the system is the common complaint. Brain or pituitary tumors leading to secondary bilateral adrenal hyperplasia, idiopathic adrenal hyperplasia or neoplasia (one or both glands) all may cause excessive cortisol release and hyperadrenocorticism. Overenthusiastic glucocorticoid therapy is the most common cause of cortisol excess.

Because exogenous, like endogenous, glucocorticoids inhibit adrenotrophic hormones, iatrogenic hyperadrenocorticism is accompanied by the paradox of atrophied adrenal glands. Sudden withdrawal of exogenous glucocorticoids leads to adrenal hypofunction. However, hypoadrenocorticism (Addison's disease) by definition includes mineralocorticoid deficiency, which does not occur in iatrogenic disease from rapid withdrawal of glucocorticoids. Addison's disease also may result from overuse of lysodren (for adrenal hyperplasia) or from idiopathic causes.

Screening tests for hyperadrenocorticism must be carefully interpreted because many dogs with nonadrenal disease such as diabetes mellitus, liver disease, or renal disease may have false-positive results. Thereafter, final diagnosis of hyperadrenocorticism are based on various positive tests performed (two out of three or three out of four tests). Conversely, if negative laboratory testing occurs with consistent clinical evidence, the animal should be retested one or two months later (if clinical signs persist).

Urinary Corticosteroids

Urine cortisol/creatinine ratio is a sensitive but not specific test to diagnose hyperadrenocorticism that allows to rule out hyperadrenocorticism. Abnormal results may appear in dogs with hyperadrenocorticism or other diseases such as diabetes, pyometra, liver failure, or hypercalcemia[28] (Procedure 8-12).

PROCEDURE 8-12

Urine cortisol/creatinine ratio

1. Obtain the urine sample avoiding stress or at home.
2. Determine cortisol and creatinine concentrations in μmol/L.
3. Results:
   a. Normal dogs ratio 1.2-6.9 $\times$ 10^{-6}
   b. Spontaneous hyperadrenocorticism ratio between 20 $\times$ 10^{-6} and 2100 $\times$ 10^{-6}
   c. Polyuria: polydipsia ratio between 8 $\times$ 10^{-6} and 150 $\times$ 10^{-6}

Corticotropin Stimulation Test (ACTH Response)

Animals with suspected hypoadrenocorticism (Addison's disease) or hyperadrenocorticism (Cushing's disease) may be evaluated with an ACTH response test. In addition, the test is indicated to distinguish among iatrogenic and spontaneous hyperadrenocorticism (Procedure 8-13). It also may test the efficacy of mitotane, ketoconazole, or metyrapone therapy. The rationale assumes that the adrenal glands will respond to exogenous ACTH stimulation by glucocorticoid release in proportion to the glands' size and development. Hyperplastic adrenal glands have exaggerated responses, whereas hypoplastic adrenal glands show diminished responses. The test, then, can detect these abnormalities but not reveal their ultimate cause.[29]

The ACTH response test is just a screening test. One potential problem exists: adrenal glands that are hyperactive from neoplasia may be insensitive to ACTH. Nonetheless, current figures indicate that the test is more than 80% accurate in diagnosing adrenocortical hyperfunction in the dog and more than 50% in the cat.[30]

PROCEDURE **8-13**

Protocol for the corticotropin stimulation test

1. Collect a plasma sample for cortisol determination.
2. Administer 5 μg/kg (dog) or 125 μg/cat of tetracosactide (synthetic ACTH Cosyntropin™ in USA or Synacthen in Europe) IV or IM.
3. Collect a second plasma sample for cortisol determination 30 (IV administration in cats) or 60 (dogs and IM administration in cats) minutes post ACTH administration.
4. Collect a third plasma sample for cortisol determination 60 (IV administration) or 90 (IM administration) minutes post-ACTH administration in cats.
5. Results:
   a. Normal pretest cortisol concentration:
      Dog: 0.5 to 4 μg/dL or 14 to 110 nmol/L
      Cat: 0.3 to 5 μg/dL or 8.3 to 138 nmol/L
   b. Normal post-ACTH cortisol concentration:
      Dog: 8 to 20 μg/dL or 220 to 552 nmol/L
      Cat: 5 to 15 μg/dL or 138 to 414 nmol/L
6. Interpretation:
   a. Exaggerated post-ACTH cortisol concentration is observed in most dogs (80%) and 51% cats (borderline increased in 16%) with hyperadrenocorticism. Cats may have increased only one of the post-ACTH cortisol determinations.
   b. Reduced post-ACTH cortisol concentration is observed, consistent, in both Addison's disease, iatrogenic Cushing's disease and, mitotane, ketoconazole, or metyrapone therapy.
   c. Normal post-ACTH cortisol concentration does not rule out Cushing's disease (occurs in 50% of dogs with adrenal-dependent Cushing's disease).

In the past, the adrenal glucocorticoid response to ACTH was monitored indirectly by following eosinophil counts. This proved inaccurate because eosinophils usually are rare in the peripheral blood. The method was largely abandoned in favor of plasma cortisol determinations. Sporadic measurements of plasma cortisol without some test challenge are diagnostically unreliable because normal and abnormal ranges overlap. Use of prednisone and prednisolone may interfere with plasma cortisol measurements.

◆ Dexamethasone Suppression

Dexamethasone suppression tests evaluate the adrenal glands differently, using the adrenal feedback loops. The low-dosage test confirms or replaces the ACTH response test for hyperadrenocorticism (Cushing's disease). The high-dosage test goes further, differentiating pituitary from adrenal causes of hyperadrenocorticism (Procedure 8-14). In cats, only a high-dose dexamethasone suppression test is suitable.

Dexamethasone, a potent glucocorticoid, suppresses ACTH release from the normal pituitary gland, resulting in a drop in plasma cortisol concentration. Hyperadrenocorticism of any etiology is usually resistant to suppression from small

---

PROCEDURE 8-14

Protocol for dexamethasone suppression tests in dogs

Low Dosage

1. Obtain a blood sample for baseline plasma cortisol determination at 8 am. (Some clinicians also do a 2- or 3-hour test as well.)
2. Immediately give dexamethasone IV at 0.01 mg/kg.
3. At 4 pm (see comment in Step 1 above), obtain postinjection plasma sample for cortisol determination.
4. Results:

Adrenal condition	Pretest cortisol level	Posttest cortisol level
Normal	1.1–8.0 μg/dl	0.1–0.9 μg/dl (<1.4)
Hyperadrenal	2.5–10.8 μg/dl	1.8–5.2 μg/dl (>1.4)

High Dosage

1. Use the same protocol as above, except the dexamethasone dosage is 0.1 mg/kg.
2. Results:
   Pituitary-dependent hyperadrenocorticism: Normal values as above
   Adrenal-dependent hyperadrenocorticism: As for hyperadrenal values above
Note: Successful suppression is defined as a 50% decrease in the plasma cortisol concentration from the baseline value. In 15% of dogs with pituitary-dependent hyperadrenocorticism, the plasma cortisol level is not suppressed by 50%. About 20% of dogs with adrenal-dependent hyperadrenocorticism have suppression of the plasma cortisol level by less than 50%, but all values remain above these considered adequate for suppression (greater than 1.5 μg/dl).

dexamethasone doses because a diseased pituitary gland is abnormally insensitive to the drug and continues elaborating excessive ACTH, although 35% of dogs with pituitary-dependent hyperadrenocorticism have a 4-hour post–dexamethasone cortisol lower than 1μg/dL or 50% of the baseline concentration. Neoplastic adrenal glands are autonomously secreting cortisol independent of endogenous ACTH control. The excessive cortisol production suppresses secretion of ACTH by the normal pituitary gland through negative feedback inhibition. Small doses of dexamethasone do not affect plasma cortisol measurements. However, such doses may complicate test results and may only differentiate normal animals from those with hyperadrenocorticism.

With larger dexamethasone doses, more differences appear. The sensitivity of a diseased pituitary gland to dexamethasone is incomplete; large dexamethasone doses overcome it and the abnormally high plasma ACTH and cortisol concentrations fall. Abnormal adrenal glands, however, continue to autonomously secrete cortisol. Thus plasma cortisol concentrations unresponsive to all dexamethasone doses are probably caused by primary adrenal gland disease. Suppression by large but not small doses suggests pituitary gland disease. The test has 73% accuracy in differentiating pituitary from adrenal causes in dogs and 75% sensitivity to diagnose hyperadrenocorticism in cats.[51]

A dual high-dosage dexamethasone test and ACTH response test are described in Procedure 8-15. Although combined protocol is a step saver, possibly ambiguous results necessitate more tests and expense. The ACTH response segment of the test is particularly prone to error. Because dexamethasone alters the adrenal responsiveness to ACTH (enhances or inhibits, depending on the duration of activity), the timing of the test is crucial. Normal standards must be newly established for any changes in protocol.

Endogenous ACTH Concentrations

Although not strictly a function test, assay of plasma ACTH concentrations may be a helpful diagnostic aid for hypoadrenocorticism and hyperadrenocorticism. Normal plasma ACTH concentrations range from 9 to 67 pg/mL (2 to 15 pmol/L) in dogs and 4.5 to 90 pg/mL (1 to 20 pmol/L) in cats. Animals with functioning adrenocortical tumors have low concentrations (less than 20 pg/ml [4.4 pmol/L]) from the negative feedback effect. Animals with pituitary-dependent hypoadrenocorticism should have higher concentrations, more than 40 to 45 pg/mL (8.8 to 9.9 pmol/L).[32]

Plasma concentration of endogenous ACTH helps also to differentiate primary (adrenal-dependent) from secondary (pituitary-dependent) hypoadrenocorticism. Low to undetectable ACTH concentrations occur in secondary Addison's disease, whereas normal (or increased) concentrations are expected in primary Addison's disease.

ACTH is a labile protein and requires special handling of the plasma sample. Aprotinin (protease inhibitor) within the EDTA tube and/or immediate freezing of the plasma may be required.

Corticotropin-Releasing Hormone (CRH) Stimulation

This test may be indicated to differentiate among pituitary-dependent and primary hyperadrenocorticism. Plasma cortisol concentration and ACTH should not be elevated

PROCEDURE 8-15

Protocol for combined dexamethasone suppression and corticotropin stimulation test

1. Collect a plasma sample for cortisol determination.
2. Administer dexamethasone 0.1 mg/kg IV.
3. Collect a plasma sample for cortisol determination 4 hours later.
4. Administer, immediately, 5 µg/kg (dog) or 125 µg/cat of tetracosactide (synthetic ACTH Cosyntropin in USA or Synacthen in Europe) IV or IM.
5. Collect a third plasma sample for cortisol determination 30 (cat IV administration) or 60 (dog and cat IM administration) minutes post-ACTH administration.
6. Collect a fourth plasma sample for cortisol determination 60 (cat IV administration) or 90 (cat IM administration) minutes post-ACTH administration (in cats).
7. Results:
   a. Normal pretest cortisol concentration:
      Dog: 0.5–4 µg/dL or 14–110 nmol/L
      Cat: 0.3–5 µg/dL or 8.3–138 nmol/L
   b. Normal post-dexamethasone cortisol concentration:
      1–1.4 µg/dL or 28–39 nmol/L
   c. Normal post-ACTH cortisol concentration:
      Dog: 8–20 µg/dL or 220–552 nmol/L
      Cat: 5–15 µg/dL or 138–414 nmol/L
8. Interpretation:
   a. Elevated post-dexamethasone and elevated post-ACTH cortisol concentration indicates hyperadrenocorticism.
   b. Elevated post-dexamethasone and normal post-ACTH cortisol concentration indicates hyperadrenocorticism.
   c. Normal post-dexamethasone and exaggerated post-ACTH cortisol concentration indicates pituitary-dependent hyperadrenocorticism.

after corticotropin-releasing hormone (CRH) stimulation in dogs with adrenal-dependent Cushing's disease.

The protocol of this test consists of obtaining a pretest sample to determine cortisol and ACTH, administering 1 µg/kg of CRH, and obtaining blood samples again 15 and 30 minutes later to evaluate cortisol and ACTH.[33]

TESTS OF THYROID FUNCTION

Thyroid hormones have pervasive effects, influencing the metabolic rate, growth, and differentiation of all body cells. Because the clinical signs of thyroid malfunction are numerous and confusing, function tests are valuable.

The thyroid glands are governed like the adrenal cortices. Thyrotropin-releasing factor (TRF) from the hypothalamus encourages the anterior pituitary to release thyrotropin or thyroid-stimulating hormone (TSH). TSH enhances thyroid growth, func-

PROCEDURE 8-16

Protocol for TSH response test

1. Collect a blood sample for baseline serum TT_4 determination.
2. Administer bovine 0.1 IU/kg (do not exceed 5 IU/dog or 1 IU/cat) TSH (bTSH) IV (IM or SC administration can also be appropriate).
3. Collect a second blood sample 4 or 6 hours after bTSH-stimulation for serum TT_4 determination.
4. Results:
   TT_4 post-bTSH stimulation in normal dogs:
   Higher than 2–2.9 μg/dL or 26–38 nmol/L
   Exceeds basal TT_4 in more than 1.5 μg/dL or 19 nmol/L

tion, and thyroxine release. Thyroxine really comprises two varieties of hormones, triiodothyronine (T_3) and thyroxine (T_4), varying in their extent of iodination. T_4 also is converted to the more active T_3 in tissues. Thyroxine completes the regulatory cycle by inhibiting TRF and TSH release.

Thyroid disease is manifested primarily as hypofunction in dogs, horses, ruminants, and swine, and hyperfunction in cats. The cause may be dietary iodine deficiency or excess, or goitrogens, most common in large animals. Primary glandular disease (neoplasia, autoimmune disease, idiopathic atrophy) comprises most cases, whereas pituitary (secondary thyroid disease) comprises 5% of hypothyroid dogs. Hypothalamic disease, or tertiary hypothyroidism, has not been described in (small) animals. In food animals, diagnosis is based on clinical signs (e.g., abortion, stillbirths, alopecia, and goiter in fetuses and neonates), serum thyroxine concentrations, serum protein-bound iodine concentrations, and pasture iodine analyses. Feeds may be examined for goitrogenic plants (*Brassicae* spp.) or excess calcium, which decreases iodine uptake.

Baseline thyroxine concentrations are used diagnostically, but normal values vary dramatically. Their diagnostic inadequacy mirrors that of plasma cortisol determinations. Some drugs, such as insulin or estrogens, may increase T_4 concentrations; others, such as glucocorticoids, anticonvulsants, antithyroid drugs, penicillins, thrimetoprim-sulfamides, diazepam, androgens, and sulfonylureas, may decrease T_4 concentrations. In addition, total T_4 (TT_4) may be increased in hypothyroid dogs as a result of the presence of anti-T_4 antibodies.

Specific determination of the active form of thyroxine non–protein-bound or free T_4 (FT_4) by equilibrium dialysis is a more accurate approach to thyroid function. Thereafter, determination of both endogenous TSH and T_4 (TT_4 or FT_4) are suitable to diagnose canine hypothyroidism.[34]

◆ TSH Response

This test is used on small animals (except in cats with hyperthyroidism) and horses and provides a reliable diagnostic separation of patients with normal *vs.* abnormal thyroid function (Procedure 8-16). Exogenous TSH challenge may sort out borderline cases and separate real hypothyroid patients from those with other illness or drug-depressed thyroxine concentrations and also may pinpoint the site of the lesions.

The test usually is used to explore canine hypothyroidism. After TSH is injected, thyroid response (usually serum T_4 levels, the most reliable index) is followed. An increase in the serum T_4 level occurs in normal animals. Primarily exhausted or insensitive thyroids do not respond to exogenous TSH. Indeed, endogenous TSH concentrations are already high from failing thyroxine inhibition. Therefore serum T_4 level is not increased in these animals. With pituitary or brain disease, however, the thyroid glands remain responsive. Such lesions result in too little endogenous thyrotropin. Although an increase in the serum T_4 level is expected in animals with pituitary lesions, 2 to 3 days of TSH challenge may be necessary before increased serum T_4 levels are seen. The extra TSH is required to overcome chronic glandular atrophy, similar to "priming the pump."

Hypothyroidism's insidious onset rarely is recognized. If it is suspected, the veterinarian must be aware that animals with early primary hypothyroidism may have some slight TSH responsiveness. Glucocorticoids seem to inhibit both TSH and thyroxine secretion, so euthyroidism with low serum T_3 levels only often accompanies Cushing's disease or vigorous glucocorticoid therapy. Fortunately, the TSH and ACTH response tests may be performed simultaneously. In such animals, the glands remain responsive to TSH but the absolute values of pre- and post-challenge serum T_4 are low or low resting with normal post-TSH values.

Feline hyperthyroidism is usually due to functional thyroid adenomas. Oddly, with exogenous TSH challenge, little or no increase occurs in the serum T_4 level, as in canine primary hypothyroidism. This phenomenon suggests that the neoplasm either functions independently of the trophic hormone or is already manufacturing and leaking thyroxine at maximum capacity. A lack of TSH responsiveness, appropriate clinical manifestations, and high baseline plasma thyroxine concentrations all attest to feline hyperthyroidism.

In horses, iodine-deficiency hypothyroidism is rare because iodized salt usually is offered free choice or in feeds. Overzealous iodine supplementation with kelp meal or vitamin-mineral mixes, however, provokes hypothyroidism and goiter. Excessive use of iodine inhibits thyroid function. In the assessment of thyroid function in horses, the normal serum T_4 values are 1 to 3 $\mu g/dl$, which is lower than in other species. Hypothyroidism should be suspected only with serum T_4 concentrations of less than 0.5 $\mu g/dl$.

Rare tumors of the *pars intermedia* of the pituitary, compressing the anterior pituitary, may cause secondary hypothyroidism in older horses. Because pituitary damage induces a plethora of signs, the TSH response test may be especially helpful.

◆ TRH Response

TRH response is used on small animals and provides a reliable diagnostic separation of patients with normal versus abnormal thyroid function. FT_4 is the fraction of thyroxine that is not bound to protein. FT_4 levels are less influenced by nonthyroidal diseases or drugs that total T_4 (TT_4) concentrations. Exogenous TRH challenge may sort out borderline cases and separate real hypothyroid and hyperthyroid patients from those with other illness or drug-depressed thyroxine concentrations. The test usually is used to explore canine hypothyroidism when TSH is not available. Baseline serum TT_4 and FT_4 concentrations are determined. Four hours after 0.1 mg/kg or 0.2 mg (total dose) of TRH are injected intravenously, thyroid response (serum TT_4 and FT_4 levels) is followed. An increase of the serum TT_4 concentration of 50% or 1μg/dL (13 nmol/L) and FT_4 (1.9 times) concentration, compared with baseline concentrations, occurs in normal animals. The evaluation of FT_4 levels allows a clearer distinction between euthyroid and hypothyroid dogs when TT_4 results are equivocal.[35] TRH response test may be used to diagnose mild to moderate feline hyperthyroidism. Baseline serum TT_4 and FT_4 concentrations are determined. About 4 hours after 0.1 mg/kg of TRH are injected intravenously, serum TT_4 and FT_4 levels are determined. An increase of the serum TT_4 less than 50%, compared with baseline concentrations, occurs in hyperthyroid cats. Increases between 50% and 60% are borderline, and increases more than 60% rule out hyperthyroidism.[36]

◆ Triiodothyronine Suppression Test

Hyperthyroidism is common in middle-age to old cats in the United States and Great Britain. Diagnosis may be based on resting thyroid hormone concentrations. Determination of both TT_4 and FT_4 may help to distinguish a nonthyroidal disease. The combination of high FT_4 value with low TT_4 is indicative of nonthyroidal illness, whereas a high FT_4 concentration and high-normal TT_4 concentration indicates hyperthyroidism. However, some cases may require a functional test to confirm or rule out the disease.

Thyroid suppression testing is based on the expected negative feedback regulation of TSH, induced by high concentrations of circulating thyroid hormone. Hyperthyroid cats should not have a normal pituitary-thyroid regulation. As a result, administration of exogenous T_3 must induce a decrease on endogenous T_4 unless feedback TSH regulation is altered.

To perform the test, a basal T_3 and T_4 determination is required. Seven T_3 doses of 25 μg *per os* q8h are administered at home. Approximately 2 to 4 hours after the seventh dose, a blood sample is obtained for T_3 and T_4 determination. Cats with hyperthyroidism have serum T_4 concentrations higher than 1.5 μg/dL or 20 nmol/L, whereas nonhyperthyroid cats have lower values. Low posttest T_3 concentrations indicate an invalid test resulting from failure of exogenous T_3 administration.[41]

⬤ TESTS OF GLUCOSE HOMEOSTASIS

The remaining endocrine function tests focus on the maintenance of blood glucose levels. This is crucial because brain cells, among others, must constantly be supplied with glucose as fuel. Accordingly, glucose metabolism is closely regulated. Glucagon, thyroxine, growth hormone, epinephrine, and glucocorticoids are all agents favoring hyperglycemia. They boost blood glucose levels by encouraging glycogenolysis, gluconeogenesis, and/or lipolysis, while discouraging glucose entry into cells. Insulin is the hypoglycemic hormone. Promoting glucose flux into its target cells, it also triggers anabolism, a process that converts glucose to other substances. This regulatory effect prevents the blood glucose concentration from exceeding the renal threshold and the spilling of glucose into the urine.

Regulation of blood glucose levels is complex. The pancreatic islets respond directly to blood glucose concentrations and release insulin (from the beta cells) or glucagon (from the alpha cells) as needed. Glucagon release also directly stimulates insulin release. Epinephrine is under direct sympathetic neural control; hyperglycemia is one aspect of the classic "flight or fight" state. The other hormones mentioned respond to hypothalamic/pituitary command. At any point in time, most of these agents are acting, shifting the blood glucose concentration up or down.

Because only insulin lowers blood glucose levels, aberrations of insulin action have the most obvious clinical effects. Hypofunction (diabetes mellitus) or hyperfunction (hyperinsulinism) can occur.

◆ Glucose Tolerance

Glucose tolerance tests directly challenge the pancreas with a glucose load and measure insulin's effect via blood or urine glucose concentrations. If adequate insulin is released and its target cells have healthy receptors, the artificially elevated blood glucose peaks 30 minutes after ingestion and begins to drop, reaching normal value within 2 hours, and no glucose appears in the urine. A normal glucose blood level at 2 hours postprandial may rule out diabetes mellitus. Prolonged hyperglycemia and glucosuria are consistent with diabetes mellitus. Profound hypoglycemia after challenge may indicate a glucose-responsive, hyperactive beta-cell tumor of the pancreas. This test may be simplified by determining a single 2-hour postprandial glucose.

The oral glucose tolerance test has been described earlier in this chapter as a test of intestinal absorption. Because test results are affected by abnormal intestinal function, such as enteritis or hypermotility, and excitement (as from gastric intubation), an IV glucose tolerance test is preferred. The IV test is the only practical option for ruminants.

With the IV glucose tolerance test (Procedure 8-17), a challenge glucose load is injected after a 12- to 16-hour fast (except in ruminants). Blood glucose is subsequently checked and its progress mapped as a tolerance curve. Results are standardized as disappearance half-lives or glucose turnover rates expressed as percent/minute:

Turnover rate = 0.693/Half-life × 100

Decreased glucose tolerance (increased half-life, decreased turnover rate) occurs in diabetes mellitus and less consistently in hyperthyroidism, hyperadrenocorticism, hyperpituitarism, and severe liver disease. Increased glucose tolerance (decreased half-life, increased turnover rate) is observed with hypothyroidism, hypoadrenocorticism, hypopituitarism, and hyperinsulinism. However, results may be erroneous. Normal animals on low-carbohydrate diets may manifest "diabetic curves." Therefore the authors recommend 2 to 3 days of high-carbohydrate meals before testing. The IV glucose tolerance test results are so variable in normal horses, depending on diet and fasting, that they are not very useful.

PROCEDURE 8-17

Protocol for the intravenous glucose tolerance test

1. Check the animal's diet. If it is low in carbohydrates, feed a high-carbohydrate diet (100 to 200 g/day for dogs) for 3 days before the test.
2. Fast the animal for 12 to 16 hours to lower the blood glucose level to 70 mg/dl in patients with suspected hyperinsulinism (do not fast ruminants). Fasting is dangerous in dogs with insulinoma!
3. Obtain a preinjection blood sample in a sodium fluoride tube for a baseline blood glucose determination.
4. Begin timing the trial at the infusion of sterile 50% glucose solution IV at 0.5 g/kg. Complete the infusion in exactly 30 seconds for small animals and within 2 to 3 minutes for large animals.
5. Obtain blood samples at 5, 15, 25, 35, 45, and 60 minutes after glucose infusion, using sodium fluoride as an anticoagulant, and submit all blood samples for glucose assay.
6. Plot glucose values on a semilog graph and determine the serum glucose half-life or turnover rate.
7. Results (values in species other than dogs and cats may be comparable):
   a. Dogs: The postinfusion blood glucose level should fall to baseline by 90 minutes. The normal half-life of glucose is 25 (8 minutes and the normal turnover time is 2.76 ± 0.91%/min. A turnover time of 2.0%/min indicates diabetes mellitus, and >2.0%/min but < 2.5%/min indicates an insulin-secreting tumor (see text).
   b. Cats: The postinfusion blood glucose level should fall to baseline by 120 to 180 minutes.

Glucose tolerance tests are usually unnecessary to obtain a diagnosis of diabetes mellitus. Persistent hyperglycemia and glucosuria, frequently with a history of polyuria, polydipsia, polyphagia, and weight loss, are sufficient to diagnose diabetes mellitus. The test may be of value in detecting hyperinsulinism because most beta-cell tumors of the pancreas are not rapidly responsive to glucose. They may even cause diabetic glucose tolerance curves because insulin-antagonist hormones are released as a result of the initial hypoglycemia. Patient stress and chemical restraint also affect glucose tolerance test results. Serum glucose measurements themselves may be erroneously low if blood samples are not subjected to anticoagulants and are allowed to sit at room temperature. However, the test is still used.

The best use for the glucose tolerance test is in animals with borderline hyperglycemia without persistent glucosuria. However, this test is not cost effective for the owner and may not result in significant therapeutic change. This dilemma is most often seen in cats in which high renal thresholds for glucose and stress-induced hyperglycemia are common and misleading.

Extra information may be obtained from the IV glucose tolerance test if immunoreactive insulin concentrations are followed simultaneously. This protocol may differentiate diabetes mellitus resulting from absolute lack of insulin (type I) from that resulting from target-cell insensitivity (type II) or inappropriate slow insulin release (type III).[37]

◆ Insulin Tolerance

This test also probes the causes of diabetes mellitus. Specifically, it checks the responsiveness of target cells to challenge with regular crystalline (short-acting) insulin 0.1 IU/kg SC or IM. Serum glucose levels are measured in blood samples obtained before insulin injection (fasting-blood glucose) and every 30 minutes after injection, for 3 hours. If the serum glucose level fails to drop to 50% of the fasting concentration within 30 minutes of insulin injection (insulin resistance), the insulin receptors are unresponsive or insulin action is being severely antagonized. The latter may occur in hyperadrenocorticism and acromegaly. Insulin resistance profoundly influences prognostic and therapeutic decisions.

If the insulin-induced hypoglycemia persists for 2 hours (hypoglycemia unresponsiveness), hyperinsulinism, hypopituitarism, or hypoadrenocorticism should be suspected. Because the test may cause this hypoglycemia, with possible weakness and convulsions, a glucose solution should always be on hand for rapid IV administration.

◆ Glucagon Tolerance

The main indications for this test are repeated normal or borderline results with the amended insulin:glucose ratio test (see below) or lack of an insulin assay. The glucagon tolerance test gives another assessment of hyperinsulinism. Glucagon stimulates the pancreatic beta cells directly and indirectly to increase the blood insulin level. In normal animals, glucagon injection (0.03 mg/kg IV up to a total of 1.0 mg in dogs and 0.5 mg in cats) transiently elevates the blood glucose level to greater than 135 mg/dl. In normal animals, this concentration level is greater than 135 mg/dl. In normal animals, this concentration returns to fasting concentrations. In normal cats, peak insulin occurs at 15 minutes, declining to basal concentration at 60 minutes. Type I diabetic cats present a flat insulin response. If the animal has a pancreatic beta-cell tumor, the serum glucose level peak is lower than normal and is followed within 1 hour by hypoglycemia (serum glucose is less than 60 mg/dl) because excessive insulin is secreted by the stimulated neoplasm.

To perform the test, the patient is fasted until the serum glucose level dips below 90 mg/dl (usually less than 10 hours). Glucagon is injected and sodium fluoride-anticoagulated blood samples are obtained before glucagon injection and 1, 3, 5, 15, 30, 45, 60, and 120 minutes after injection to monitor the glucose response. Unfortunately, the test is insensitive and may cause hypoglycemia convulsions up to 4 hours later. Patients must be fed immediately after the test and observed for hours.

◆ Amended Insulin:Glucose Ratio

The cause of hyperinsulinism may be assessed by taking simultaneous measurements of serum glucose and insulin levels in a fasting animal. Hypoglycemia normally inhibits insulin secretion. Pancreatic beta-cell tumors, hyperactive and unresponsive to glucose, secrete an abundance of insulin inappropriate to the prevailing blood glucose concentration. Although fasting serum insulin concentrations are often normal in hyperinsulinism, ratios of insulin to glucose concentrations are usually aberrant.

The absolute ratio of insulin to glucose can be amended to increase diagnostic accuracy. The amended insulin:glucose ratio (AIGR) subtracts 30 from the serum glucose concentration (Procedure 8-18). At a serum glucose level of 30 mg/dl or less, insulin is normally undetectable, so this discriminant puts the zero of both the glucose and insulin scale at the same physiologic place. Because abnormally high insulin concentrations are more obvious at low serum glucose concentrations, the AIGR is most valuable in animals with a confirmed hypoglycemia of less than 60 mg/dl. Insulin and glucose have to be measured from the same serum sample. Then serial determinations may be performed to select an insulin concentration in hypoglycemia. However, the test is not totally dependable. If the results are unconvincing, the procedure should be repeated or other tests tried. Specifically, diagnostic imaging and insulin-like growth factor tests should be tried to rule out or confirm paraneoplastic hypoglycemia.[38]

PROCEDURE 8-18

Protocol for amended insulin:glucose ratio determination

1. Feed the patient a normal meal at 8 AM, then begin fast.
2. Obtain a blood sample in a sodium fluoride tube every 2 to 3 hours for blood glucose assays. Save any samples with blood glucose values less than 60 mg/dl* for the immunoreactive insulin assay (usually occurs within 6 to 10 hours). Stop the test. If an immediate blood glucose assay is unavailable, obtain blood samples for 8 hours and then stop the test. Instruct the laboratory to measure the serum insulin concentration on the sample with the lowest blood glucose value. If the blood glucose value does not fall below 60 mg/dl in 8 to 10 hours, feed the patient at 5 pm, 8:30 PM and 12 PM and repeat the test by beginning fasting at midnight and obtaining blood samples from 8 AM to 5 PM the next day (if necessary).
3. Feed the patient several small meals over the next 2 hours after testing to avoid postprandial reactive hypoglycemia.
4. Compute the AIGR:

$$\text{AIGR} = \text{Plasma Insulin Level (U/ml)} \times \frac{100}{\text{Plasma Glucose Level (mg/dl)} - 30}$$

5. *Results:* A normal AIGR for dogs is 8.2 to 25.6.[†] Some authors suggest any ratio less than 30 is normal. If the animal is insulinopenic (insulin concentration less than 6 U/ml), it probably does not have a pancreatic beta-cell tumor, regardless of the AIGR.

Patients with hyperinsulinism usually do not exhibit clinical signs at this level of hypoglycemia.

[†]*Varies with the laboratory.*

◆ Miscellaneous Tests of Insulin Release

When results of a glucagon response test or AIGR are equivocal, glucose, epinephrine, leucine, tolbutamide, or calcium challenges may be attempted. These substances, like glucagon, may provoke a hyperinsulinemic response from pancreatic islet-cell tumors, resulting in decreased serum glucose levels. However, tumors vary in their sensitivity to these agents and false negatives (no response) can occur. These tests are also dangerous because they can precipitate severe, prolonged hypoglycemia.

◉ PITUITARY FUNCTION TESTS

Diagnosis of canine acromegaly may be based on documentation of elevated growth hormone (GH). Serial GH determinations (three to five samples taken at 10-minute intervals) are performed because affected dogs have constant levels of GH instead of fluctuating GH concentrations. In addition, affected dogs do not respond to stimulation with GH-releasing hormone (GHRH). This test requires intravenous administration of 1µg/kg GHRH or 10 µg clonidine. Posttest plasma GH in normal dogs increases 5 to 15 µg/L or 13 to 25 µg/L, respectively.[39,40]

References

1. Youngberg CA et al: Radiotelemetric determination of gastrointestinal pH in four healthy Beagles, *Am J Vet Res* 46:1516-21, 1985.
2. Zerbe CA, Washabau RJ: Gastrointestinal endocrine disease. In Ettinger SJ, Feldman EC, editors: *Textbook of veterinary internal medicine,* ed 5, Philadelphia, WB Saunders, p 1500-8, 2000.
3. Williams DA et al: Fecal proteolytic activity in clinically normal cats and in a cat with exocrine pancreatic insufficiency, *J Am Vet Med Asoc* 197:210-2, 1990.
4. Williams DA et al: Fecal proteolytic activity in clinically normal cats and a cat with exocrine pancreatic insufficiency, *J Am Vet Med Assoc* 197:210-3, 1990.
5. Williams DA, Reed SD: Comparison of methods for assay of fecal proteolytic activity, *Vet Clin Pathol* 19:20-4, 1990.
6. Melgarejo T et al: Enzyme-linked immunoabsorbant assay for canine alpha₁-protease inhibitor (a₁-PI), *J Vet Intern Med* 7:133-7, 1993.
7. Barton CL et al: The diagnosis and clinicopathologic features of canine protein-losing enteropathy, *J Am An Hosp Assoc* 14:85-91, 1978.
8. Merritt AM, Duely P: Phloroglucinol microassay for plasma xylose in dogs and horses, *Am J Vet Res* 44:2184-5, 1983.
9. Edwards DF, Russell RG: Probable vitamin K-deficient bleeding in two cats with malabsorption syndrome secondary to lymphocytic-plasmacytic enteritis, *J Vet Int Med* 1:97-101, 1987.
10. Emm SG et al: The rate of D-xylose absorption in normal cats, *Aust Vet J* 60:30-2, 1983.
11. Hawkins EC et al: Digestion of bentiromide and absorption of xylose in healthy cats and absorption in cats with infiltrative intestinal disease, *Am J Vet Res* 47:567-9, 1986.
12. Elwood CM et al: A novel method of assessing canine intestinal permeability and function using a multiple sugar test, *J Vet Intern Med* 7:131-6, 1993.
13. Rutgers HC et al: Small intestinal bacterial overgrowth in dogs with chronic intestinal disease, *J Am Vet Med Assoc* 206:187-93, 1995.

14. Williams DA, Batt R: Diagnosis of canine exocrine pancreatic insufficiency by the assay of serum trypsin like immunoreactivity, *J Small Anim Pract* 24:583-8, 1983.

15. Steiner JM et al: Development and validation of a radioimmunoassay for feline trypsin-like immunoreactivity, *Am J Vet Res* 57:1417-20, 1996.

16. Washabau RJ et al: Evaluation of intestinal carbohydrate malabsorption in the dog by pulmonary hydrogen gas excretion, *Am J Vet Res* 47:1402-6, 1986.

17. Center SA: Editorial: BSP-a retired test revisited, *J Vet Intern Med* 14:557-9, 2000.

18. Flatland B et al: Evaluation of the bromosulfophthalein 30-minute retention test for the diagnosis of hepatic disease in dogs, *J Vet Intern Med* 14:560-8, 2000.

19. Center: Pathophysiology, laboratory diagnosis, and diseases of the liver. In Ettinger SJ, Feldmn EC, editors: *Textbook of veterinary internal medicine,* ed 4, Philadelphia, 1995, WB Saunders, p 1261-1312.

20. Tenant BC: Hepatic function. In Kaneko J, Harvey J, Bruss M: *Clinical biochemistry of domestic animals,* ed 5, New York, 1997, Academic Press, p 327-52.

21. Rothuizen J: Rectal ammonia tolerance test in the evaluation of portal circulation in dogs with liver disease, *Res Vet Sci* 33:22-5, 1982.

22. Callery S et al: Hepatic insufficiency after portacaval shunting is prevented by prior intraportal pancreatic islet autotransplantation, *Surgery* 106:257-6, 1989.

23. Lumsden J et al: Contribution of delta bilirubin to the interpretation of hyperbilirubinemia in the horse—a pilot study, *Can Vet J* 32:169-172, 1991.

24. Moe L, Heiene R: Estimation of glomerular filtration rate in dogs with [99M]-Tc-DTPA and iohexol, *Res Vet Sci* 58:138-43, 1995.

25. Haller H et al: Single-injection inulin clearance—a simple method for measuring glomerular filtration rate in dogs, *Res Vet Sci* 64:151-6, 1998.

26. Di Bartola S: Clinical approach and laboratory evaluation of renal disease. In Ettinger SJ, Feldmn EC, editors: Textbook of veterinary internal medicine, ed 4, Philadelphia, 1995, WB Saunders p1706-19.

27. Holt PE: Investigation and therapy of incontinent animals, *Eur J Compan An Pract (EJCAP)* 10:111-6, 2000.

28. van Vonderen IK et al: Influence of veterinary care on the urinary corticoid:creatinine ratio in dogs, *J Vet Intern Med* 12:431-5, 1998.

29. van Lic CH et al: Comparison of results of adrenocorticotropic hormone stimulation and low-dose dexamethasone suppression test with necropsy findings in dogs: 81 cases (1985-1995), *J Am Vet Med Assoc* 21:322-5, 1997.

30. Zerbe CA: Screening tests to diagnose hyperadrenocorticism in cats and dogs, *Comp Cont Ed Pract Vet* 22:17-31, 2000.

31. Duesberg C, Peterson ME: Adrenal disorders in cats, *Vet Clin North Am (Sm An Pract)* 27:321-47, 1997.

32. Kempainen RJ, Clark TP: CVT update: sample collecting and testing protocols in endocrinology. In Kirk R, Bonagura, editors: *Kirk's current veterinary therapy XII,* Philadelphia, 1995, WB Saunders, pp 335-9.

33. Zerbe CA: Differentiating tests to evaluate hyperadrenocorticism in dogs and cats, *Comp Cont Ed Pract Vet* 22:149-57, 2000.

34. Dixon RM et al: Epidemiological, clinical, haematological and biochemical characteristics of canine hypothyroidism, *Vet Rec* 145:481-7, 1999.

35. Sparkes AH et al: Assessment of dose and time responses to TRH and thyrotropin in healthy dogs, *J Sm An Pract* 36:245-51, 1995.

36. Peterson ME: Hyperthyroidism. In Ettinger SJ, Feldman EC, editors: *Textbook of veterinary internal medicine,* ed 5, Philadelphia, 2000, WB Saunders, pp 1400-19.

37. Kaneko JJ: Carbohydrate metabolism and its diseases. In Kaneko JJ, Harvey JW, Bruss ML, editors: *Clinical biochemistry of domestic animals,* ed 5, San Diego, 1997, Academic Press, pp 517-51.

38. Tobin RL et al: Outcome of surgical versus medical treatment of dogs with beta-cell neoplasia: 39 cases (1990-1997), *J Am Vet Med Assoc* 15:226-30, 1999.

39. Mol JA, Rijnberk AD: Pituitary function. In Kaneko JJ, Harvey JW, Bruss ML, editors: Clinical biochemistry of domestic animals, ed 5, San Diego, 1997, Academic Press, pp 517-51.

40. Rijnberk AD, Mol JA: Progestin induced hypersecretion of growth hormone—an introductory review, *J Reprod Fertil Suppl* 51:107-9, 1997.

Immunology and Serology

9

ELOYES HILL

A nimals in the recovery phase of an infectious disease are resistant to reinfection. *Immunity* (from the Latin *immunis,* meaning "safe") is the word used to describe this state of heightened resistance.

The goal of the body's immune response is to combat the effects of foreign substances on vital bodily processes. To accomplish this, the body must be able to recognize minute differences among foreign substances and between foreign substances and itself. After a substance is recognized as foreign, the body must have a means of responding to it physiologically, which eliminates or limits any harmful effects of the agent. Memory components for the foreign material facilitate a future immune response to an encounter with the same agent.

Occasionally, the immune system malfunctions, resulting in such disorders as allergy, immunodeficiency, neoplasia, or autoimmune disease. This chapter reviews the basic principles of immunity and the immune response and the practical applications of immunology that have been developed, including vaccination and immunodiagnostic procedures.

THE IMMUNE RESPONSE

Vertebrate species have two major internal defense systems: the *innate* or *nonspecific immune system* and the *acquired* or *specific immune system.* Foreign bodies, such as bacteria, viruses, and fungi, first encounter barriers of the innate immune system. These barriers include the skin; physical and biochemical components in the nasopharynx, gut, lungs, and genitourinary tract; and the body's inflammatory response. The body also has populations of commensal bacteria that compete with invading pathogens.

Another major function of the innate system is phagocytosis, a nonspecific response. Phagocytic cells (the chief phagocyte is the macrophage) ingest and destroy inert particles, viruses, bacteria, and cellular debris. Macrophages are found throughout the body.

In the blood they are called *monocytes*. From the blood they migrate to various tissues and organs and are then called *macrophages* or other specialized names. They locate in connective tissue, liver, brain, lung, spleen, bone marrow, and lymph nodes and together make up the mononuclear phagocytic system.

If foreign bodies evade the innate immune system, they then encounter the acquired immune system, which is more sophisticated. The acquired immune system is divided into two components: the humoral immune system and the cell-mediated immune system. The acquired immune system has the ability to respond specifically to foreign substances. These substances, or antigens, may be bacterial, viral, fungal, or altered endogenous cells of the host's body. Their presence initiates humoral and cellular responses that neutralize, detoxify, and eliminate these foreign materials from the host.

Lymphocytes and their progeny are the cell types largely responsible for the acquired immune system. This line of defense is not, however, divorced from the innate immune system. Macrophages process antigens and present them to antigen-committed lymphocytes. That is, they act as antigen-presenting cells.

Lymphoid stem cells develop first in the yolk sac and then in the fetal liver (Figure 9-1). The bone marrow assumes this responsibility near parturition and serves as the source of these cells throughout postnatal life. The lymphoid stem cells are destined to further mature in one of two places: the bone marrow or the thymus. B-lymphocytes mature in the bone marrow, whereas T-lymphocytes mature in the thymus.

◆ Humoral Immune System

Lymphocytes that mature in the bone marrow (B-cells) are concerned chiefly with production and secretion of immunoglobulin (Ig) molecules, which are also known as *antibodies*. Their maturation process consists of three stages: the lymphoblast, the prolymphocyte, and the mature lymphocyte. The mature cells leave the bone marrow to seed secondary lymphoid organs, chiefly the spleen and lymph nodes, where they encounter antigens. The humoral immune system can recognize billions of different antigens because as B-cells mature, each B-cell develops a specific receptor molecule to a specific antigen. When an antigen enters the body, a mature B-cell is committed to and reacts with that particular antigen. Stimulation of that B-cell to produce antibodies is a complex process, usually requiring the help of macrophages and specialized T-lymphocytes called *helper T-cells*. The antigen stimulated B-cell then quickly divides and produces a clone of identical B-cells that all produce the same type of antigen-specific antibody. These antibody-secreting B-cells are now called *plasma cells*. Some of the antigen stimulated B-cells differentiate into memory B-cells, which respond faster to a second exposure of that antigen (see Figure 9-1).

Antibodies (immunoglobulins) are proteins consisting of two distinct functional portions. One portion of the antibody molecule, the variable portion, is specific for the antigen. The other portion of the antibody molecule, the constant portion, is the same in all antibodies of the same class. When an appropriate antibody encounters an antigen, the antibody binds to the antigen to form a complex.

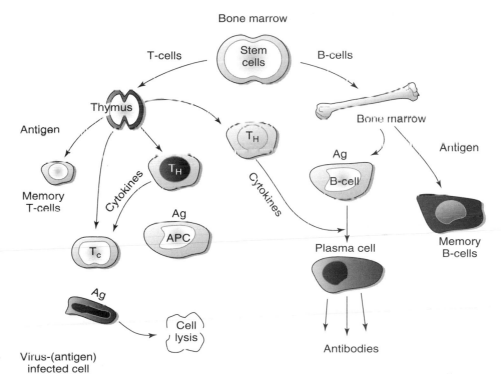

Figure 9-1
Pathways of lymphoid cells in the immune response. Stem cells in the bone marrow give rise to T- and B-lymphocytes. Lymphocytes mature in the thymus and bone marrow. Memory and effector cells differentiate and proliferate upon interaction with antigens. *Ag,* antigen. *TH,* T-helper lymphocytes. *TC,* T-cytotoxic lymphocyte. *APC,* antigen-presenting cell.

Immunoglobulins are divided into distinct classes, each with unique biologic properties. The most abundant of these classes is IgG, the major immunoglobulin in serum. It plays the major role in humoral immunity.

IgM, the largest antibody, is the first antibody to appear in response to exposure to an antigen. Its concentration rapidly declines, followed by an increase in IgG concentration, which is also specific for the same antigen. Functions of IgG and IgM include bacterial toxin neutralization, activation of complement, and phagocytic enhancement.

IgA prevents attachment of pathogens to mucosal surfaces and is important in protection of the respiratory, intestinal, and urogenital tracts. High levels of IgE are found in allergic and parasitized individuals. IgD is a B-lymphocyte surface antigen receptor in some species.

◆ Cell-Mediated Immune System

Lymphoid stem cells that mature in the thymus develop into T-cell lymphocytes. Like that of B-cells, their maturation process consists of three morphologically distinct stages: lymphoblast, prolymphocyte, and lymphocyte. As these cells mature, they also develop receptors to specific antigens and become *immunocompetent* or *antigen-committed* T-lymphocytes. Then, after contact with their specific antigens, these cells proliferate and differentiate into either clones of memory cells or clones of effector cells against those antigens.

Memory cells recognize antigens to which they have previously been exposed. On a subsequent encounter, they elicit a more rapid immune response.

Different types of T-effector cells exist, such as helper T-cells (CD4+) and cytotoxic T-cells (CD8+). CD4+ and CD8+ refer to surface molecules, or markers, found on helper T (T_H) and cytotoxic T (T_C) lymphocytes, respectively. HIV (human immunodeficiency virus), the AIDS virus, has a special affinity for the T_H (CD4+) lymphocytes.

T-helpers, in addition to their function in humoral immunity, affect the actions of other cells, such as cytotoxic T-cells. In this process an antigen-processing cell, such as a macrophage, may pick up an antigen, process it, and bring the antigenic portion of the antigen to its surface. A T-helper can then recognize the antigen and release cytokines, which help to activate cytotoxic T-cells. Cytotoxic T-cells attach to antigen-infected cells and destroy them. Virus-infected cells, tumor cells, and cells of foreign tissue graft all may be eliminated in this manner (see Figure 9-1).

Passive Immunity

Animals become passively resistant to disease by receiving maternal antibodies in the colostrum or by receiving preformed antibodies by injection. These antibodies have been produced in a donor animal. A donor animal is vaccinated with a pathogen. When its serum antibodies reach a high concentration, the animal is bled and the globulin portion containing the antibodies is separated and purified. The protection that an animal receives from an injection of this immune globulin is short lived but immediate.

Immunization

Animals become actively resistant to disease by having the disease and developing antibodies, or by being vaccinated or immunized, in which case they also develop their own antibodies. Immunization is accomplished by injecting a suspension of microorganisms into an animal for the purpose of eliciting an antibody response but not causing the disease. The microorganisms may be either attenuated (weakened but still alive) or inactivated (killed). Attenuated vaccines normally cause a longer-lasting, more potent immune response. Inactivated vaccines are generally safer and have no ability to cause disease. An adjuvant may be added to the vaccine to enhance the normal immune response. Some adjuvants do this by simply slowing the rate of antigen elimination from the body so that the antigen is present longer to stimulate antibody production.

Vaccines may be given subcutaneously or intramuscularly, depending on the vaccine. Other vaccines are aerosolized and given intranasally. Some vaccines are put in the feed or drinking water. Veterinary technicians working at fish hatcheries may vaccinate fish by putting the vaccine into their water.

DISORDERS OF THE IMMUNE SYSTEM

Some immune responses have an adverse effect on the host animal. Among hypersensitivity reactions are allergies; anaphylactic shock, a severe reaction that may occur within seconds after an antigen enters the circulation; autoimmune hemolytic anemia, a condition causing destruction of red blood cells by the host itself; glomerulonephritis, caused by deposition of antibody-antigen complexes in the kidney; and contact hypersensitivity reactions, such as reactions to contact with poison ivy.

In addition to the hypersensitivity reactions just described, the immune system also may show deficiencies. A deficiency may exist in phagocytes or in immunoglobulins. A condition called *combined immunodeficiency* affects animals in early life, after serum levels of maternally derived antibodies have declined. Arabian foals with this disease often die from opportunistic infection resulting from an absence or deficiency of immunoglobulins.

Lymphoma, a type of tumor characterized by uncontrolled proliferation of lymphocytes, is another abnormality of the immune system. The immune system normally recognizes and destroys cancer cells before they become established in the body, but sometimes the cancer seems to become resistant and escapes the immune defense mechanisms.

PRINCIPLES OF COMMON IMMUNOLOGIC LABORATORY TESTS

◆ Tests of Humoral Immunity

The science of detection and measurement of antibodies or antigens is called *serology*. Detection depends on the binding of antibodies and antigens. Unfortunately, this binding phenomenon is ordinarily invisible. Visualization, and thus detection, of the antigen-antibody reaction depends on secondary events by which the union is easily detected and therefore of diagnostic use in veterinary practice.

Commercial production of monoclonal antibodies to many different antigens has resulted in a variety of test kits for use in the veterinary laboratory. Specific antibodies to many different antigens can be produced and used in the laboratory for rapid identification of disease-producing organisms.

Immunization with viruses, bacteria, or other entities stimulates antibody production in an animal. The antibody-secreting, transformed lymphocytes (plasma cells) may be isolated from the animal and chemically fused with a type of "immortal" cell that propagates indefinitely, such as mouse myeloma cells. The antibodies these hybrid cells produce, called *monoclonal antibodies,* are collected. Because each monoclonal antibody attaches to only one specific part of one type of molecule (antigen), use of these antibodies in diagnostic kits makes the tests specific and greatly reduces interpretation problems of the result. For example, the feline leukemia virus antigen only reacts with the feline leukemia virus antibody. A specific reaction is diagnostically significant for this complicated disease. In addition to their specificity, these procedures allow rapid identification of the pathogen.

Many serologic tests use monoclonal antibodies. Enzyme immunoassay, latex agglutination, immunodiffusion, and rapid immunomigration are methodologies used in veterinary laboratories. Other methods, such as complement fixation, immunofluorescence, immunoelectron microscopy, virus neutralization, and polymerase chain reaction (PCR) DNA amplification are used in veterinary reference laboratories and research facilities and are not included in this discussion. Many of the principles are the same, however, and understanding a few procedures gives readers a good basis for understanding others.

Reference laboratories offer myriad serologic tests specifically developed for veterinary samples. Tests for blood types, allergies, bovine leukemia virus, reproductive hormones, Lyme disease, and brucellosis are a few of the diagnostic tests available (Table 9-1).

Figure 9-2
A critical step in the microwell enzyme immunoassay is washing away the unbound enzyme-labeled antibodies. (Pet Check Heartworm PF Antigen Test Kit, courtesy IDEXX Laboratories, Westbrook, ME.)

Figure 9-3
Kit to detect progesterone levels in canine serum (ICG Status Pro; Synbiotics) based on the ELISA membrane format. (Courtesy Synbiotics Corporation, San Diego, CA.)

ELISA

ELISA is an acronym for *enzyme-linked immunosorbent* assay. This enzyme immunoassay has been adapted to many agents commonly tested for in the veterinary laboratory (Figures 9-2 to 9-5 and Table 9-1). Using monoclonal antibodies, the specificity of ELISA is high; that is, little cross-reactivity occurs with other agents. This phenomenon makes ELISA an accurate way to detect specific antigens, such as viruses, bacteria, parasites, or hormones in serum. ELISA also may be used to test for an antibody in the serum, in which case the test kit contains the specific antigen. Some of the available ELISA kits detect heartworms, feline leukemia virus, feline immunodeficiency virus, canine parvovirus, and progesterone (Procedures 9-1 to 9-3).

Text continued on p. 414

Figure 9-4
With the ELISA wand format to test for FeLV (Assure/FeLV; Synbiotics), a positive reaction is indicated by color development in the tube on the left. The wands have been removed from both tubes. (Courtesy Synbiotics Corporation, San Diego, CA.)

Figure 9-5
Enzyme immunoassay for heartworm antigen (Snap Whole Blood Heartworm Antigen Test; IDEXX). **A,** Negative reaction. **B,** Weak positive reaction. **C,** Strong positive reaction. (Courtesy IDEXX Laboratories, Westbrook, ME.)

TABLE 9-1

Some commercially available immunologic test kits

Disease/Condition	Product Name	Manufacturer	Type of Test	Use
Allergies	Equitec	DMS Laboratories*	ELISA	For semiquantitative determination of allergen-specific IgE antibodies in equine serum
Blood Group Test	RapidVet-H	DMS Laboratories*	Monoclonal antibody agglutination test	To classify dogs as DEA 1.1 or cats types A, B, or AB
Borreliosis (Lyme disease)	Lymechek	Synbiotics†	ELISA	For detection of *Borrelia burgdorferi* antibodies in dogs
Bovine leukemia virus infection	Herdchek:Anti-BLV Antibody Test Kit	IDEXX‡	Enzyme immunoassay	For detection of antibodies to bovine leukemia virus in cattle
Brucellosis	CITE *Brucella abortus* antibody	IDEXX‡	Enzyme immunoassay	For detection of antibodies to *Brucella abortus* in cattle
Equine infectious anemia	Lab-EZ/EIA	Synbiotics†	Agar-gel immunodiffusion	For detection of infectious anemia anti-bodies in horses
Equine infectious anemia	Diasystems EIA CELISA Antibody Test Kit	IDEXX‡	CELISA	For detection of infectious anemia anti-bodies in horses
Failure of passive transfer	CITE Foal IgG Test Kit	Blue Ridge§	ELISA	For semiquantitative measurement of IgG levels in equine serum, plasma, or whole blood
Feline infectious peritonitis (FIP)	Diasystems CELISA-FIP Antibody Test Kit	IDEXX‡	CELISA	For detection of antibodies to FIP virus in cats
Feline immunodeficiency virus (FIV) infection	PETChek Anti FIV Antibody Test Kit	IDEXX‡	Enzyme immunoassay	For detection of antibodies to FIV in cats
Feline leukemia virus (FELV) infection	Assure/FeLV	Synbiotics†	ELISA	For detection of FeLV antigens in cats
	PROBE FeLV Antigen Test Kit	IDEXX‡	ELISA	For detection of FeLV antigens in cats
	Virachek	Synbiotics†	ELISA	For detection of FeLV antigens in cats
	Witness FeLV	Synbiotics†	RIM	For detection of FeLV antigens in cats

Disease/Condition	Product	Manufacturer	Method	Description
Feline leukemia virus and immunodeficiency virus infection	SNAP Combo FeLV Ag/FIV Ab	IDEXX‡	ELISA	For detection of FeLV antigens and FIV antibodies in cats
Heartworm infection	Assure/CH	Synbiotics†	ELISA	For detection of heartworm antigens in dogs
	Dirochek	Synbiotics†	ELISA	For detection of heartworm antigens in dogs
	Heska Solo Step FH	Heska‖	Lateral flow immunoassay	For detection of heartworm antibodies in cats
Heartworm infection	VetRED	Synbiotics†	RBC agglutination	For detection of heartworm antigens in dogs
	Witness HW	Synbiotics†	RIM	For detection of heartworm antigens in dogs
Johne's disease	Herdchek Mycobacterium paratuberculosis Antibody Test Kit	IDEXX‡	Enzyme-linked immunosorbent assay	For detection of antibody to M. paratuberculosis in bovine serum or plasma
	Rapid Johne's Test	ImmuCell¶	Agarose gel immunodiffusion	For detection of antibodies to M. paratuberculosis in bovine serum
Mycoplasma species	Mycoplasma gallisepticum nobilis Antigen Test Kit	Intervet#	Plate agglutination test	To detect Mycoplasma antibodies in poultry; screening method
Neospora caninum	Herdchek Neospora caninum Antibody Test Kit	IDEXX‡	Enzyme immunoassay	For detection of antibodies to Neospora caninum in bovine serum
Newcastle disease	Flockchek: Anti-NDV	IDEXX‡	Enzyme immunoassay	For detection of antibodies to Newcastle disease virus in chicken serum
Ovulation timing	icg Status–LH	Synbiotics†	Immunochromatographic assay	For the semi-quantitative measurement of luteinizing hormone levels in dogs

Continued

TABLE 9-1

Some commercially available immunologic test kits—cont'd

Disease/Condition	Product Name	Manufacturer	Type of Test	Use
Parvovirus infection	PROBE Canine Parvovirus Antigen Test Kit	IDEXX‡	ELISA	For detection of parvovirus antigens in canine feces
Progesterone	Target Canine Ovulation Kit	BioMetallics**	Immunoassay	For the determination of the optimum time for fertilization
Pseudorabies	Herdchek Pseudorabies Virus Antibody Test Kit	IDEXX‡	Enzyme immunoassay	For detection of pseudorabies virus antibodies in the serum of pigs
Rheumatoid arthritis	CRF	Synbiotics†	Latex aggulation	For detection of rheumatoid arthritis factor in canine serum
Salmonellosis	Flockchek SE Test Kit	IDEXX‡	Enzyme immunoassay	For detection of antibodies to *Salmonella enteritidis* in chicken serum or egg yolk
Tuberculosis	Tuberculin PPD	Synbiotics†	Intradermal test	For intradermal testing of cattle for bovine TB
von Willebrand factor deficiency	vWF ZYMTEC	DMS Laboratories*	ELISA	For determination of vWF in multiple species

*DMS Laboratories, Inc., 2 Darts Mill Road, Flemington, NJ 08822.

†Synbiotics Corporation, 11011 Via Frontera, San Diego, CA 92127.

‡IDEXX Laboratories, One Idexx Drive, Westbrook, ME 04092.

∥Blue Ridge Pharmaceuticals, Inc., 4249-105 Piedmont Parkway; Greensboro, NC 27410.

|Heska Corporation, 1613 Prospect Parkway; Fort Collins, CO 80525.

¶ImmuCell Corporation, 56 Evergreen Drive, Portland, ME 04103.

#Intervet Inc., 405 State Street, P.O. Box 318, Millsboro, DE 19966.

**Biometallics, Inc., Veterinary Science Division, P.O. Box 2251, Princeton, NJ 08543.

PROCEDURE 9-1

Protocol for microwell ELISA

1. Plastic wells come precoated with antibodies specific for the antigen being tested.
2. Add samples (which may contain antigen) and a second antibody, labeled with an enzyme, to the wells.
3. Antigen, if present, binds to both the solid phase (wells) and enzyme-labeled antibodies.
4. Unbound enzyme-labeled antibodies are washed away.
5. Add chromogenic substrate, which reacts with the enzyme, causing a color to develop.
6. Development of a color indicates the presence of the antigen in the sample.

PROCEDURE 9-2

Protocol for membrane ELISA

1. Add sample to a membrane, which is precoated with antibodies specific for the antigen being tested.
2. Any antigens in the sample are captured by the antibodies on the membrane.
3. Typically, positive-control spots containing the antigen also have been precoated on the membrane.
4. Add a second antibody, enzyme-labeled, to the membrane. This antibody also binds to the captured patient antigen and the control antigen. The antigen is now "sandwiched" between two antibodies.
5. Wash unbound enzyme-labeled antibodies away.
6. Add chromogen to the membrane, which reacts with the enzyme on the second antibody to produce a color.
7. Color appears where the positive control and patient antigens are present on the membrane.

PROCEDURE 9-3

Protocol for wand ELISA

1. The bulbous ends of plastic wands come precoated with antibodies specific for the antigen being tested.
2. Any antigens in the sample are captured by the antibodies on the wand.
3. Incubate a second antibody, labeled with an enzyme, with the sample and wand. These antibodies also bind with the antigen.
4. Any unbound enzyme-labeled antibody is washed away and a chromogenic reagent is added.
5. The reagent reacts with the enzyme-labeled antibodies that are bound to the antigens, producing a color reaction.

For the ELISA antigen detection system, monoclonal antibody is bound to the walls of wells in a test tray, to a membrane, or to a plastic wand. Antigen, if present in the sample, binds to this antibody, and to a second enzyme-labeled antibody that is added to aid in detection of the antigen. When a chromogenic (color-producing) substrate is added to the mixture, it reacts with the enzyme to develop a specific color, indicating the presence of antigen in the sample. If the sample contained no antigen, the second antibody would be washed away in a rinsing process and no color reaction would develop.

A similar procedure is used for ELISA antibody detection. In this procedure, antigen is bound to the wells, membrane, or wand, and the patient sample is assayed for the presence of a specific antibody.

CELISA

CELISA is an acronym for *competitive enzyme-linked immunosorbent assay*. If used to test for patient antigen, this assay uses an enzyme-labeled antigen as well as monoclonal antibodies. Patient antigen, if present, competes with enzyme-labeled antigens for the antibodies coating the test wells. Color developer reacts with the enzyme to produce a color. The intensity of the color produced varies with the concentration of the patient antigen (Procedure 9-4). Feline infectious peritonitis (FIP) antibodies may be detected in cat serum with a CELISA test.

Latex Agglutination

This test uses small, spherical latex particles coated with antibody (or antigen) and suspended in water. If serum containing the corresponding antigen is added to the

---

PROCEDURE 9-4

Protocol for CELISA

1. Test wells come precoated with monoclonal antibodies.
2. Patient samples (that may contain antigen) are added to test wells.
3. Enzyme-labeled antigens are then added to the same test wells.
4. The two antigens compete for antibodies on the test wells. The antigen in higher concentration binds more antibodies.
5. After incubation, rinse the wells to wash away excess enzyme-labeled antigens.
6. Add color developer, which reacts with the enzyme on the enzyme-labeled antigen.
7. If the sample contains low levels of patient antigen, most of the antigen bound to the antibodies on the test wells is enzyme-labeled antigen and a deep color develops.
8. If the sample contains high levels of patient antigen, most of the antigen bound to the antibodies on the test wells is antigen from the patient and little color develops.

mixture, formation of antibody-antigen complexes causes agglutination (clumping). Agglutination changes the appearance of the latex suspension from smooth and milky to clumpy because the latex particles have clustered together. If no antigen is present in the sample, the mixture of latex and serum remains evenly dispersed. Serum for canine rheumatoid factor may be tested using this method (Figure 9-6, Table 9-1, and Procedure 9-5).

RIM

RIM is an acronym for *rapid immunomigration*. Historically, this technology has been called *immunochromatography* or *lateral flow immunoassay*. The "signal-generating" component of this test is colloidal gold. Its counterparts in other technologies are enzymes and color reagent or agglutinated latex particles. All three types of components create a positive result.

In this type of procedure colloidal gold is conjugated to antibodies specific for the antigen being tested. These conjugated antibodies are present in the membrane of the test cassette where patient sample is applied. If antigens are present in the patient

Figure 9-6
Clumped latex particles, representing antigen-antibody complexes. Samples *1*, *2*, and *3* indicate a positive reaction. Samples *4*, *5*, and *6*, showing no clumping, indicate a negative reaction. (Canine RF Test; courtesy Synbiotics Corporation, San Diego, CA.)

PROCEDURE 9-5

Protocol for latex agglutination

1. Use a dark glass slide to read the agglutination reactions.
2. Deposit positive and negative reference sera (positive contains antibodies being tested) and patient sera (with possible antibodies) separately on the glass slide.
3. Add a suspension of latex particles that has been coated with antigens that react with the test antibodies to each sample on the slide.
4. Rotate the slide and observe for the appearance of visible agglutination. Agglutination indicates a positive result.

sample, they bind to the conjugated antibodies and the antibody-antigen complexes migrate along the membrane to another area of the cassette where the results are read. Buffer may be added to aid the migrational flow of the antibody-antigen complexes. In the reading area a second antibody is present in the membrane. If antigen is in the sample, it is captured along with the first antibody and the colloidal gold, by the second antibody. The accumulation of colloidal gold in that area causes a color change.

To ensure quality results, control antigen is present in another area of the membrane strip. The conjugated first antibody binds to the antigen in the control area. Its accumulation also causes a color change and occurs whether or not antigen is present in the patient sample. A positive patient result will show two areas of color change, one for the patient and one for the quality control antigen. If the control antigen area does not change color, the test is considered invalid regardless of color change in the patient area. Heartworm test kits (e.g., Witness HW, Synbiotics) that use rapid immunomigration are available. (Figure 9-7, Table 9-1, and Procedure 9-6).

Figure 9-7
Witness HW utilizes rapid immunomigration, a reliable one-way flow of sample and reagent, giving accurate answers in minutes. (Witness HW test; courtesy Synbiotics Corporation, San Diego, CA.)

PROCEDURE 9-6

Protocol for RIM

1. Apply patient sample to an area on the membrane that contains colloidal gold conjugated with antibodies to the test antigen.
2. If antigen is present in the patient sample, it binds to the conjugated antibodies and flows along the membrane to a reading area.
3. The reading area of the membrane contains capture antibodies to the test antigen.
4. If the patient sample contains antigen, it will be captured along with the bound conjugated antibody, by the second antibody in the reading area.
5. The accumulation of colloidal gold (now complexed with the first antibody, the antigen and the capture antibody) causes a color change.

Immunodiffusion

In this procedure, patient serum samples (possibly containing antibodies) and the antigen to this antibody (supplied in the test kit) are placed into separate wells in an agar gel plate. Both components diffuse into the agar and form a visible band of precipitation when they combine. If no band forms, no antibody exists in the patient's serum sample or the patient's antibody levels are insufficient to cause precipitation in the gel. Diseases that may be detected by immunodiffusion are equine infectious anemia and Johne's disease (Figure 9-8, Table 9-1, and Procedure 9-7).

Coombs' Test

The direct Coombs' test is used for diagnosis of autoimmune hemolytic anemia, in which erythrocytes become coated with antibodies and are subsequently removed

---

PROCEDURE 9-7

Protocol for immunodiffusion

1. Use an agar plate with one central well and multiple surrounding wells.
2. Place antigens from the test kit in the center well.
3. Place patient serum samples (with possible antibodies) and positive controls (with antibodies) in alternating surrounding wells. Use control samples for comparison.
4. Antigen from the center well and antibodies from the surrounding wells migrate through the agar toward each other.
5. Where the antigens and antibodies meet, a line of visible precipitation forms. A line of precipitate in front of a patient well indicates antibodies present in the patient serum.

Figure 9-8
Agar plate showing lines of precipitation. No lines of precipitation are evident near negative patient wells. (EIA Immunodiffusion, courtesy Synbiotics Corporation, San Diego, CA.)

from circulation by the mononuclear phagocytic system. The causative antibodies can be detected on the surface of RBCs by using antiserum specific for the antibodies on the RBCs.

Intradermal Tests

Skin tests are used to diagnose various allergies to allergens in the environment and in food or water. Allergies are mediated by IgE antibody molecules and can be detected by using allergenic extracts of grasses, pollens, ragweed, and other possibly offending antigens. The extracts are injected intradermally, and the injection sites are monitored for allergic reactions. A positive reaction indicates the presence of antibodies, meaning that the animal is allergic to that antigen.

◆ Tests of Cell-Mediated Immunity

Whereas tests of humoral immunity involve detection of circulating antibodies, evaluation of cell-mediated immunity is much more difficult.

Tuberculin Skin Test

The tuberculin skin test correlates with a specific cell-mediated immune reaction. Animals infected with *Mycobacterium* species bacteria develop characteristic delayed hypersensitivity reactions when exposed to purified derivatives of the organism called *tuberculin.*

In the tuberculin skin test, tuberculin is injected intradermally at a site in the cervical region or in a skin fold at the base of the tail in large animals (see Table 9-1). A delayed, local inflammatory reaction is observed if the animal has been exposed to mycobacteria. The reaction to injection is delayed because it takes a day or more for the T-lymphocytes to migrate to the foreign antigen injected into the dermis.

COLLECTING SAMPLES FOR SEROLOGIC TESTING

Nearly all serologic tests require serum or plasma as the sample. Whole blood should not be sent to the diagnostic laboratory when serum or plasma is specified. The most practical method of collection is the Vacutainer System (Becton-Dickinson, Rutherford, NJ), commonly available from many veterinary and medical supply companies. A red-top vacuum tube is used when serum is required and a lavender-top tube is used to collect plasma, unless heparinized plasma (green-top tube) is specifically requested.

Reference laboratories have strict requirements concerning specimen type, quality, and handling. If any uncertainty exists, the laboratory should be contacted for specific details. For each test, the requirements should be read carefully and exactly what is requested should be submitted. If a blood sample is to be collected in a syringe, a 5-ml syringe and 20-gauge needle combination should be used; it causes the least hemolysis.

HANDLING SEROLOGIC SAMPLES

When serum is to be submitted, the blood sample is allowed to clot for 20 to 30 minutes at room temperature and then is centrifuged for 10 minutes at a speed not faster than 1500 rpm. If little serum has separated after centrifuging, "rimming" the tube with a wooden applicator stick to loosen the clot may help; however, this also may cause hemolysis. If plasma is desired, the sample may be centrifuged immediately after collection.

After centrifugation, a small pipette is used to aspirate the serum or plasma (upper layer) off the packed erythrocytes. The aspirate is placed into a transfer tube or other sealable test tube and labeled clearly. The serum or plasma may be tested immediately or may be frozen or refrigerated for later use.

Samples for most serologic tests need not be frozen but should be shipped cold, especially during hot weather. The major problem with shipping tubes is breakage. The tubes must be packed firmly in place so that they do not move around when the package is jarred. The tubes should be packed tightly with paper towels, packing material, or even newspaper. Each sample must be labeled clearly and correctly and the pertinent paperwork enclosed to facilitate proper reporting of the results from the laboratory.

References

Entriken T: *Veterinary pharmaceuticals and biologicals,* ed 12, Lenexa, Kan, 2001/2002, Veterinary Healthcare Communications.

Goldsby RA et al: *Kuby immunology,* ed 4, New York, 2000, WH Freeman.

Lewis RM, Picut CA: *Veterinary clinical immunology: from classroom to clinic,* Philadelphia, 1989, Lea & Febiger.

McKenzie SB: *Textbook of hematology,* ed 2, Philadelphia, 1996, Lippincott, Williams & Wilkins.

Roitt I, Brostoff J, Male D: *Immunology,* ed 6, St Louis, 2001, Mosby.

Tizard IR: *Veterinary immunology: an introduction,* ed 6, Philadelphia, 2000, WB Saunders.

Tortora GJ, Funke BR: *Microbiology: an introduction,* ed 7, Redwood City, Calif, 2000, Benjamin/Cummings Publishing.

Turgeon: *Fundamentals of immunohematology,* ed 2, Baltimore, 1995, Williams & Wilkins.

Necropsy

10

CHARLES M. HENDRIX

This chapter on necropsy (postmortem examination) is intended to help veterinary technicians better understand the procedures involved in establishing a diagnosis. Information obtained from a properly performed necropsy often is correlated with clinical and laboratory findings to establish a final diagnosis.

Necropsy is an underused veterinary diagnostic technique. Necropsies should be used to help clarify disease pathogenesis and to distinguish one disease from another. A skillfully performed necropsy, with proper specimen processing, yields a wealth of diagnostic information.

Necropsy technique and specimen processing are easy to mismanage and difficult to perform well. A necropsy carelessly done or attempted by improperly trained individuals is likely to provide misinformation or no information. Before lesions can be studied adequately, they must be obtained properly through a systematic plan and an orderly necropsy technique. An excellent beginning can be made by learning the technique for necropsy on a dog; appropriate procedural modifications then can be applied to other domestic animals.

The organizational concept of necropsy and supportive laboratory procedures should stress a "collect and do" approach rather than a "collect and send" philosophy. Even though a veterinary practice may not be located near reference laboratories, many laboratory procedures can be performed easily, especially with the help of diagnostic kits. A common mistake is omitting laboratory procedures or performing difficult, rarely needed tests without first perfecting the techniques for simple tests that are supportive, inexpensive, and more rewarding.

The veterinary technician can contribute to the diagnostic process by performing the necropsy, recording the findings, and performing cytologic, clinical chemistry, and microbiologic procedures.

The authors recognize and appreciate the original work of Albert C. Strafuss, on whose research this chapter is based.

REASONS FOR NECROPSY

Necropsies are performed for a number of reasons. A necropsy is a diagnostic tool that is aided by the history, clinical signs, and laboratory findings. Apart from diagnosis, necropsies play a vital role in clarifying the process and pathogenesis of disease. In disease surveillance, data from necropsies may provide answers to management problems in herd or flock problems. Necropsy also can serve as an early warning system that allows a disease trend to be corrected before it becomes catastrophic. Finally, a necropsy has legal significance when forensic tests are performed on valuable, insured animals that have died suddenly.

NECROPSY PROTOCOL

To gain confidence in performing a necropsy, the technician first should become skilled in necropsy of dogs and cats. These cadavers are easily manipulated, and the digestive tracts are short and simple. Also, the procedural sequence for dogs and cats can be applied to other species. Some procedures are common to necropsy of all species. For example, all animal species except horses are placed on their left side for necropsy (horses are placed on their right side). A midline skin incision is made from the lips to the cranial brim of the pelvis, superficial to the linea alba. The lower jaw, tongue, and organs of the neck are removed, along with the thoracic organs. Pelvic skeletal cuts, removal of the pelvic organs and urogenital male or female tract, and removal of the brain and spinal cord are all done in the same manner in the various species. The anatomic variations of the different species' gastrointestinal tracts, however, require a different sequence in removal of abdominal viscera.

An informative necropsy requires a knowledge of the general and specific pathologies of organs and organ systems. More important, the development of a standardized necropsy protocol ensures that pathologic conditions are not overlooked. Each organ system is grossly observed in turn. Thoroughness eventually becomes routine and allows for neatness and precision. A standardized necropsy protocol allows for uniform, rapid, systematic, and complete necropsies, which are the key to accurate interpretation of lesions. Shortcuts lead to an incorrect diagnosis or no diagnosis at all.

Sequential removal of tissues from the cadaver allows for proper evaluation of gross lesions and tissues. Visualization of gross lesions at necropsy often is not sufficient for definitive diagnosis; such lesions or tissues must be submitted for diagnostic tests. The necropsy therefore becomes crucial to the selection of appropriate samples for adjunctive histopathologic, microbiologic, toxicologic, virologic, and parasitologic examinations. Careful selection of tissues is necessary to arrive at a pathologic diagnosis.

The history is vital and, when submitted with animals for necropsy, enables the diagnostician to make a more accurate and complete diagnosis. Failure to submit a history may lead to incorrect diagnosis. The history is an integral part of the necropsy procedure, one that guides the prosector in the proper selection of tests.

⬤ SPECIMEN COLLECTION AND SUBMISSION

Test results from the diagnostic laboratory directly reflect the quality and consideration given to selection and handling of specimens. If tissues for submission are handled improperly, the time and effort expended on the necropsy may be wasted. Careful selection and collection of specimens are among the most important steps in the necropsy procedure. The appropriate specimens must arrive at the laboratory in good condition. The veterinarian submitting the specimens is primarily responsible for properly collecting, packaging, and sending them to the laboratory, but in many instances the technician performs these duties.

Tissues from autolyzed or frozen birds usually are unrewarding in laboratory procedures. Because dry plumage slows the escape of body heat and accelerates autolysis, recently dead birds should immediately be soaked with water and detergent containing a germicide. This reduces the insulating capability of plumage and allows body heat to escape more rapidly. Dead birds should be chilled in a refrigerator before they are packaged and transported to the laboratory.

The quality of specimens submitted for laboratory tests has more of an influence on the diagnosis than the history or clinical findings. Considering all the tests that are performed, it follows that appropriately selected and properly handled specimens are more likely to provide an accurate diagnosis than samples not so treated.

Each tissue in a specimen container is an island of information unto itself; therefore great care should be taken to package the specimen properly. The common practice of submitting intestine (even if tied off) and parenchymatous organs together in the knotted arm of an obstetric sleeve should be avoided. Bacterial contamination spreads rapidly when tissues lack proper refrigeration and tissue fluids are present in the container. Packaging intestines with parenchymatous organs typically prevents the diagnostic laboratory from extracting useful information from all of the commingled specimens.

When an animal is euthanized, tissues can be collected and refrigerated immediately. This allows more tests to be performed on the specimen, especially enzymatic analysis.

Tissues collected from animals found dead have limited value, because autolysis precludes enzymatic or other chemical analyses. Agonal changes cause breakdown of macrophages and the reticuloendothelial system by enzymatic digestion. The reticuloendothelial system may then release bacteria, leading to contamination of organs. While an animal is alive, bacteria are continually cleared from the bloodstream by the reticuloendothelial system. After the animal dies, these bacteria are released in many organs.

In ruminants, bacteria are present in the rumen in great numbers and continue to multiply after death. This increases the cadaver temperature and accelerates tissue liquefaction and gas production.

Factors such as humidity and temperature also influence the rapidity of cadaver decomposition after death. When animals die suddenly from lightning strike, blackleg, or poisoning, bacteria in the digestive tract continue to generate heat and accelerate tissue autolysis. Stopping the putrefactive processes as soon as possible after death is a high priority.

Tissue specimens should be refrigerated immediately and cooled for 3 to 4 hours before they are packed for shipment. Sufficient fixative should be added to samples to be submitted for histopathologic examination. For shipping, the specimens are packed in a sturdy container and surrounded by cooling packets and insulating material. The transport system used should be able to deliver the specimens to the diagnostic laboratory within 24 hours. The quicker the specimens are delivered and processed, the better the results. Poor specimen handling results in hemolyzed blood samples, toxic serum samples, and bacterial infiltration of organs.

◉ SHIPPING OF SPECIMENS TO THE LABORATORY

It is essential to submit a complete, detailed history along with tissues, including gross lesions observed during the necropsy. Specimens may be delivered to the laboratory by bus, postal service, air, or private courier.

Veterinary clinical diagnostic specimens are considered to be Hazard Class 6, Division 6.2. Specimens is this category include "any human or animal material including, but not limited to, excreta, secreta, blood, blood components, tissues, and tissues fluids that have been collected and are being mailed to a medical or forensic laboratory for the purpose of diagnosis." The staff of the veterinary clinic should consult with local postal authorities to learn the U.S. Postal Service regulations. Mailing of clinical specimens is prohibited unless items are properly prepared for mailing and handling in transit. Clinical specimens must be packaged in a securely sealed primary container with sufficient absorbent material to take up the contents in case of leakage. The primary container then is placed in an outer shipping container with secondary leakproof material, so that if the primary container leaks during shipment, the contents will not escape from the outer shipping container. Shock-resistant material should be used that can withstand conditions incident to ordinary handling in transit, such as shock and pressure changes. If any doubt exists about proper packaging, postal authorities should be consulted. It is in the best interest of the veterinary profession to comply with these regulations.

Many diagnostic laboratories can supply the veterinary clinic with preaddressed mailers for submission of diagnostic specimens ranging from test tube samples to fresh tissue for microbiologic evaluation. Clinic staff members should consult nearby reference laboratories and should check with postal authorities to determine the types of containers acceptable for mailing.))

◉ METHODS OF EUTHANASIA

It is best to collect tissues from a cadaver immediately after death. Necropsy done immediately after euthanasia helps ensure more accurate results.

No one method of euthanasia is the best or only method for all circumstances. Several options are available, and the prosector must consider the ethical repercussions before selecting the method. Most animals are killed by rapid intravenous injection of euthanasia solution. To ensure proper and humane euthanasia of animals and to reduce the chance of drug abuse, the American Veterinary Medical Association has recommended that the drugs on the Drug Enforcement Administration's schedule of controlled substances for euthanasia of animals be used *only* under the supervision of a licensed veterinarian. Veterinarians (and their technicians) are required to keep accurate records of the amounts of solution used and the cases in which the solution is administered.

A gas chamber can be used for small animals. The size of animals that can be euthanized in a chamber depends on the size of the chamber. An overdose of a gaseous anesthetic is administered until the animal is dead. For most small animals, a cylinder of carbon dioxide can be connected to the chamber. For small birds or "pocket pets" (e.g., mice, rats, or gerbils), a cotton ball can be saturated with ether or chloroform and placed in a container (bell jar) with the animal. A larger chamber may be constructed from a trash can, with a tube entering the lid. Halothane is more expensive but creates less excitement for the animal.

In addition to intravenous injection, large animals may be humanely killed with a captive-bolt gun. The gun is placed against the animal's forehead at the intersection of two imaginary lines drawn from the base of the ear to the opposite medial canthus of the eye.

POSTMORTEM CHANGES

Immediately after euthanasia, the jugular vein, axillary vessels (in the axillary space), or femoral vessels (through disarticulation of the coxofemoral joint) can be severed to exsanguinate (bleed out) the cadaver. Exsanguination is important, because excessive blood in tissues or body cavities tends to obscure lesions; it is best to allow as much blood as possible to escape from the vascular system.

In cases of natural death, the necropsy should be performed as soon as possible after death. Postmortem destruction of tissues by the body's own enzymes begins immediately after death. Antemortem fever or high ambient temperature hastens decomposition of the carcass by speeding up the rate of enzyme reactions. Obese animals or those with a dense haircoat (wool) decompose more quickly as a result of heat entrapment. Ruminants with active rumen fermentation at the time of death generate gas and heat, enhancing postmortem changes.

Postmortem changes, or changes that occur after death, have profound effects on normal and diseased tissues. If postmortem changes are not recognized in tissues, they may be mistaken for antemortem lesions. For example, hemoglobin staining of intestinal contents, a postmortem change, often is mistaken for hemorrhagic enteritis. The diffuse red coloration tends to obscure interpretation of antemortem lesions of hyperemia and hemorrhage. Postmortem changes are found to varying degrees and may be confusing when present concurrently. A detailed description of postmortem changes can be found elsewhere in the literature.

DISPOSAL OF DEAD ANIMALS

Proper disposal of dead animals is becoming increasingly difficult. Fewer and fewer landfill sites are available, especially near metropolitan areas. Local ordinances may forbid the use of landfills for disposal of dead animals because rodents and insects could carry diseases to residential areas. Although certain chemicals can be applied to carcasses to speed the breakdown of body tissue and to kill infectious agents in tissues, chemical contamination of underground water supplies may be a problem in certain types of soil. Also, the cost may be prohibitive.

Rendering plants can be used for large animal disposal. These plants are designed for carcass disposal and are inspected by government authorities. Disposal of small animal carcasses often can be arranged locally through municipal incineration units or preexcavated burial pits. A crematorium is a prohibitively expensive item for most veterinary hospitals.

 ## COSMETIC NECROPSY

A cosmetic necropsy is restrictive because it limits examination of the animal to the extent that the client will tolerate. However, the internal organs usually can be examined with near completeness by means of a ventral midline incision from the xiphoid cartilage to the cranial brim of the pubis. The thoracic organs usually can be removed by cutting the diaphragm and pulling the organs caudally to the exterior. Splitting the sternum allows the thoracic cage to be pulled apart for removal of the lungs and heart. These incisions can be sutured after the organs have been examined and replaced, or the thoracic and abdominal cavities can be filled with paper to absorb fluids and maintain the shape of the cavities.

If the brain is to be removed, an incision should be made on the dorsum of the neck, extending rostrally over the calvarium and reflecting the skin laterally to the zygomatic process and eye. The calvarium and then the brain should be removed. The skull should be replaced and the skin sutured over the calvarium, leaving only a suture line. An inverted suture pattern probably is most desirable for this area.

 ## NECROPSY OF RABIES SUSPECTS

Any animal with clinical signs of viral encephalitis or one that shows abnormal behavior patterns must always be considered a rabies suspect. Proper protective clothing and gloves must be worn when handling a dead or live animal that has shown abnormal behavior. Clients should be instructed not to touch or handle live animals in pain under any circumstances so as to avoid possible exposure. They should be instructed to call animal control authorities to handle such cases or to contact public health officials or the local government veterinarian to help them evaluate the situation. The veterinarian should always instruct clients or individuals who have been exposed to possibly rabid animals to call their physician for proper treatment. The veterinarian should also call the reference laboratory for specific instructions on submitting specimens for rabies examination. Under all circumstances, the local rabies control authority or public health official must be contacted regarding suspected rabies cases.

NECROPSY EQUIPMENT

Necropsy does not require elaborate equipment. Frequently technicians or veterinarians are judged more on the way in which they conduct a necropsy than on their knowledge of disease. The client probably will formulate an opinion more from the veterinarian's tools of the trade than from the science of diagnosis; therefore it is logical to assume that the owner and others viewing the necropsy will judge the prosector by the expertise shown in opening the cadaver and removing organs.

Necessary equipment includes shears for cutting bones, enterotome scissors for incising the gut, and a knife for cutting skin and muscle. A sharp knife is the most important tool for necropsy; it is as important to the prosector as a scalpel is to a surgeon. A necropsy should never be attempted with a dull knife; a sharp knife is imperative. A scalpel, scissors, and forceps are desirable for dissecting small caged birds or pocket pets. A supply of sterile syringes and needles, vials for liquid specimens, and petri dishes for microbiologic samples should be at hand.

NECROPSY PROCEDURE

A cadaver is examined to determine the pathologic processes in relation to the history and clinical findings regarding the cause of death. The necropsy procedure should be planned, with the various specimens collected according to the diagnosis anticipated.

All animals except horses should be placed in left lateral recumbency. (Horses are placed in right lateral recumbency to accommodate the anatomic differences of the equine gastrointestinal tract; these differences necessitate a different sequence for removal of abdominal viscera.) Placing most animals in the same position for necropsy helps familiarize the examiner with the normal relative location of the viscera.

Before starting a necropsy, the prosector should perform an external examination to assess the animal's position at the time of death; the general appearance of the carcass (bloat, rigor, postmortem decomposition, dehydration); the body condition or nutritional status (obese, cachectic); the condition of the haircoat and whether external parasites are present; the color and appearance of visible mucous membranes; the presence or absence of discharges from body openings and the mammary glands; and any evidence of swelling, wounds, hernias, or fractures.

There is no single correct way to perform a necropsy. The procedure detailed here is an efficient approach.

NECROPSY OF DOGS AND CATS

Dogs and cats are placed on their left side. The specimen should be thoroughly rinsed in water to soak the haircoat, because this reduces the number of stray hairs that might contaminate the field of the necropsy procedure. The prosector faces the ventral abdomen to perform the necropsy.

◆ Opening the Cadaver

A paramedian ventral skin incision is started at the sternum and extended to the symphysis of the mandible. The incision is extended from the sternum caudally to the groin, lateral to the umbilicus, mammary gland, or external male genitalia (Figure 10-1).

The front leg is lifted, the muscle attachments are cut close to the thorax, and the leg is reflected dorsolaterally. The skin is reflected dorsolaterally from the midline incision of the neck to the base of the ear. The proximal rear leg is grasped, and the adductor, gracilis, and quadratus muscles are incised. The coxofemoral joint is disarticulated, and the leg is reflected dorsolaterally so that it lies flat on the surface of the table. The abdominal skin is reflected dorsolaterally from the paramedian incision to the transverse processes of the spinal column (Figure 10-2).

The legs (front and rear) and the integument of the cadaver are reflected dorsolaterally as one unit. The legs are not removed from the cadaver or from the abdominal skin. The skin of the left side of the body is reflected laterally for about 5 cm along the entire length of the initial incision.

To remove the lower jaw, the masseter muscle is cut by inserting the knife at the commissure of the lip just lateral to the ramus (Figure 10-3). The cut is extended to the angle of the ramus, and the masseter muscle is severed from the lateral surface of the angle of the ramus. The mandibular symphysis is cut with pruning shears or a saw. The right ramus then is grasped and pulled caudally. The muscles are cut caudal to the molar teeth, and cutting continues through the muscle attachments medial to the ramus and around the caudal border of the angle of the ramus. The right

Figure 10-1
An initial paramedian ventral skin incision is extended from the sternum to the mandibular symphysis and then to the groin. (Strafuss AC: *Necropsy procedures and basic diagnostic methods for practicing veterinarians,* Springfield, Ill, 1988, Charles C Thomas.)

ramus is pulled caudally by rotating it laterally in one movement to disarticulate it. The disarticulated ramus is twisted, and the remaining muscle attachments are cut to allow it to be removed. The tongue is grasped and cut loose from the medial surface of the left ramus. Cutting continues caudal to the hard palate and around the pharynx to the level of the hyoid bones (Figure 10-4). The hyoid bones are disarticulated, and the tongue, pharynx, esophagus, and trachea are reflected to the thoracic inlet (Figure 10-5).

Figure 10-2
The rear leg is disarticulated, and the legs and skin are reflected dorsolaterally as a unit. (Strafuss AC: *Necropsy procedures and basic diagnostic methods for practicing veterinarians,* Springfield, Ill, 1988, Charles C Thomas.)

Figure 10-3
The knife is inserted just lateral to the ramus of the mandible. (Strafuss AC: *Necropsy procedures and basic diagnostic methods for practicing veterinarians,* Springfield, Ill, 1988, Charles C Thomas.)

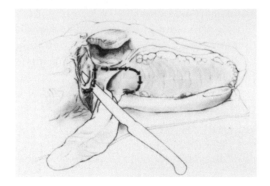

Figure 10-4
The tongue is cut loose with an incision around the pharynx to the level of the hyoid bones. (Strafuss AC: *Necropsy procedures and basic diagnostic methods for practicing veterinarians,* Springfield, Ill, 1988, Charles C Thomas.)

Figure 10-5
The hyoid bones are disarticulated, and the tongue, pharynx, esophagus, and trachea are pulled caudally. (Strafuss AC: *Necropsy procedures and basic diagnostic methods for practicing veterinarians,* Springfield, Ill, 1988, Charles C Thomas.)

    The abdomen is opened by cutting the muscles along the costal arch, from the transverse process of the spinal column to the sternum and caudally along the linea alba to the brim of the pelvis (Figure 10-6). The inguinal canal is examined for evidence of cryptorchidism, incarcerated hernia, infarcted spermatic cord, or hemorrhage from faulty castration.

    The rib cage is removed by cutting the ribs with rib shears (or pruning shears or a cleaver) along the line of proposed cuts. The cuts are made from the xiphoid cartilage cranially to the thoracic inlet (just ventral to the esophagus, trachea, and tongue, which have been reflected to the thoracic inlet). The next cut begins from the most dorsal aspect of the first rib (dorsal to the reflected neck organs) and extends caudally to the transverse process of the first lumbar vertebra. In heavily muscled animals, the muscles of the rib cage are reflected along the proposed cuts. After the ribs have been detached, the color of the exposed tissues and organs is noted because it may indicate hemorrhage, congestion, postmortem imbibition, or autolysis. Before the organs are removed, their anatomic relationships are examined for signs of volvulus, torsion, intussusception, hernia, or other anomalies. The presence of hydropericardium and hydrothorax or hydroperitoneum also is noted, along with the characteristics of any fluid.

Figure 10-6
The abdomen is opened with an incision caudal to the costal arch that proceeds caudally along the linea alba. (Strafuss AC: *Necropsy procedures and basic diagnostic methods for practicing veterinarians,* Springfield, Ill, 1988, Charles C Thomas.)

Specimens for microbiologic culture or direct microscopic examination should be collected at this time, before any organ is contaminated by manipulation or handling of viscera. Pericardial, pleural, or abdominal effusions, fluid from cysts, bile, and urine are best collected before the organs are handled.

The tongue, esophagus, and trachea then are grasped, and the thoracic organs (heart, lungs, and thymus) are pulled from the thoracic cavity. The esophagus is opened and checked for ulcers or parasites. The thyroid and parathyroid glands, which lie adjacent to the trachea and caudal to the larynx, are examined. The trachea is opened, and the incision is extended into the bronchi and bronchioles. Each lung lobe is palpated and then incised to allow inspection for lesions. *The heart is not detached from the lungs.*

◆ Examining the Heart

The thoracic organs are laid out so that the tongue, esophagus, and trachea are to the examiner's right. The pericardial sac is then opened. The heart is held in the left hand with the apex toward the examiner. With scissors, a cut is made in the right ventricle adjacent to the septum and extended caudodorsally into the caudal vena cava (Figure 10-7). The initial cut in the right ventricle then is extended craniodorsally, adjacent to the septum, and continued out to the conus arteriosus and pulmonary artery (Figure 10-8). All valves and openings of the right auricle and ventricle are examined.

Figure 10-7
The right ventricle is opened near the inter-ventricular septum, and the incision is extended into the caudal vena cava. (Strafuss AC: *Necropsy procedures and basic diagnostic methods for practicing veterinarians,* Springfield, Ill, 1988, Charles C Thomas.)

Figure 10-8
The right ventricular incision is extended to the conus arteriosus and pulmonary artery. (Strafuss AC: *Necropsy procedures and basic diagnostic methods for practicing veterinarians,* Springfield, Ill, 1988, Charles C Thomas.)

The heart then is rotated counterclockwise until the left auricle is uppermost. The examiner holds the heart in the left hand with the thumb over the left auricle. The left ventricle is bisected near the apex, and the cut is extended dorsally into the pulmonary veins (Figure 10-9). The left atrioventricular (AV) valve is examined.

With the left index finger and thumb, the examiner grasps the left half of the left ventricle and, with scissors in the right hand, cuts through the left ventricle, going beneath the left AV valve (Figure 10-10). The incision is extended distally to the aorta. The origins of the coronary, subclavian, and brachycephalic arteries are examined (Figure 10-11).

◆ Removing the Gastrointestinal Tract

The duodenum and pancreas are grasped and reflected dorsolaterally over the vertebral column. The omentum then is grasped and pulled ventrally. The cecum usually is visible as an inflated, comma-shaped structure surrounded by intestine and ventral to the right kidney. After the ileum has been located at the apex of the

Figure 10-9
The left ventricle is bisected near its apex, and the incision is extended into the pulmonary veins. (Strafuss AC: *Necropsy procedures and basic diagnostic methods for practicing veterinarians,* Springfield, Ill, 1988, Charles C Thomas.)

Figure 10-10
Scissors are used to cut through the left ventricle. (Strafuss AC: *Necropsy procedures and basic diagnostic methods for practicing veterinarians,* Springfield, Ill, 1988, Charles C Thomas.)

cecum, the small intestine is cut from its mesenteric attachment to the caudal duodenum; the incision stops where the duodenum loops under the large intestine (Figures 10-12 and 10-13).

Holding the cecum in the left hand, the prosector cuts craniodorsally to the cecum and the mesenteric lymph node. The cecum, terminal ileum, colon, and mesenteric lymph node then are pulled toward the examiner while the mesenteric attachments are cut (Figure 10-14).

Figure 10-11
The origins of the coronary, subclavian, and brachycephalic arteries are examined. (Strafuss AC: *Necropsy procedures and basic diagnostic methods for practicing veterinarians,* Springfield, Ill, 1988, Charles C Thomas.)

Figure 10-12
The small intestine is cut from its mesenteric attachment to the caudal duodenum. (Strafuss AC: *Necropsy procedures and basic diagnostic methods for practicing veterinarians,* Springfield, Ill, 1988, Charles C Thomas.)

Figure 10-13
The mesenteric incision is extended to the point where the duodenum loops under the large intestine. (Strafuss AC: *Necropsy procedures and basic diagnostic methods for practicing veterinarians,* Springfield, Ill, 1988, Charles C Thomas.)

Figure 10-14
The mesenteric attachments of the cecum, terminal ileum, colon, and mesenteric lymph nodes are cut, and the duodenum is severed at the tail of the pancreas. (Strafuss AC: *Necropsy procedures and basic diagnostic methods for practicing veterinarians,* Springfield, Ill, 1988, Charles C Thomas.)

Figure 10-15
Incisions are made to free the kidneys, adrenal glands, and ureters. (Strafuss AC: *Necropsy procedures and basic diagnostic methods for practicing veterinarians,* Springfield, Ill, 1988, Charles C Thomas.)

The caudal duodenum is grasped, cut loose from any remaining attachments, and laid down outside the abdominal cavity. The pancreas can be examined *in situ* (in its natural position) in the abdominal cavity. The duodenum is cut at the tail of the pancreas, and the small intestine is removed for examination. The cecum, terminal ileum, colon, and mesenteric lymph nodes are reflected over the paralumbar region.

The right kidney is grasped, and a cut is made craniolateral to the kidney and adrenal gland. The right kidney, adrenal gland, and ureter are reflected caudally to the pelvic inlet and laid dorsally over the paralumbar region. This procedure is repeated for the left kidney, adrenal gland, and ureter (Figure 10-15).

The patency of the bile duct is checked by squeezing the gallbladder and noting whether bile flows into the opened duodenum. The stomach is removed by cutting it from the hilus of the liver; the spleen, duodenum, and pancreas are removed with the stomach (Figure 10-16). The liver and diaphragm are removed together by cutting the diaphragm from its costal attachment.

◆ Pelvic Cuts and Removal of the Urogenital Tract

Before the genital tract, urinary system, and caudal alimentary tract can be removed, the lateral aspects of the pelvis must be removed. Three cuts are required, and all are made close to the exposed coxofemoral joint (Figure 10-17).

The first cut is made from the cranial brim of the pelvis to the obturator foramen. The second cut is made from the obturator foramen to the ischial arch, parallel to the long axis of the vertebral column. The third cut is made across the shaft of the ileum, cranial to the disarticulated coxofemoral joint. The ligaments and muscles surrounding the detached lateral bony pelvis are then cut, and the detached bony pelvis is removed from the cadaver.

In females, the kidneys, attached adrenal glands, ureters, uterus, and large intestine are grasped and reflected caudally to the level of the ischial arch; all attachments close to the abdominal wall and bony pelvis are cut. The fascial attachments are cut from the ventral floor of the pelvis, and the cut is extended adjacent to the ischial arch to remove the vulva with the internal reproductive tract intact (Figure 10-18). A gravid uterus with full-term fetuses may be examined *in situ* or cut at the cervix and removed separately.

Figure 10-16
The spleen, duodenum, and pancreas are removed with the stomach. (Strafuss AC: *Necropsy procedures and basic diagnostic methods for practicing veterinarians,* Springfield, Ill, 1988, Charles C Thomas.)

Figure 10-17
Three cuts are made to remove the lateral aspects of the pelvis. (Strafuss AC: *Necropsy procedures and basic diagnostic methods for practicing veterinarians,* Springfield, Ill, 1988, Charles C Thomas.)

Figure 10-18
The reproductive tract of females is removed intact. (Strafuss AC: *Necropsy procedures and basic diagnostic methods for practicing veterinarians,* Springfield, Ill, 1988, Charles C Thomas.)

In males, the kidneys, attached adrenal glands, ureters, and large intestine are grasped, and their pelvic attachments are cut at a point just cranial to the ischial arch. The external genitalia are reflected caudally (scrotum included) to near the caudoventral border of the ischial arch. The external genitalia and reflected pelvic organs are then grasped, and the ligaments and crura are cut close to the caudal border of the symphysis of the pubis and ischial arch; reflection continues ventrally around the anus. The urogenital organs and large intestine are removed together (Figure 10-19). This step permits removal of an intact internal and external urethra for examination.

Figure 10-19
In males, the urogenital organs and large intestine are removed together. (Strafuss AC: *Necropsy procedures and basic diagnostic methods for practicing veterinarians,* Springfield, Ill, 1988, Charles C Thomas.)

◆ Collecting Cerebrospinal Fluid

A cut is made caudal to the angle of the mandible, deep to the caudal border of the occipital condyle, exposing the foramen magnum (Figure 10-20). Cerebrospinal fluid may be removed at this time for microbiologic and clinicopathologic examination (Figure 10-20, *inset*).

◆ Removing the Brain

The brain should be examined in all cases in which the clinical history suggests neurologic disturbances.

The head is left attached to the spinal column, and the skin is reflected from the head. The brain can be removed easily through a ventral paramedian incision, about 1 to 2 cm to one side of the ventral midline. With a saw, the incision is begun on the ventral side of the head and extended caudally to the level of the occipital condyle (Figure 10-21). After the calvarium and brain have been exposed, each half is removed by gentle traction and passive gravitational force. The brain typically peels out of the calvarium after the cranial nerves and dural attachments have been cut with curved, pointed scissors. *The brain should not be squeezed or handled roughly; it is easily damaged.*

As an alternative, the head may be removed from the cadaver and the brain removed through a dorsal approach. A dorsal midline cutaneous incision is made from the frontal prominence to a point caudal to the occiput. The skin is reflected back on either side to expose the temporal muscles to the zygomatic arch. The temporal muscles are cut free from their proximal attachments and from the bone over the dorsolateral surfaces of the skull in the temporal fossa. The head is removed by making a deep transverse cut through the extensor muscles immediately caudal to the occipital protuberance to the atlantooccipital articulation.

Figure 10-20
The foramen magnum is exposed with an incision deep to the caudal border of the occipital condyle. Cerebrospinal fluid may then be collected *(inset)*. (Strafuss AC: *Necropsy procedures and basic diagnostic methods for practicing veterinarians,* Springfield, Ill, 1988, Charles C Thomas.)

Figure 10-21
The brain can be exposed through a ventral paramedian incision. (Strafuss AC: *Necropsy procedures and basic diagnostic methods for practicing veterinarians,* Springfield, Ill, 1988, Charles C Thomas.)

After the head has been removed, three cuts are made through the calvarium to open the cranial cavity. Sawing proceeds on a line from the dorsolateral periphery of the foramen magnum, cutting the dorsal one third of the occipital condyle and medial to the orbit. The incision is extended rostrally on a line to the medial canthus of the opposite eye. This cut is repeated for the other side.

The frontal bone is cut transversely at the rostral limit of the cranial cavity (the line varies with species, age, and breed) on a line caudal to the supraorbital process. The severed calvarium is lifted or pried off the cerebral hemispheres and cerebellum. With scissors, the meninges and falx cerebri (the dura between the cerebral hemispheres and the cerebellum) are cut, and the meninges are reflected from the dorsal aspect of the brain. The head then is inverted so that gravity helps ease the brain out of the cranial cavity. Cutting the cranial nerve roots and ventral dural attachments allows the brain to be removed easily from the cranial cavity. The brain must be handled carefully, because it easily becomes an amorphous mass if mishandled.

The brain may be sectioned immediately or placed *in toto* (whole) in 10% buffered neutral formalin and sectioned after preliminary fixation for 12 to 24 hours. The brain may be placed in a container to which concentrated formalin (37% w/v) is added until the brain floats. This rapidly makes the brain firm for sectioning. To section a fresh brain, the organ is placed on its ventral surface, and the olfactory lobes are pressed against a block or the lip of the table. The knife is moistened in physiologic saline or water before each cut so that tissue does not adhere to it. A series of transverse cuts (1 cm apart) is carefully made through both lobes. When diffuse changes or large focal lesions are present, sectioning when the brain is fresh provides better fixation. Small focal lesions are best detected grossly in fixed brains. Lesions in fixed brain tissue are grossly observed as darkened foci and are often easily distinguishable.

◆ Removing the Spinal Cord

The muscles and tendons are cut from the dorsal, ventral, and transverse processes of the spinal column. In large animals, a cleaver or an ax may be used to chip away the exposed transverse processes along the vertebral column. Chipping continues parallel to the transverse process until the right side of the vertebral column has been removed and the spinal cord is exposed. In small animals, a rongeur may be used to accomplish the same end. An oscillating Stryker saw may be used if the examiner is not adept at handling a cleaver or an ax. Starting at the atlantooccipital joint, the spinal cord is removed by grasping the meninges with forceps to hold the spinal cord at an obtuse angle. The dorsal and ventral nerve roots are cut to free the cord from the vertebral column. *Care must be taken not to squeeze, mash, or pull the spinal cord at acute angles from the spinal column.*

After the cord has been removed from the spinal column, the meninges are cut along the entire length of the spinal cord and examined grossly. The cord is placed in 10% buffered neutral formalin to fix for 24 hours before sectioning. Gentle handling and a sharp knife may be used in making transverse cuts in the fresh cord, allowing examination for lesions.

◆ Opening Limb Joints

A medial skin incision is made over the joint; the skin is reflected; and the joint is opened so that the type and amount of fluid can be assessed and the articular surfaces can be examined for erosions.

Any of three approaches is recommended if joint fluid is to be cultured. According to one method, the examiner saws across the long bone midshaft proximal and distal to the joint and sends the joint intact to a diagnostic laboratory for culture. In the second method, the skin is reflected from the joint surface, and a sterile syringe and needle are used to aspirate joint fluid or exudate for culture. In the third method, the skin is reflected from the joint surface; the tissue surface is seared; and the joint is opened with a sterile blade. A sterile loop then is used to streak a sample of joint contents directly onto a blood agar plate, or a sample is taken with a sterile swab, and the specimen is sent to the diagnostic laboratory.

NECROPSY OF SWINE

The same procedures described for dogs and cats are used for opening swine cadavers (see Figures 10-1 to 10-6) and for examining the heart (see Figures 10-7 to 10-11). However, the entire pharynx must be removed because the tonsil of swine is a flattened structure embedded in the pharynx and is easily overlooked.

◆ Removing the Gastrointestinal Tract

The ileum is grasped near its entry into the cecum, and the small intestine is cut away from its mesenteric attachment to the point where the small intestine courses under the large intestine. At this point the ileum and caudal duodenum are severed, and the small intestine is removed (Figure 10-22, *bottom*). Cutting the small intestine close to its mesenteric attachment frees the attached border so that the intestine is easily opened for examination.

Figure 10-22
Incisions are made at the ileum and caudal duodenum to remove the small intestine *(bottom)*. The colon is severed near the right kidney, and the duodenum is severed caudal to the gallbladder *(top)*. (Strafuss AC: *Necropsy procedures and basic diagnostic methods for practicing veterinarians,* Springfield, Ill, 1988, Charles C Thomas.)

The rectum and colon are bluntly dissected cranially from the pelvic inlet to the right kidney. The colon is severed and placed over the paralumbar fossa (Figure 10-22, *top*). The pancreas is examined; the duodenum is severed caudal to the gallbladder; and the duodenum is bluntly dissected from the stomach (see Figure 10-22, *top*). The large intestine (spiral colon) is grasped in the left hand and pulled taut from its mesenteric attachments, then severed and removed from the abdominal cavity.

The kidneys, adrenal glands, ureters, and urinary bladder, and a nongravid uterus, are reflected caudally to the pelvic inlet and placed over the paralumbar region. A gravid uterus with fetuses may be examined *in situ* or removed at the cervix.

The patency of the bile duct is checked by squeezing the gallbladder, and the stomach, spleen, and duodenum then are removed together. The costal attachments of the diaphragm are severed, and the liver and diaphragm are removed.

Pelvic cuts and removal of the urogenital organs, caudal gastrointestinal tract, brain, and spinal cord are the same as for dogs and cats (see Figures 10-17 to 10-19).

NECROPSY OF CATTLE, SHEEP, AND GOATS

All ruminants are placed on their left side with the prosector facing the ventral abdomen. The same procedures described for dogs and cats are used for opening ruminant cadavers (see Figures 10-1 to 10-6) and for examining the heart (see Figures 10-7 to 10-11).

◆ Removing the Gastrointestinal Tract

The ileum is grasped with the left thumb and index finger near its entry into the cecum, and the small intestine is cut away from its mesenteric attachment to the point where the small intestine disappears beneath the large intestine (duodenojejunal flexure). The small intestine is cut close to its mesenteric attachment because this frees the attached border, allowing the intestine to be easily straightened and opened for examination. The small intestine is severed and removed. The duodenum is cut caudal to the gallbladder; the patency of the bile duct is checked by squeezing the gallbladder; and the duodenum is bluntly dissected to the abomasum (Figure 10-23, *bottom*). The rectum is bluntly dissected cranially from the pelvic inlet to the right kidney and then severed and placed over the paralumbar region (Figure 10-23, *top*).

The large intestine is grasped in the left hand and pulled taut from its mesenteric attachments, then severed and removed from the abdominal cavity. The kidneys, adrenal glands, ureters, and urinary bladder, and a nongravid uterus, are reflected caudally to the pelvic inlet and placed over the paralumbar fossa. Near-term fetuses in the uterus can be removed and the uterus examined *in situ*. As an alternative, the uterus may be severed at the cervix and removed.

The area between the reticulum and the diaphragm is palpated for lesions associated with foreign bodies before the rumen is removed. The dorsal attachments of the rumen are severed from the abdominal wall, and the rumen is pulled counterclockwise. The attachments between the liver and the omasum are severed, and the omasum and abomasum are pulled ventrally and clockwise from the abdominal cavity.

Figure 10-23
The ileum and duodenum are severed to remove the small intestine *(bottom)*. The rectum is severed near the right kidney *(top)*. (Strafuss AC: *Necropsy procedures and basic diagnostic methods for practicing veterinarians,* Springfield, Ill, 1988, Charles C Thomas.)

The caudodorsal area of the rumen is grasped; the remaining dorsal attachments are severed; and the rumen is pulled counterclockwise out of the abdominal cavity. The spleen lies on top of the rumen and can be examined. The costal attachments of the diaphragm then are severed, and the liver and diaphragm are removed.

Pelvic cuts and removal of the urogenital tract, caudal gastrointestinal tract, brain, and spinal cord are the same as for dogs and cats (see Figures 10-17 to 10-19).

◉ NECROPSY OF HORSES

Horses are placed on their right side with the prosector facing the ventral abdomen. The same procedures described for cats and dogs are used for opening equine cadavers (see Figures 10-1 to 10-6) and for removing and examining the thoracic organs (see Figures 10-7 to 10-11).

◆ Removing the Gastrointestinal Tract

The spleen is ligated and removed (ligation prevents blood from flowing over the abdominal viscera). The small colon is grasped and laid over the paralumbar area.

The pelvic flexure of the great colon is grasped and pulled out of the abdominal cavity so that it is at right angles to the long axis of the cadaver. The ileum is located adjacent to the cecum. The small intestine is cut from the mesenteric attachment cranially to the point where the duodenum disappears beneath and is attached to the transverse colon. The small intestine is cut close to its mesenteric attachment so that the intestine can be easily straightened and opened for examination (Figure 10-24, *bottom*).

The duodenum (usually ventral to the left kidney) is grasped and bluntly torn loose from its mesenteric attachments and from the large intestine cranial to the stomach. The stomach is pulled cranially, and the esophageal portion is cut loose from the diaphragm. The duodenum then is grasped at the pylorus and bluntly dissected from its mesenteric attachments caudally until it is free. The duodenum is severed near the right kidney, and the proximal end is tied in a knot. The stomach is grasped, and it and the first portion of the duodenum are pulled cranially from the abdominal wall. The small colon is severed and ligated 4 cm caudal to the transverse colon and laid over the paralumbar region (Figure 10-24, *top*).

A cut is made lateral to the left kidney, and the kidney is reflected medially. The incision is extended craniomedially so that the left adrenal gland, left kidney, and left ureter can be removed as a unit by pulling them caudally (Figure 10-25). These organs are laid over the cranial brim of the pelvis or over the paralumbar region. Major ab-

Figure 10-24
The small colon is severed and ligated 4 cm caudal to the transverse colon *(top)*. The small intestine is cut near its mesenteric attachment to remove it from the abdomen *(bottom)*. (Strafuss AC: *Necropsy procedures and basic diagnostic methods for practicing veterinarians,* Springfield, Ill, 1988, Charles C Thomas.)

dominal blood vessels are checked for thrombi. Starting at its most cranial aspect, the abdominal aorta is opened to its termination (the internal and external iliacs). The celiac, cranial mesenteric, and renal arteries are opened, and the three major branches of the cranial mesenteric artery are examined.

The abdominal aorta is severed caudal to the cranial mesenteric artery, and this section is removed, along with the large colon, from the abdominal cavity (Figure 10-26). *When the large colon is reflected, the right kidney and adrenal gland should not be removed with it.* The right kidney and adrenal gland lie partly beneath the liver and may be torn loose when the large intestine and abdominal aorta are removed.

A cut is made craniolateral to the right kidney and adjacent adrenal gland (beneath the liver), and these organs are reflected caudally to the cranial brim of the pelvis. The left kidney, adrenal gland, and ureter, and a nongravid uterus, are reflected caudally to the pelvic inlet and placed over the paralumbar region. A gravid uterus with a full-term fetus can be examined *in situ,* or the gravid uterus may be removed at the cervix.

The costal attachments of the diaphragm are severed, and the liver and diaphragm are removed. Pelvic cuts and the removal of the urogenital organs, caudal gastrointestinal tract, brain, and spinal cord are the same as for dogs and cats (see Figures 10-17 to 10-19).

Figure 10-25
The left kidney, adrenal gland, and ureter are removed as a unit. (Strafuss AC: *Necropsy procedures and basic diagnostic methods for practicing veterinarians,* Springfield, Ill, 1988, Charles C Thomas.)

Figure 10-26
A section of the caudal aorta is removed with the large colon. (Strafuss AC: *Necropsy procedures and basic diagnostic methods for practicing veterinarians,* Springfield, Ill, 1988, Charles C Thomas.)

NECROPSY OF EXOTIC PETS

◆ Pocket Pets, Cage Birds, Ornamental Fish, Reptiles, and Assorted Arthropods

The veterinarian and the veterinary technician must remember that because of the diverse nature of twenty-first century society, many clients may not favor the traditional canine and feline pets. Pets of many different species may arrive in the reception area of today's veterinary clinics. Veterinarians and their technicians may be called on to observe and treat many different classes of animal species, ranging from spiders to centipedes, parakeets to ostriches, snakes to crocodiles, or mice to potbellied pigs. The selection of a pet often is left to the whim of the pet owner; unfortunately, the uniqueness of the pet may hamper adequate veterinary care.

The veterinary technician must understand that a knowledge of what is normal for an exotic species is the groundwork for developing an understanding of the abnormal. The pet owner must learn to recognize the exotic pet's normal behavior, normal morphology, and normal function and must inform the veterinary team of these facts. The veterinarian and the staff should make the most of opportunities to learn as much as possible about these atypical pets, taking both mental and physical notes about real life situations. Fortunately, with the explosion of access to the "information superhighway," the Internet, many veterinary technicians can become almost experts in the care and feeding of exotic pets.

Veterinarians and technicians can acquire invaluable information by using the Internet to communicate with information specialists at nearby colleges and universities, with veterinarians in continuing education settings, with veterinary specialty groups, and with state and local veterinary authorities in regional diagnostic laboratories. These resources can provide indispensable assistance in establishing expertise in the treatment and care of a wide variety of classes of pet animals.

When such pets expire, the veterinarian and the technician may be called upon to perform a necropsy on one of these different species. It is virtually impossible to describe the unique procedures for every species of exotic animal that might be submitted for necropsy examination. In many instances these cases should be referred to a regional (state or provincial) diagnostic laboratory, where skilled veterinary pathologists have the expertise to handle such examinations.

◆ Necropsy Examination

In many instances the pet owner may believe that the small size of an exotic pet might preclude the necropsy examination. It is important to remember that recently deceased pocket pets are subject to rapid decomposition of the body. These tiny pets should be necropsied as soon as possible after death.

Under laboratory conditions or in laboratory colonies, an affected specimen (e.g., a laboratory mouse or rat) usually is sacrificed, and the pathologic etiology is determined for the entire colony. However, this situation does not usually present itself in companion animal practice, and pocket pets would not fall under this precept.

The veterinarian and the veterinary technician must be on guard to ensure that the caged bird or pocket pet is an individual pet and not part of a colony of laboratory animals. The same holds true for poultry. In any commercial poultry operation, several affected chickens often are sacrificed to determine the etiology of a disease process. The same sacrificial procedure and resulting necropsy obviously would not be performed on a pet chicken. Again, in such cases communication between the veterinary clinic staff and the client is of utmost importance.

Because of postmortem changes that often occur, the speed with which a cadaver is submitted to the diagnostic facility is critical. The referring veterinarian should act as liaison for specimen submission.

The following procedures are the tip of the iceberg with respect to procedural necropsy examinations. Because it is not possible to include the precise necropsy for every type of pocket pet, representative examples of procedures are given for some common pocket pets (small caged birds, small mammals, ornamental fish, reptiles, and arthropod/invertebrates). Veterinary technicians are encouraged to seek outside sources (e.g., reference materials, short courses, and the Internet) to become proficient at pocket pet necropsy. On-line training is available on the Internet; the veterinary technician should visit the website http://www.ncifcrf.gov/vetpath/necropsy.html, where a virtual mouse necropsy can be performed.

◆ Caged Bird Necropsy

Necropsies for caged birds are routinely performed in both state and provincial veterinary diagnostic laboratories. The referring veterinarian may perform an avian necropsy in the veterinary clinic. A necropsy in this setting is often necessary to respond to a distraught client's concerns or demands. The veterinarian should remember that diagnostic laboratories accept an entire bird for necropsy examination.

After a general examination of the carcass, the veterinarian should place the bird on its back. The skin on the medial thigh is incised, and the hips are disarticulated laterally. The skin from the chest is reflected and incised along the neck to the beak. The abdomen is incised, and the abdominal cavity is exposed. The ribs and the shoulder bones are then removed to reveal the cavity of the chest. All internal organs are exposed. The brain is removed by excising the head and removing the calvarium using hardware shears or used scissors. Representative tissues for culture and histopathologic examination should be submitted from any lesion. The following tissues should be submitted for histopathologic study in 10% neutral buffered formalin: brain, esophagus, trachea, thyroid gland, crop, proventriculus, gizzard, duodenum, pancreas, lower intestine, liver, heart, kidney, gonads, skeletal muscle, and skin with feathers. Specimens for culture should be stored in culturettes; samples of infected tissues for culture should be packed in whirlpaks and chilled (not frozen) in an insulated container with enough cold packs or ice to last until delivery to the diagnostic facility. The client must understand that freezing damages tissues for histopathologic examination and may also impair diagnosis of bacterial infections, including chlamydial agents. Again, a sacrificial procedure and resulting necropsy would not be performed on a pet chicken.

◆ Ornamental Fish Necropsy

Many of the clinical signs exhibited by ornamental fish are common to a variety of diseases. Inappetence, lethargy, color changes, fin clamping, and swelling of the abdomen and eyes can be caused by a variety of infectious agents. Some specific symptoms, such as irritation and "flashing," or respiratory distress, may suggest certain disease syndromes; in most situations, however, a more definitive diagnosis requires a necropsy in conjunction with laboratory analysis.

The extent of laboratory analysis often depends on the problem under investigation and the value of the fish to the owner. For a relatively inexpensive fish, such as a "run of the mill" goldfish, it is quite appropriate to sacrifice a few affected individuals to complete a thorough clinical investigation. However, this would not be the case if the pathogen involves a small number of highly valued individuals, such as expensive Japanese show koi.

For the most conclusive necropsy to be carried out, the client must understand that only very *fresh* specimens should be examined. This is necessary when histopathologic examination is required because fish tissue degenerates so rapidly that taking samples even 1 hour after death could yield results of no diagnostic value. Live affected fish or fish in the process of dying should be sacrificed for necropsy examination. Clients should be informed that tissue samples taken from frozen fish are useless. Gill squashes, skin scrapings, examinations, histopathologic examinations, bacteriologic examinations, virologic samplings, blood samplings, and toxicologic determinations are other procedures that veterinarians may use to determine the pathogens involved. For details of specific necropsy procedures, veterinarians and technicians may consult the reference on fish necropsy.

◆ Reptilian Necropsy

Reptiles differ significantly from mammals and birds with regard to the anatomy, physiology, and husbandry. Veterinarians and their technicians who serve the devotees of snakes, lizards, chelonians, and crocodilians should consult specific anatomic guides to assist in the reptilian necropsy procedure. To assist novices, a reptilian necropsy protocol has been designed to include all information relevant to reptile postmortem evaluation. All information related to husbandry should be recorded. Age and gender are important relative to the frequency and occurrence of neoplastic diseases. The type of cage, substrate, temperature, photoperiod, and disinfectants used should be recorded; these parameters are important with respect to environmental disorders. The diet (whole animal, whether dead or alive, and source) should be noted. In many cases the clinical signs exhibited by reptiles are subtle and go unnoted by the owner. The exotic pet owner must understand that knowledge of what is normal for the species is a necessity for understanding the abnormal. The owner must learn to recognize normal reptilian behavior, normal reptilian morphology, and normal reptilian function.

As with all exotic species, every reptilian necropsy must be performed in a routine, systematic manner. An excellent form for the reptilian necropsy is provided in Figure 10-27. Radiography of the entire specimen may be necessary to rule out impactions or possible fractures or dislocations. A website is available for detailing necropsy procedures on a seaturtle (document presently under construction).*

◆ Arthropodan and Invertebrate Necropsy

Postmortem examination of invertebrates (e.g., tarantulas, centipedes, and hissing cockroaches) has potential as a diagnostic veterinary procedure; however, there is little published information on this subject. A gross necropsy examination can provide some useful data, such as whether an animal has received a traumatic injury or is demonstrating a retained exoskeleton during the molting process. It is important to remember that microbiologic culture may reveal a number of interesting organisms, but the significance of these organisms usually is unclear. Most of the organisms cultured are environmental contaminants. Fungi, rickettsiae, and viruses have been reported and are characterized histologically by damage to the internal organs, especially the hepatopancreas. In most instances, if the veterinarian or the technician does not have the expertise, the cadaver may be placed in a jar of 95% alcohol or 10% formalin, and the specimen can be referred to an arthropodologist (entomologist or arachnologist) at a nearby college or university. However, it is important to remember that a spider lying on its back is probably not dead, but molting. The owner should not rush to dispose of the carcass or to drop the spider into the alcohol or formalin solution.

---

*http://www.vetmed.ufl.edu/sacs/wildlife/zoologicalmedicine.htm research seaturtles

Necropsy forms:

I. History — Accession no. _____
Date _____ Pathologist _____
Submitted — Owner _____
by _____

Name _____ Name _____
Address _____ Address _____
Phone no. _____ Phone no. _____

Taxonomic information:
Common name _____
Family _____
Order _____ Genus _____
— Species (subsp.) _____

Wild or from a collection _____
If wild, where collected and date _____
_____
If from collection, how long in captivity_____
_____
Age _____ Sex _____ Weight _____
Snout to vent length _____
Vent to tail length _____
For chelonians, length of carapace (straight line)
_____
Length of plastron _____
No. submitted _____
No. housed with _____
If housed with different species list _____
_____
Environmental conditions (temperature, humidity,
photoperiod, type of cage, substrate, disinfectants
used for cleaning):

Diet (if whole animal state whether offered dead or
alive and source):
Disease duration:
Medications:
Previous history of disease:
Clinical signs:

II. Gross necropsy observations
Time of death _____
General appearance and physical condition:
Integument (condition of scales or scutes):
Eyes:
Oral cavity:
Nares:

Tongue:
Cloaca:
Subcutis:
Musculature:
Skeletal system and articulations:
Peritoneum:
Circulatory system:
  Heart:
Pericardium:
  Blood vessels:
Respiratory system:
  Nasal cavity:
  Trachea:
Bronchi:
  Lungs:
  Air-sacs:
Digestive system:
  Oral cavity: — Stomach: — Pancreas:
Pharynx: — Small intestine:
Esophagus: — Cecum:
Colon: — Gallbladder:
Cloaca:
Liver:
Spleen:
Thymus:
Urinary system:
Kidneys:
Ureters:
Bladder:
Reproductive system:
Nervous system:
Any additional findings:

III. Processing of specimens
Tissues for histopathologic evaluation (include
fixative):
Tissues for E.M. (include fixative):
Tissues for virology, bacteriology, and
toxicology (circle):
Parasites submitted for identification:
Blood samples:
Blood smears _____
Hematology _____
Blood chemistry _____
Photographs:
Diagnosis:

Figure 10-27
Necropsy form for a reptile. (Courtesy E.R. Jacobson, DVM, Gainesville, Florida.)

◆ Veterinary Technicians and Lifelong Learning

The veterinary technician who desires to learn more about exotic pet husbandry, physiology, anatomy, and necropsy techniques should be encouraged to develop a close working relationship with any licensed source of exotic pets. Whenever exotic pets die unexpectedly in pet stores and are to be properly disposed of, the veterinary technician should be contacted to pick up the fresh cadaver to perform a practice necropsy. In this manner, necropsy skills and expertise are developed. Veterinary technicians should be discouraged from collecting "road kill" animals and using them to practice necropsy techniques. First, collecting the specimen puts a person in danger of becoming a traffic fatality. Second, the animal may have been rabid at the time of death or may be infected with one of a myriad of zoonotic diseases.

In some areas of the country, the veterinary technician may be able to visit a wharf where fishing boats dock to acquire an intact, fresh fish on which to practice necropsy procedures. In addition, sport fishermen may be contacted to supply freshly caught specimens for necropsy practice. Under no circumstances should live fish be procured from a pet store and subjected to gross dissection. Fish (and all vertebrate animals) must be euthanized humanely. Many pet stores are willing to provide fish that have recently died, and these specimens are perfect for practicing the art of anatomic prosection and specimen collection.

Recommended Reading

Andrews J: Necropsy techniques, *Vet Clin North Am Food Anim Pract* 2:1 *et seq,* 1986.

Brown LJ: Necropsy techniques in small animal medicine, *Vet Tech* 16:409-19, 1995.

Cooper JE: A veterinary approach to spiders, *J Small Anim Pract* 28:229-39, 1987.

Cooper JE: Feeding exotic and pocket pets, *J Small Anim Pract* 31:482-8, 1990.

Feldman RG: Necropsy, *Proc Ann Mtg AAHA,* pp 542-7, 1973.

Jacobson ER: Reptile necropsy protocol, *J Zoo An Med* 9:7-13, 1978.

Jones TC, Gleiser CA: *Veterinary necropsy procedures,* Philadelphia, 1954, Lippincott.

Malley AD, van der Hage MH: The pet rabbit in companion animal practice. VI. Necropsy procedure, *Irish Vet J* 49:488-90, 1996.

Monlux WS: Routine necropsy procedure in the bovine, *Southwestern Vet* 5:121-9, 1952.

Rooney JR: *Autopsy of the horse: technique and interpretation,* Huntington, NY, 1970, Williams & Wilkins.

Runnells RA et al: *Principles of veterinary pathology,* ed 7, Ames, Iowa, 1965, Iowa State University Press.

Sheahan BJ: The necropsy in small animal practice, *J Small Anim Pract* 16:569-74, 1975.

Southgate PJ, Branson EJ: Autopsy procedures and laboratory techniques. In Butcher RL, editor: *Manual of ornamental fish,* Gloucestershire, England, 1992, British Small Animal Veterinary Association.

Strafuss AC: *Necropsy procedures and basic diagnostic methods for practicing veterinarians,* Springfield, Illl, 1988, Charles C Thomas.

Van Kruiningen HJ: Veterinary autopsy procedure, *Vet Clin North Am* 1:163-9, 1971.

C H A P T E R

Cytologic Examination

11

RICK L. COWELL
K.E. DORSEY

⬤ COLLECTION AND SMEAR PREPARATION

Cytologic samples may be collected by swabbing, scraping, and/or aspirating the lesion. The technique(s) used to collect cytologic samples and prepare slides vary, depending on the anatomic location, characteristics of the tissue being sampled, and characteristics of the patient (e.g., tractability).

When possible, several smears should be prepared and some left unstained so that smears are available for special stains if necessary. General considerations for collection and preparation of cytologic samples are discussed in this chapter. Cytology texts should be consulted for more information on procedures for cytologic examination of specific tissues.

◆ Imprints

Imprints for cytologic evaluation may be prepared from external lesions on the living animal or from tissues removed during surgery or necropsy. They are easy to collect and require minimal restraint, but they collect fewer cells than scrapings and usually contain a greater amount of contamination (bacterial and cellular) than fine-needle aspiration biopsies (FNABs). As a result, imprints from superficial lesions often reflect only a local secondary bacterial infection and/or inflammation-induced tissue dysplasia. In many instances, the bacteria and tissue dysplasia markedly hinder making an accurate diagnosis of neoplasia.

Ulcers should be imprinted before they are cleaned. The lesion should then be cleaned with a saline-moistened surgical sponge and reimprinted and/or scraped. A fine-needle aspirate of the tissue underlying the surface of the lesion should also be collected. In some conditions, such as *Dermatophilus congolensis* (streptothricosis), *Sporothrix schenckii* (sporotrichosis), *Blastomyces dermatitidis* (blastomycosis), and *Coccidioides immitis* (coccidioidomycosis) infections, impressions from the uncleaned lesion often contain more organisms than impressions from cleaned lesions and samples collected by FNAB. Imprints of the underside of the scabs from *Dermatophilus congolensis* lesions are usually most rewarding. Other conditions may yield more information on the imprints from cleaned lesions than the imprints from uncleaned lesions.

To collect imprints from cleaned cutaneous lesions or tissues collected during surgery or necropsy, blood and tissue fluid first should be removed from the surface of the lesion being imprinted by blotting with a clean absorbent material. Excessive blood and tissue fluids inhibit tissue cells from adhering to the glass slide, producing a poorly cellular preparation. Also, excessive fluid inhibits cells from spreading and assuming the size and shape they usually have on air-dried smears. The middle of a clean glass microscope slide is then touched against the blotted surface of the tissue to be imprinted. Although multiple imprints generally are made on each slide, one imprint per slide usually is sufficient. Several slides are imprinted so that slides are available for special stains if necessary.

◆ Scrapings

Smears of scrapings may be prepared from tissues collected during necropsy or surgery or from external lesions on the living animal. Scraping has the advantage of collecting many cells from the tissue and therefore is advantageous when the lesion is firm and yields few cells. The major disadvantages of scrapings are that they are more difficult to collect and they collect only superficial samples. As a result, scrapings from superficial lesions often reflect only a secondary bacterial infection and/or inflammation-induced tissue dysplasia, which markedly hinders their use in diagnosis of neoplasia.

Veterinary technicians may prepare a scraping by holding a scalpel blade perpendicular to the lesion's cleaned and blotted surface and pulling the blade toward themselves several times. The material collected on the blade is transferred to the middle of a glass microscope slide and spread by one or more of the techniques described under preparation of smears from aspirates of solid masses.

◆ Swabs

Generally, swabs are collected only when imprints, scrapings, and aspirates cannot be made, such as with fistulous tracts and vaginal collections. The lesion is swabbed with a moist, sterile cotton swab. Sterile isotonic fluid, such as 0.9% saline, should be used to moisten the swab. Moistening the swab helps minimize cell damage during sample collection and smear preparation. If the lesion is moist, the swab need not be moistened. After sample collection, the swab is gently rolled along the flat surface of a clean glass microscope slide. The swab should not be rubbed across the slide surface because this causes excessive cell damage.

◆ Aspiration of Masses

Fine-needle aspiration biopsies may be collected from masses, including lymph nodes, nodular lesions, and internal organs. For cutaneous lesions, they avoid superficial contamination (bacterial and cellular) but collect fewer cells than scrapings.

Selection of Syringe and Needle

Fine-needle aspiration biopsies are collected with a 21- to 25-gauge needle and a 3- to 20-ml syringe. The softer the aspirated tissue is, the smaller the needle and syringe used. Using a needle larger than 21 gauge for aspiration is seldom advantageous, even for firm tissues, such as fibromas. When larger needles are used, tissue cores tend to be aspirated, resulting in a poor yield of free cells suitable for cytologic preparation. Also, larger needles tend to cause greater blood contamination.

The size of syringe used is influenced by the consistency of the tissue being aspirated. Softer tissues, such as lymph nodes, often may be aspirated successfully with a 3-ml syringe. Firm tissues, such as fibromas and squamous-cell carcinomas, require a larger syringe to maintain adequate suction for sufficient collection of cells. Because the ideal size of the syringe is not known for many masses before aspiration, a 12-ml syringe is a useful size.

Preparation of the Site for Aspiration

If microbiologic tests are to be performed on a portion of the sample collected or a body cavity, such as peritoneal and thoracic cavities and joints, is to be penetrated, the area of aspiration is surgically prepared. Otherwise, skin preparation is essentially that required for a vaccination or venipuncture. An alcohol swab may be used to clean the area.

Aspiration Procedure

The mass to be aspirated is held firmly to aid penetration of the skin and mass and to control the direction of the needle. The needle, with syringe attached, is introduced into the center of the mass and strong negative pressure is applied by withdrawing the plunger to about three fourths the volume of the syringe (Figure 11-1). Several areas of the mass should be sampled, but aspiration of the sample into the barrel of the syringe and contamination of the sample by aspiration of tissue surrounding the mass must be avoided. To accomplish this, when the mass is large enough to allow the needle to be redirected and moved to several areas in the mass without danger of the needle's leaving the mass, negative pressure is maintained during redirection and movement of the needle. However, when the mass is not large enough for the needle to be redirected and moved without danger of the needle's leaving the mass, negative pressure is relieved during redirection and movement of the needle. In this situation, negative pressure is applied only when the needle is static. Often high-quality collections do not have aspirate material visible in the syringe and sometimes not even in the hub of the needle.

When material is observed in the hub of the needle or after several areas are sampled, the negative pressure is relieved from the syringe and the needle is withdrawn from the mass and skin. Next the needle is removed from the syringe and air is drawn into the syringe. Then the needle is replaced onto the syringe and some of the tissue in the barrel and hub of the needle is expelled onto the middle of a glass microscope slide by rapidly depressing the plunger. When possible, several preparations should be made as described in the following sections.

Figure 11-1
A, Fine-needle aspiration from a solid mass. **B,** Negative pressure is placed on the syringe by rapidly withdrawing the plunger (usually one half to three fourths the volume of the syringe). The needle is redirected several times while negative pressure is maintained, if this can be accomplished without the needle's point leaving the mass. **C,** Before removing the needle from the mass, the plunger is released, relieving negative pressure on the syringe.

Nonaspirate Procedure (Capillary Technique, Stab Technique)

The technique described here is a modification of the procedure first described by Drs. Menard and Papageorges. Technically, this technique is easier to perform than aspiration because it does not involve directing the syringe and needle and pulling the plunger with the same hand. A 22-gauge needle is attached to a 10-ml syringe prefilled with air. The mass to be sampled is held firmly to aid penetration of the skin and mass and to help direct the needle. Some technicians like to grasp the syringe barrel as if holding a throwing dart, whereas others believe grasping at the base of the needle gives one better control. The needle, with syringe attached, is introduced into the mass. The needle is moved rapidly back and forth through the mass five to six times along the same tract. Aspiration is not necessary because the cells are collected by shearing and capillary action. The needle is removed from the mass, and the material is expelled onto a clean glass microscope slide by rapidly depressing the plunger. The expelled material should be smeared using one of the techniques described under preparation of smears.

Generally, enough material is collected to make only one smear. Therefore the procedure should be repeated two or three times in different sites of the mass to have adequate slide numbers and areas of the mass to evaluate.

◆ Preparation of Smears from Aspirates of Solid Masses

Several methods may be used to prepare smears for cytologic evaluation of solid masses, including lymph nodes and internal organs. The experience of the person preparing the smears and characteristics of the sample influence the choice of smear preparation technique. The authors suggest a combination of slide preparation techniques. Some cytologic preparation techniques are described in the following sections.

Combination Technique

One combination procedure involves spraying the aspirate onto the middle of a clean glass microscope slide, or prep slide. Keeping the prep slide on a flat, solid, horizontal surface, the technician should pull another slide, called the *spreader slide,* backward at a 45-degree angle to the first slide until it contacts about one third of the aspirate (Figure 11-2). Then the spreader slide is slid smoothly and rapidly forward, as if making a blood smear. Next, the spreader slide is placed horizontally over the back one third of the aspirate at a right angle to the prep slide. The weight of the spreader slide (top slide) is allowed to spread the material, resisting the temptation to compress the slides manually. Keeping the spreader slide flat and horizontal, the technician quickly and smoothly slides it across the prep slide.

This procedure makes a squash preparation (see following) of the back third of the aspirate. The middle third of the aspirate is left untouched. This procedure leaves the front third of the aspirate gently spread. If the aspirate is of fragile tissue, this area should contain sufficient intact cells to evaluate. The back third of the aspirate has been spread with the shear forces of a squash preparation. If the aspirate contains clumps of cells that are difficult to spread, some clumps should be sufficiently spread in the back one third of the preparation. If the aspirate is of low cellularity, the middle third remains more concentrated and is the most efficient area to study.

Squash Preparation

In expert hands, the squash preparation can yield excellent cytologic smears. However, in less experienced hands, it often yields unreadable cytologic smears because too many cells are ruptured or the sample is not sufficiently spread. A squash preparation is made by expelling the aspirate onto the middle of one slide and then gently placing a second slide (spreader slide) over the aspirate horizontal with and at right angles to the first slide (prep slide) (Figure 11-3). The spreader slide is then quickly and smoothly slid across the prep slide. Downward pressure should not be placed on the spreader slide because this may cause excessive cell rupturing, making the sample unable to be interpreted.

Other Spreading Techniques

A modification of the squash preparation that has less tendency to rupture cells is to lay the second slide over the aspirate, rotate the second slide 45 degrees, and lift it upward (Figure 11-4).

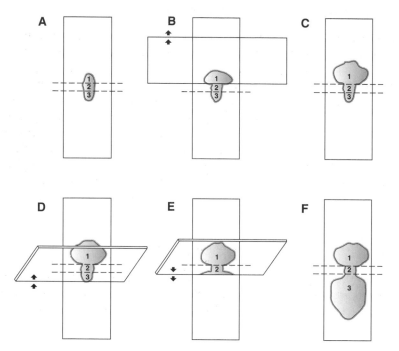

Figure 11-2
Combination cytologic preparation. **A,** A portion of the aspirate is expelled onto a glass microscope slide (prep slide). **B,** Another glass microscope slide is placed over about one third of the preparation. If additional spreading of the aspirate is needed, gentle digital pressure can be used. Excessive pressure should be avoided. **C,** The spreader slide is smoothly slid forward. This procedure makes a squash prep of about one third of the aspirate (*area 1*). The spreader slide also contains a squash prep (*not depicted*). Next, the edge of a tilted glass microscope slide (second spreader slide) is slid backward from the end opposite the squash prep until it contacts about one third the expelled aspirate (**D** and **E**). **F,** Then the second spreader slide is slid rapidly and smoothly forward. These steps produce an area (3) that is spread with mechanical forces like those of a blood smear preparation. The middle area (2) is left untouched and contains a high concentration of cells.

Another technique for spreading aspirates is to drag the aspirate peripherally in several directions with the point of a syringe needle, producing a starfish shape (Figure 11-5). This technique tends not to damage fragile cells but does allow a thick layer of tissue fluid to remain around the cells. Sometimes the thick layer of fluid prevents the cells from spreading well and interferes with evaluation of cell detail. Usually, however, some acceptable areas are present.

◆ Preparation of Smears from Fluids

Cytologic smears should be prepared immediately after fluid collection. When possible, fluid samples for cytologic examination should be collected in ethylenediaminetetra-

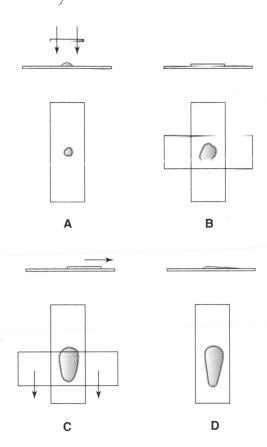

Figure 11-3
Squash preparation. **A,** A portion of the aspirate is expelled onto a glass microscope slide. **B,** Another slide is placed over the sample, spreading the sample. If the sample does not spread well, gentle digital pressure can be applied to the top slide. Care must be taken not to place excessive pressure on the slide, causing the cells to rupture. **C,** The slides are smoothly slid apart, which usually produces well-spread smears (**D**) but may result in excessive cell rupture.

acetic acid (EDTA) tubes. Smears may be prepared directly from fresh, well-mixed fluid or from the sediment of a centrifuged sample by blood smear (Figure 11-6), line smear (Figure 11-7), and squash preparation techniques (see Figure 11-3). The cellularity, viscosity, and homogeneity of the fluid influence the selection of smear technique.

The squash preparation technique often spreads viscous samples and samples with flecks of particulate material better than the blood smear and line smear techniques. The blood smear technique usually produces well-spread smears of sufficient cellularity from homogeneous fluids containing at least 5000 cells/μl but often produces smears of insufficient cellularity from fluids containing less than 5000 cells/μl. The line smear technique may be used to concentrate fluids of low cellularity but often does not sufficiently spread cells from highly cellular fluids. In general, translucent fluids are of

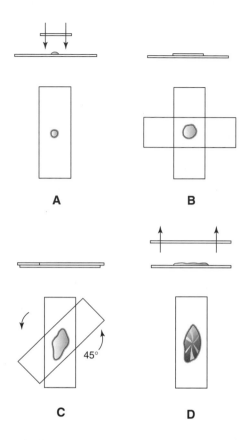

A   **B**

C   **D**

Figure 11-4
Modification of the squash preparation. **A,** A portion of the aspirate is expelled onto a glass microscope slide. **B,** Another slide is placed over the sample, causing the sample to spread. If necessary, gentle digital pressure can be applied to the top slide to spread the sample more. Care must be taken not to place excessive pressure on the slide, causing the cells to rupture. **C,** The top slide is rotated about 45 degrees and lifted directly upward, producing a squash preparation with subtle ridges and valleys of cells (**D**).

Figure 11-5
Needle spread or "starfish" preparation. **A,** A portion of the aspirate is expelled onto a glass microscope slide. **B,** The tip of a needle is placed in the aspirate and moved peripherally, pulling a trail of the sample with it. This procedure is repeated in several directions, resulting in a preparation with multiple projections.

A   **B**

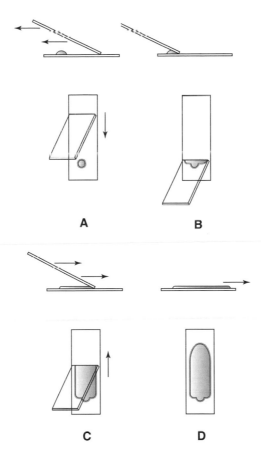

Figure 11-6
Blood smear technique. **A,** A drop of fluid sample is placed on a glass microscope slide close to one end, then another slide is slid backward to contact the front of the drop (**B**). When the drop is contacted, it rapidly spreads along the juncture between the two slides. **C** and **D,** The spreader slide is then smoothly and rapidly slid forward the length of the slide, producing a smear with a feathered edge.

low to moderate cellularity, whereas opaque fluids usually have high cellularity. Therefore translucent fluids often require concentration, either by centrifugation or by the line smear technique. When possible, concentration by centrifugation is preferred.

To prepare a smear by the blood smear technique, a small drop of the fluid is placed on a glass slide about 1.0 to 1.5 cm from the end (see Figure 11-6). Another slide is pulled backward at a 30- to 40-degree angle until it contacts the drop. When the fluid flows sideways along the juncture between the slides, the second slide is quickly and smoothly pushed forward until the fluid has all drained away from the second slide. This procedure makes a smear with a feathered edge.

To concentrate fluids by centrifugation, the fluid is centrifuged 5 minutes at 165 to 360 G with a centrifuge with a radial arm length of 14.6 cm (the arm length of most urine centrifuges) at 1000 to 1500 rpm. After centrifugation, the supernatant is separated from the sediment and analyzed for total protein concentration. The sediment is resuspended in a few drops of supernatant by gently thumping the side of the tube. A drop of the resuspended sediment is placed on a slide, and a smear is made by the blood smear or squash preparation technique. When possible, several smears should be made by each technique.

When the fluid cannot be concentrated by centrifugation or the centrifuged sample is of low cellularity, the line smear technique may be used to concentrate cells in the smear (Figure 11-7). A drop of fluid is placed on a clean glass slide and the blood

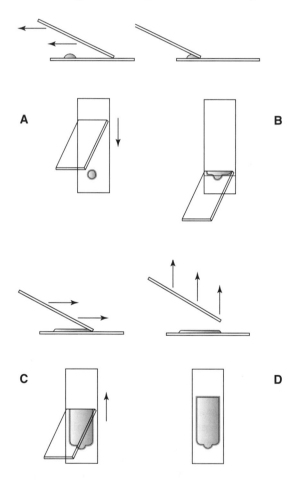

Figure 11-7
Line smear concentration technique. **A,** A drop of fluid sample is placed on a glass microscope slide close to one end, then another slide is slid backward to contact the front of the drop (**B**). When the drop is contacted, it rapidly spreads along the juncture between the two slides. **C,** The spreader slide is then smoothly and rapidly slid forward (**D**). After the spreader slide has been advanced about two thirds to three fourths the distance required to make a smear with a feathered edge, the spreader slide is raised directly upward. This procedure produces a smear with a line of concentrated cells at its end, instead of a feath-

smear technique is used, except the spreading slide is raised directly upward about three fourths of the way through the smear, yielding a line containing a much higher concentration of cells than the rest of the slide. Unfortunately, an excessive amount of fluid also may remain in the "line" and prevent the cells from spreading well.

STAINING

◆ Types of Stains

Several types of stains have been used for cytologic preparations. The two general types most commonly used are the Romanowsky-type stains (Wright's, Giemsa, Diff-Quik, DipStat) and Papanicolaou stain and its derivatives, such as Sano's trichrome. The advantages and disadvantages of both types of stains are discussed. However, because the Romanowsky-type stains are more rewarding, practical, and readily available in practice situations, the remainder of this discussion deals predominantly with Romanowsky-stained preparations.

Romanowsky Stains

Romanowsky stains are inexpensive, readily available, and easy to prepare, maintain, and use. They stain organisms and the cytoplasm of cells excellently. Although nuclear and nucleolar detail cannot be perceived as well with Romanowsky stains as with Papanicolaou stains, nuclear and nucleolar detail usually is sufficient for differentiating neoplasia and inflammation and for evaluating neoplastic cells for cytologic evidence of malignant potential (criteria of malignancy).

Smears to be stained with Romanowsky stains are first air dried. Air drying partially preserves ("fixes") the cells and causes them to adhere to the slide so that they do not fall off during the staining procedure.

Many Romanowsky stains are commercially available, including Diff-Quik (Dade Behring, Deerfield, IL), DipStat (Medichem, Inc., Santa Monica, CA), and other quick Wright's stains. Most, if not all, Romanowsky stains are acceptable for staining cytologic preparations. Diff-Quik stain does not undergo the metachromatic reaction. As a result, granules of some mast cells do not stain. When mast-cell granules do not stain, the mast cells may be misclassified as macrophages, which may lead to confusion in examination of some mast-cell tumors. Also, in evaluation of blood smears or bone marrow aspirates, Diff-Quik does not stain polychromatophilic RBCs well and occasionally does not stain basophils. The variations among different Romanowsky stains should not cause a problem once the evaluators become familiar with the stain they use routinely.

Each stain usually has a unique recommended staining procedure. These procedures should be followed in general but should be adapted to the type and thickness of smear being stained and to the evaluator's preference. The thinner the smear and the lower the total protein concentration of the fluid, the less time needed in the stain. The thicker the smear is and the greater the total protein concentration of the fluid, the more time needed in the stain. As a result, fluid smears with low protein and low cellularity, such as abdominal fluid, may stain better using half or less of the recommended time. Thick smears, such as smears of neoplastic lymph nodes, may need to be stained twice the recommended time or longer. Each person tends to have a different preferred staining technique. By trying variations in the recommended time intervals for stains, the evaluator can establish which times produce the preferred staining characteristics.

New Methylene Blue Stain

New methylene blue (NMB) stain is a useful adjunct to Romanowsky stains. It stains cytoplasm weakly, if at all, but gives excellent nuclear and nucleolar detail. Because NMB stains cytoplasm weakly, often the nuclear detail of cells in cell clumps may be visualized. Generally, red blood cells (RBCs) do not stain with NMB but may develop a pale blue tint. As a result, marked RBC contamination of smears does not obscure nucleated cells.

Papanicolaou Stains

The delicate Papanicolaou stains give excellent nuclear detail and delicate cytoplasmic detail. They allow the viewer to see through layers of cells in cell clumps and to evaluate nuclear and nucleolar changes well. They do not stain cytoplasm as strongly as Romanowsky stains and therefore do not demonstrate cytoplasmic changes as well as Romanowsky stains. They also do not demonstrate bacteria and other organisms as well as Romanowsky stains.

Papanicolaou staining requires multiple steps and considerable time. Also the reagents often are difficult to locate, prepare, and maintain in practice. Papanicolaou stains and their derivatives require the specimen to be wet-fixed (i.e., the smear must be fixed before the cells have dried). The veterinary technician achieves wet-fixing by spraying the smear with a cytologic fixative or placing it in ethanol immediately after preparation. When the smear is to be placed in ethanol, it should be made on a protein-coated slide, which prevents the cells from falling off the slide when it is immersed.

◆ Staining Problems

Poor stain quality often perplexes the novice and experienced cytologist. Most staining problems can be avoided if the following precautions are taken:
- New slides; fresh, well-filtered (if periodic filtration is required) stain(s); and fresh buffer solution (if a buffer is required) should be used.
- Cytologic preparations should be stained immediately after air-drying.
- The surface of the slide or smear should not be touched at any time by human hands.

Occasionally a sample may be contaminated with a foreign substance, such as K-Y Jelly, that alters the specimen's staining. Table 11-1 gives some of the problems that can occur with Romanowsky stains and some proposed solutions to these problems.

TABLE 11-1

Some possible solutions to problems seen with common Romanowsky stains

Problem	Solution
Excessive Blue Staining (RBC May Be Blue-green)	
Prolonged stain contact	Decrease staining time
Inadequate wash	Wash longer
Specimen too thick	Make thinner smears if possible
Stain, diluent, buffer, or wash water too alkaline	Check with pH paper and correct pH
Exposure to formalin vapors	Store and ship cytologic preps separate from formalin containers
Wet fixation in ethanol	Air dry smears before fixation
Delayed fixation	Fix smears sooner if possible
Surface of the slide was alkaline	Use new slides
Excessive Pink Staining	
Insufficient staining time	Increase staining time
Prolonged washing	Decrease duration of wash
Stain or diluent too acidic	Check with pH paper and correct pH; fresh methanol may be needed
Excessive time in red stain solution	Decrease time in red stain solution
Inadequate time in blue stain solution	Increase time in blue stain solution
Mounting coverslip before preparation is dry	Allow preparation to dry completely before mounting coverslip
Weak Staining	
Insufficient contact with one or more of the stain solutions	Increase staining time
Fatigued (old) stains	Change stains
Another slide covered specimen during staining	Keep slides separate
Uneven Staining	
Variation of pH in different areas of slide surface (may be due to slide surface being touched or slide being poorly cleaned)	Use new slides and avoid touching their surface before and after preparation
Water allowed to stand on some areas of the slide after staining and washing	Tilt slides close to vertical to drain water from the surface or dry with a fan
Inadequate mixing of stain and buffer	Mix stain and buffer thoroughly
Precipitate on Preparation	
Inadequate stain filtration	Filter or change the stain(s)
Inadequate washing of slide after staining	Rinse slides well after staining
Dirty slides used	Use clean new slides
Stain solution dries during staining	Use sufficient stain and do not leave it on slide too long

Continued

TABLE 11-1

Some possible solutions to problems seen with common Romanowsky stains—cont'd

Problem	Solution
Miscellaneous	
Overstained preparations	Destain with 95% methanol and restain; Diff-Quik-stained smears may have to be destained in the red Diff-Quik stain solution to remove the blue color; however, this damages the red stain solution
Refractile artifact on RBC with Diff-Quik stain (usually result of moisture in fixative)	Change the fixative

MICROSCOPIC EVALUATION

A detailed discussion of microscopic evaluation and cytologic interpretation is beyond the scope of this book. Reference sources contain detailed information. However, the basic principles are as follows.

After the smear has been stained and dried, it is scanned at low magnification (4× to 10× objective) to determine if all areas of the smear are stained adequately and to detect any localized areas of increased cellularity or areas with unique staining features. If the smear is inadequately stained, it may be restained. However, not all areas of a slide must be adequately stained. For example, even if only the edges of thick smears are stained adequately, they still may be adequately evaluated.

Any areas of increased and/or unique cellularity should be mentally noted for later evaluation. Also, large objects, such as crystals, foreign bodies, parasites, and fungal hyphae, may be seen during a scan of the slide at low magnification. When proper staining is ensured and all areas of increased and/or unique cellularity are recognized, magnification is increased to the 10× or 20× objective. An impression of the cellularity and cellular composition (e.g., inflammatory cells, epithelial cells, or spindle cells) of the smear and of cell size usually is developed at this magnification. Areas of increased cellularity and/or unique cellularity are evaluated.

Next the smear is viewed with the 40× objective. To improve resolution by decreasing light diffraction, a drop of oil may be placed on the smear; then a coverslip is placed over the drop of oil. At this magnification, individual cells are evaluated and compared with other cells in the smear. Usually, nucleoli and the chromatin pattern may be discerned. With experience, the veterinary technician can see most organisms that are visible microscopically with the 40× objective. However, using the 100× (oil-immersion) objective may be necessary to identify some organisms and inclusions and to confirm the identity of organisms seen with the 40× objective. Cell morphology (nuclear chromatin pattern, nucleoli, etc.) is evaluated in detail with the 100× (oil-immersion) objective.

Cell types encountered depend on the origin of the specimen. Familiarity with the appearance of erythrocytes, neutrophils, lymphocytes, plasma cells, eosinophils, mast cells, macrophages, mesothelial cells, squamous (keratinized and nonkeratinized) epithelial cells (Figures 11-8 and 11-9), and neoplastic cells is required. Appreciation of the difference between pyknosis, karolysis, and mechanical disruption of cells (smear artifact) is mandatory for proper interpretation (Figure 11-10). Pyknosis represents slow cell death (aging) and refers to a small, condensed, dark nucleus that may fragment (called *karyorrhexis*) (Figure 11-11). Karolysis represents rapid cell death, as in some septic (bacterial) inflammatory reactions, and appears as a swollen, ragged nucleus with reduced staining intensity (Figure 11-12). Macrophages and neutrophils should be noted as nonphagocytic, phagocytic (with a description of the ingested material), nonvacuolated, or vacuolated (see Figure 11-11).

Neoplastic cells are classified as cytologically benign or malignant. As a generalization, a cytologically benign neoplasm has a uniform population of cells, whereas a cytologically malignant neoplasm tends to have a pleomorphic population of cells, with cells, nuclei, and nucleoli tending to be large, usually with a disproportionately large nucleus

Figure 11-8
Large binucleate mesothelial cell in equine peritoneal fluid. Cytoplasmic "pseudopods" around the cell are an artifact of slide preparation. (Wright's stain, 1140×)

Figure 11-9
A raft of mesothelial cells (*R*) in peritoneal fluid from a horse with resolving peritonitis. Several neutrophils and erythrocytes, a phagocytic macrophage, and a mesothelial cell (*M*) are also present. (Wright's stain, 810×)

Figure 11-10
Blood smear artifact. Most neutrophils are intact, with normal morphology. However, the nucleus of one cell (*A*) has been mechanically disrupted. (Wright's stain, 780×)

Figure 11-11
Peritoneal fluid smear from a horse with resolving peritonitis. Numerous neutrophils with normal morphology are present. One neutrophil nucleus (*PK*) is pyknotic (condensed and has increased affinity for stain) and karyorrhexic (fragmented). A macrophage that has phagocytosed cellular debris also is present (*M*). (Wright's stain, 780×)

Figure 11-12
Peritoneal fluid smear from a dog with acute, septic, suppurative peritonitis, secondary to a ruptured bile duct. All nuclei are karyolytic (swollen, with decreased affinity for stain). Bacteria (*B*) and bile pigment (*P*) are also present. (Wright's stain, 780×)

(referred to as a high nucleus/cytoplasm ratio). In addition, malignant neoplastic cells frequently have multiple, pleomorphic, bizarre (angular) nucleoli with active (basophilic) cytoplasm (Figure 11-13, Table 11-2).

Histopathologic verification of cytologic findings is important for most tumors (whether cytologically benign or malignant). Also, cytologically benign cells may be obtained from malignant tumors. Histopathologic examination offers the advantage

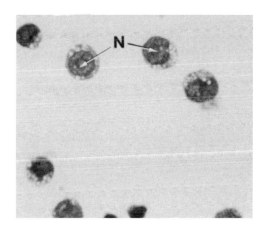

Figure 11-13
Smear of feline thoracic effusion resulting from lymphoblastic lymphosarcoma. Note the large immature lymphocytes with prominent nucleoli *(N)*. (Wright's stain, 780×)

TABLE 11-2

Easily recognized general and nuclear criteria of malignancy

Criteria	Description	Schematic Representation
General Criteria		
Anisocytosis and macrocytosis	Cell size varies, with some cells ≥ 1.5 times larger than normal.	
Hypercellularity	Cell exfoliation is increased as a result of decreased cell adherence.	
Pleomorphism (except in lymphoid tissue)	Size and shape varies in cells of the same type.	
Nuclear Criteria		
Macrokaryosis	Increased nuclear size. Cells with nuclei larger than 10 μ in diameter suggest malignancy.	RBC
Increased nucleus: cytoplasm ratio (N:C)	Normal nonlymphoid cells usually have an N:C of 1:3 to 1:8, depending on the tissue. Ratios ≥ 1:2 suggest malignancy.	See "Macrokaryosis"
Anisokaryosis	Variation in nuclear size. This is especially important if the nuclei of multinucleated cells vary in size.	

Continued

TABLE 11-2

Easily recognized general and nuclear criteria of malignancy—cont'd

Criteria	Description	Schematic Representation
Multinucleation	Multiple nucleation in a cell. This is especially important if the nuclei vary in size.	
Increased mitotic figures	Mitosis is rare in normal tissue.	Normal Abnormal
Abnormal mitosis	Chromosomes are improperly aligned.	See Increased mitotic figures
Coarse chromatin pattern	The chromatin pattern is coarser than normal. It may appear ropy or cord-like.	
Nuclear molding	Nuclei are deformed by other nuclei within the same cell or adjacent cells.	
Macronucleoli	Nucleoli are increased in size. Nucleoli $\geq$ 5 μ strongly suggest malignancy. For reference RBC are 5 to 6 μ in cats; 7 to 8 μ in dogs.	RBC
Angular nucleoli	Nucleoli are fusiform or have other angular shapes, instead of their normal round to slightly oval shape.	
Anisonucleoliosis	Nucleolar shape or size varies (especially important if the variation is within the same nucleus).	See "Angular nucleoli"

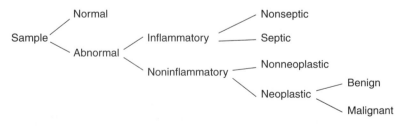

Figure 11-14
Steps involved in making a general cytologic diagnosis.

of enabling assessment of factors such as local tissue infiltration and vessel or lymphatic invasion by tumor cells. These characteristics of malignant tumors are not evident cytologically.

The cytology report should indicate the cell types present, their appearance, and relative proportions. The flow chart in Figure 11-14 shows the steps taken to arrive at a general cytologic diagnosis. Obviously such a diagnosis must be interpreted relative to other findings in that animal.

SUBMISSION OF CYTOLOGIC PREPARATIONS AND SAMPLES FOR INTERPRETATION

When in-house evaluation of a cytologic preparation does not furnish sufficient reliable information for managing a case, the preparation may be submitted to a veterinary clinical pathologist/cytologist for interpretation, or an alternative procedure, such as biopsy and histopathologic evaluation, may be performed. If possible, the person to whom the cytologic preparation is sent should be contacted, and specifics concerning sample handling should be discussed, such as the number of smears to send or whether to fix or stain the smears before mailing. The following discussion gives some general guidelines for submitting cytologic preparations for interpretation.

When possible, two or three air-dried unstained smears, and two or three air-dried Romanowsky-stained smears should be submitted. Pathologists may stain the air-dried unstained smears with the Romanowsky or new methylene blue stains of their choice. The Romanowsky-stained smears are a safety factor. Some tissues stain poorly when air dried but not stained for several days. Also slides occasionally are shattered during transport and cannot be stained upon receipt. Sometimes microscopic examination of shards from the broken prestained smears allows diagnosis. If only a couple of smears can be prepared from the sample, one should be submitted air dried and unstained and the other submitted air dried and stained. Smears should be well labeled with alcohol-resistant ink or another permanent labeling method. If a Papanicolaou stain is to be used, several wet-fixed smears should be submitted.

Fluid samples should have smears prepared from them immediately. Direct smears and concentrated smears should be submitted. Also, an EDTA (lavender top) and sterile serum tube (red top) fluid sample should be submitted. A total nucleated cell count and total protein concentration can be performed on the EDTA tube sample and, if necessary, chemical analyses can be performed on the serum tube sample.

Slides must be protected when mailed. Simple cardboard mailers do not provide sufficient protection to prevent slide breakage if they are mailed in unpadded envelopes. Marking the envelope with phrases such as "Fragile," "Glass," "Breakable," and "Please Hand Cancel" has little success. Placing a pad of bubble-paper or polystyrene on each side of the slide holder usually prevents slide breakage. Also, slides may be mailed in plastic slide holders or innovative holders, such as small pill bottles.

Slides should not be mailed with formalin-containing samples and should be protected against moisture. Formalin fumes alter the staining characteristics of smears and water causes cell lysis.

SUBMISSION OF SAMPLES FOR CULTURE

Culture results are strongly influenced by sample collection, preparation, and transport (see Chapter 4). The following procedures are suggested to optimize success in culturing lesions and fluids:

- The laboratory is contacted before collecting the sample.
- The sample is collected as aseptically as possible.
- Fresh samples are submitted for culture.
- Proper equipment is used for collection and transport of the sample.
- A timely courier service is used.

◆ Precollection Contact with the Laboratory

Each laboratory has its own preferred techniques, media, and days when cultures are read or subcultures are performed, among other things. Precollection contact with the laboratory to which the sample is submitted allows discussion of topics such as optimum sample type, transport medium, and day of the week to submit the sample. Also, some laboratories furnish culture supplies. Expensive and/or quickly outdated supplies, such as blood culture tubes, may be ordered from the laboratory as needed. Early communication with the laboratory also allows the laboratory to prepare for the sample and ensure that any special media required are available.

◆ Collect Samples as Aseptically as Possible

All samples should be collected as aseptically as possible. Even samples collected from lesions that naturally are exposed to secondary contamination, such as cutaneous ulcers, should be protected from further contamination. When samples are collected from more than one lesion, care should be taken not to cross-contaminate the samples. Finding the same organism in several different lesions is strong evidence that the organism is involved in development of the lesions. Therefore cross-contamination of samples from different lesions may lead to misinterpretation of culture results. When fluids are collected, anticoagulant and serum tubes should not be assumed sterile. Also, EDTA, through its effect on bacterial cell walls, may be bacteriostatic or bactericidal.

◆ Submission of Fresh Samples

Samples should be submitted as soon after collection as possible. Fluid aspiration, resection of lesions to be cultured, exploratory surgeries during which culture is anticipated, and other procedures that may produce samples to be cultured should be scheduled to allow immediate transport of samples to the laboratory. During transport, samples should be kept cool but not frozen.

Tissue and fluid samples usually are more rewarding than swab samples for isolation of a causative agent. Individual tissue samples submitted for culture should be about 4 cm square or larger. Whirl-Pak bags (NASCO, Ft. Atkinson, WI), which are sealable and sterile, are excellent for tissue biopsies that must be kept free of contaminants. Zippered or heat-sealed plastic bags that are not sterile are fine for submitting tissue samples that have normal microbial flora or contaminated surfaces. Tissues for anaerobic culture should be shipped in self-contained atmosphere-generating anaerobic bags such as Gas-Pak Pouch (Becton-Dickinson, Rutherford, NJ). Samples such as abscesses and skin, known to contain bacteria, must be packaged separately from other tissues. Culturette-type transport systems should be used to prevent small biopsies from drying during transport. Shipping biopsies in sterile saline should be avoided because it may cause negative culture results.

Fluid samples, such as urine, milk, joint fluid, thoracic fluid, abdominal fluid, and abscess aspirates, may submitted in sterile Vacutainer tubes, small Whirl-Pak bags, or sterile disposable syringes. Fluids for anaerobic cultures should be collected in syringes, with air expelled, and then capped and transported immediately to the laboratory for culture. However, for optimal results or if a time delay is anticipated, the fluid should be placed in a transport system that supports aerobic and anaerobic bacteria. These systems often can be obtained from the laboratory performing the culture. Containers, such as Port-A-Cul Vials (BBL, Microbiology Systems, Cockeysville, MD), are commercially available for fluid samples. These systems usually support a wide variety of anaerobic and aerobic organisms for up to 72 hours at 20° to 25° C.

When biopsies or aspirates are not obtainable or warranted, swabs are useful for sample collection, especially swabs of mucosal surfaces and deep within soft tissue lesions. Culturette-type transport swabs such as Culture Collection and Transport Tube (Curtis Matheson Scientific, Burbank, CA) containing Amies medium with charcoal, is suggested for aerobic cultures. These swabs seem to be excellent transport and holding media for fastidious bacteria. Anaerobic swab systems, such as the Marion Scientific Anaerobic Culturette (Marion Scientific, Kansas City, MO), have prereduced Cary-Blair transport medium and are necessary for transport of swabs for anaerobic culture. Swabs without medium may dry out in transport, resulting in false-negative results, whereas swabs submitted in broth medium often are overgrown by contaminants. Separate swabs should be submitted if additional cultures for fungi and/or viruses are desired.

In general, samples submitted for fungal culture, with the exception of dermatophyte suspects, should be collected and transported in the same manner as samples for bacterial culture. Again, tissues and body fluids are preferred to swabs. Swab samples never should be submitted for dermatophyte cultures. Suspect dermatophyte lesions should be cleaned gently with 70% alcohol to decrease bacterial contamination before plucking hair and scraping keratin scales from the periphery of the lesion. Dermatophyte samples must be kept dry to inhibit growth of skin contaminants. Therefore hair and scales should be transported in clean, dry, breathable containers such as envelopes or other paper containers. Tightly sealed glass or plastic tubes or containers often have condensate formation during transport and should not be used. If unsure about proper sample submission or transport for fungal cultures, veterinary technicians should contact their chosen laboratory.

References

Cowell RL, Tyler RD: *Diagnostic cytology and hematology of the horse,* ed 2, St Louis, 2002, Mosby.

Cowell RL, Tyler RD, Meinkoth JH: *Diagnostic cytology and hematology of the dog and cat,* ed 2, St Louis, 1999, Mosby.

DeNicola DB: Diagnostic cytology, collection techniques, and sample handling, *Proc 4th Ann Mtg ACVIM,* pp 15-25, 1987.

Menard M, Papageorges M: Technique for ultrasound-guided fine-needle biopsies, *Vet Radiol Ultrasound* 36:137-8, 1995.

Meyer DJ, Franks P: Clinical cytology, management of clinical specimens, *Mod Vet Pract* 67:255-9, 1986.

Meyer DJ: Management of cytology specimens, *Compend Cont Ed Pract Vet* 9(1):10-7, 1987.

O'Rourke LG: Cytology techniques, *Mod Vet Pract* 64:185-9, 1983.

Miscellaneous Laboratory Techniques

BRUCE W. PARRY

The information in this chapter is divided into four general categories: cytology, detection of fecal occult blood, toxicology, and skin biopsy. Also included in this chapter are aspects of collecting, preparing, handling, and evaluating specimens.

BIOPSY

Tissue biopsy is the sampling of a piece of tissue for cytologic and/or histopathologic examination. Many organs or tissues, including kidney, liver, lung, lymph node, prostate, skin, spleen and thyroid, or masses (tumors) may be biopsied. Biopsy techniques include gentle abrasion with a blade, needle aspiration, and excision. The technique used varies with the tissue to be biopsied. Considerations include its location, accessibility, and nature. Methods for making cytologic preparations from biopsy specimens have been described in Chapter 11.

Tissue samples for histopathologic examination often are fixed in 10% formalin. To ensure adequate fixation, slabs of tissue no more than 1 cm wide should be placed in fluid-tight jars containing formalin at about 10 times the specimen's volume.

EXFOLIATIVE CYTOLOGY

Exfoliative cytology is the study of cells shed from body surfaces. Therefore in its broadest sense, it refers to examination of cells present in body fluids (such as cerebrospinal, peritoneal, pleural, and synovial fluids), on mucosal surfaces (such as the trachea or vagina), or in secretions (such as semen, prostatic fluid, and milk). Samples typically are collected by imprint, swab, or aspiration. Common laboratory procedures used in conjunction with cytology in evaluation of these samples are presented in the following sections.

Certain gross characteristics of body fluids should be recorded at collection, including ease of sample collection, color, and turbidity. Subsequently, total nucleated cell counts, cell types, and their morphology are determined.

◆ Ease of Collection

Ease of collection may reflect the volume of fluid present and/or the pressure within that body cavity. It also is influenced by the technical proficiency of the operator and, in the case of conscious animals, the cooperation of the animal.

◆ Color and Turbidity

Color and turbidity are influenced by protein concentration and cell numbers. Gross discoloration, with increased turbidity, may be due to iatrogenic contamination with peripheral blood, recent or old hemorrhage, inflammation, or a combination of these.

Perforation of superficial vessels during collection may result in contamination with peripheral blood. Such admixture of blood with the sample may be obvious as a streak of blood in otherwise clear fluid at some stage during collection. Blood-tinged fluid also may be due to recent or old hemorrhage into the body cavity being sampled. Both peripheral blood contamination and recent hemorrhage result in a clear supernatant and a red (erythrocyte-rich) sediment after centrifugation. Recent hemolysis imparts a reddish discoloration to the supernatant. Hemorrhage that occurred at least 2 days previously generally causes a yellowish supernatant (because of hemoglobin breakdown products), usually with little erythrocytic sediment.

Cytologic examination of the fluid also may assist in determining the time of hemorrhage. Clumps of platelets may be observed in recent, often iatrogenic (operator-induced) hemorrhage (Figure 12-1). These clumps are not obvious after approximately an hour.

Blood must be present in the cavity for several hours before macrophage ingestion of erythrocytes becomes evident (erythrophagocytic macrophages, Figure 12-2). If the hemorrhage occurred a day or so before collection, hemoglobin-breakdown products, such as hemosiderin, may be seen in the macrophages (Figure 12-3).

Figure 12-1
Synovial fluid from a dog. Recent hemorrhage, probably at collection, is indicated by the clumped platelets. (May Grünwald Giemsa stain, 400×)

Figure 12-2
Synovial fluid from a dog. The erythro-phagocytic macrophage indicates hemor-rhage before collection. (May Grünwald Giemsa stain, 1000×)

Figure 12-3
Prostatic wash fluid from a dog. The hemosiderin-laden macrophages indi-cate chronic hemorrhage. (May Grün-wald Giemsa stain, 1000×)

Inflammation also may discolor body fluids, with the degree of turbidity reflecting leukocyte numbers. Color may vary from an off-white or cream to a red-cream or dirty brown, depending on the number of erythrocytes also involved and the integrity of the cells present.

CEREBROSPINAL FLUID ANALYSIS

Analysis of cerebrospinal fluid (CSF) is useful in evaluation of some neurologic dis-orders. Fluid is collected aseptically from the anesthetized animal by percutaneous insertion of a spinal needle through either the atlantooccipital or lumbosacral space, into the subarachnoid space of the spinal column. Care must be taken not to advance the needle too far and consequently damage the spinal cord. If the animal is in lateral recumbency, CSF pressure can be measured with a spinal manometer. Fluid is collected by free flow, not aspiration, into an ethylenediaminetetraacetic acid (EDTA) tube and perhaps a serum (plain) blood tube. The plain tube of CSF should be centrifuged and the supernatant (with normal CSF little sediment exists) used for biochemical tests, such as protein, glucose, lactate, and creatine kinase (CK) determinations.

◆ Color and Turbidity

Normal CSF is colorless and transparent (it looks like distilled water, and newsprint is easily read through it) because it has a low protein concentration and few cells. About 500 cells/μl must be present before turbidity is noticeable. Gross discoloration (with increased turbidity) most frequently is due to iatrogenic contamination with peripheral blood. Interpretation of discolored fluid is discussed earlier in this chapter. Yellow CSF is referred to as *xanthochromia,* which generally is due to erythrocytic breakdown products (predominantly bilirubin). It may sometimes be due to a markedly elevated serum-conjugated bilirubin concentration, with passive diffusion of the water-soluble molecule into the CSF.

◆ Cell Counts

Cells in CSF are thought to deteriorate rapidly after collection. It generally is recommended that total and differential nucleated cell counts be performed within 15 minutes (at latest, within 30 minutes) of collection in EDTA. Somewhat longer delays are possible, especially if the sample is kept cool. However, if the sample will not be processed within several hours, the sample may be diluted 1:1 with 40% to 50% ethanol to help preserve cells. This dilution should be taken into account in subsequent calculations.

Nucleated cell counts may be performed using a leukocyte pipette. A suitable diluting fluid is Rosenthal's solution (made by adding 0.1 g of crystal violet to a mixture of 10 ml of glacial acetic acid and 90 ml of distilled water). It should be filtered before use to remove debris that could be confused with cells. The pipette is filled to the 1 mark with diluting fluid and then to the 11 mark with CSF. After thorough mixing, the first few drops are discarded and both sides of a Neubauer hemacytometer chamber are charged with fluid. After 2 minutes (to allow erythrocytes to lyse and nucleated cells to settle), all nucleated cells within the entire boxed area of both sides are counted. The count is multiplied by 0.6 to give the number of cells/μl. (If ethanol-diluted CSF was used, the count is multiplied by 1.2.)

Normal CSF contains virtually no erythrocytes. Erythrocytes may be counted by charging a Neubauer hemacytometer with a well-mixed sample of undiluted and unstained CSF. All cells in the entire boxed area of one side are counted. With this method both erythrocytes and nucleated cells are observed. It usually is possible to distinguish between these two groups of cells but not to subcategorize the nucleated cells, as often may be done if Rosenthal's solution is used. Cell counts for undiluted CSF are multiplied by 1.1 to give the total number of cells/μl. (If ethanol-diluted CSF is used, the cell counts are multiplied by 2.2.)

If difficulty is experienced distinguishing erythrocytes from nucleated cells in unstained CSF, the total number of cells counted using the latter method may be subtracted from the number of nucleated cells counted, using Rosenthal's solution, to calculate the erythrocyte count.

Interpretation

As a cross-species generalization, normal CSF contains no erythrocytes and less than 25 nucleated cells/μl (usually 0 to 10/ l). Pleocytosis is an elevated CSF nucleated cell count.

Use of various "correction factors" has been advocated to adjust CSF nucleated cell counts for any peripheral blood leukocytic contamination. As normal CSF contains no erythrocytes, the observed nucleated cell count may be corrected if the number of erythrocytes/μl of CSF is known. The simplest approach is to consider that each 500 to 1000 erythrocytes would be accompanied by one leukocyte. A more complicated method is to use the following equation:

$$\textbf{Corrected nucleated cell count} = \frac{\textbf{Observed nucleated cell count}}{\textbf{WBC blood} \times \textbf{RBC CSF/RBC blood}}$$

However, this equation requires values for blood leukocyte (WBC blood) and erythrocyte (RBC blood) counts, and a CSF erythrocyte count (RBC CSF). Despite its complexity, it is no more accurate than the preceding approximation. Ideally, CSF samples should be free of iatrogenic peripheral blood contamination. Use of the previous "correction factor" is, at best, a rough guide to the uncontaminated CSF nucleated cell count.

◆ Cytologic Examination

With experience, especially when total nucleated cell counts are normal, one can perform a preliminary differential cell count on the fluid in the counting chamber, if Rosenthal's solution (or another stain) is used.

When a cytologic smear is to be made of fluid with a cell count below 500/μl, concentration of cells is mandatory. (Such concentration may be helpful even at higher cell counts.) Four methods have been described.

Low-Speed Centrifugation

Cells may be concentrated by low-speed centrifugation (about 1500 rpm for 5 minutes). The supernatant is removed carefully, and a direct smear is made from the sediment after resuspension in a small quantity of CSF supernatant or cell-free plasma from the same animal. Because CSF normally has a low protein concentration, addition of plasma may help cells adhere to the microscope slide. After air drying, the slide may be stained with a Romanowsky stain. Because of the small numbers of cells in normal CSF, few cells may be present in these smears.

Gravitational Sedimentation

Gravitational sedimentation is another method used to concentrate cells. One method uses a glass cylinder (which can be made by cutting the end off a test tube) attached to a microscope slide with paraffin wax. (The smooth tube end is dipped in melted wax and placed on a warm slide.) The cells in about 1 ml of CSF are allowed about 30 minutes to settle. The supernatant then is removed carefully with a pipette and the tube detached. (Excess CSF may be gently removed with absorbent paper.) The slide is air dried and residual paraffin carefully scraped off. The slide may be stained with a Romanowsky stain.

Membrane Filtration

Membrane filtration of alcohol-diluted CSF also may be used to concentrate cells. A membrane pore size of 5 is usually satisfactory. Filter holders that attach to a syringe are available. The CSF is permitted to gravity-feed from the syringe barrel, or it is gently injected through the filter at no more than 1 drop/second. The filter paper must be kept horizontal to evenly distribute the cells. Increased resistance to filtration suggests that the pores are becoming obstructed by cells and/or protein, and no more CSF should be forced through the filter. Filtration of another, smaller volume of CSF through fresh filter paper results in a less crowded preparation.

After removal from the syringe holder, the filter is fixed in 95% ethanol for at least 30 minutes. Holders are available for easy handling of the filter paper during fixation and staining. A trichrome-type stain must be used. Romanowsky stains are unsuitable because they stain the filter paper too intensely. A satisfactory staining procedure is as follows.

The filter paper is immersed for 2 minutes in each of the following (in order): 80%, 70%, 50%, and 30% ethanol and then distilled water, then 4 minutes in hematoxylin, 5 minutes in running tap water, 4 minutes in Pollak's stain, 1 minute in 0.3% acetic acid, 1 minute in 95% ethanol, 2 minutes in n-propyl-alcohol (propanol), 2 minutes in a 1:1 mixture of propanol and xylene, and finally three rinses of 2 minutes each in xylene. At all stages the filter must be treated gently to avoid dislodging cells. Depending on the size of the filter, it may need to be cut to a suitable size before placement on a microscope slide (cell side up). The filter is then flooded with a mounting medium with a refractive index similar to that of filter paper (about 1.5) and a coverslip applied.

Cytologically, the cells trapped by the membrane filter are rounder than those seen after sedimentation (and therefore may be harder to distinguish), and they are in slightly different planes of focus. Further, the filter produces a patterned background that may be distracting. This distraction is minimized by ensuring the sample is not overstained and by using the appropriate mounting medium. The pore size generally used is far too large to trap free bacteria. Quantitatively, more cells are collected by filtration than by the two sedimentation methods.

Cytocentrifugation

As with any fluid of low cellularity, a cytocentrifuge (e.g., Shandon cytospin; Figure 12-4) can be used for preparation of CSF cytologic smears. Such equipment is generally too expensive for a veterinary practice to justify purchasing. However, it often is used in a referral laboratory. This technique allows cells to be concentrated within a small, circular area on the slide.

Interpretation

Normal CSF contains 95% to 100% mononuclear cells, almost all of which are lymphocytes (Figure 12-5). Bacterial infections involving CSF generally cause marked pleocytosis, mostly because of neutrophils. Inflammation associated with viruses, fungi, neoplasia, or degenerative conditions generally causes less dramatic pleocytosis, with a significant proportion of mononuclear cells (often lymphocytes). Eosinophils sometimes are seen, especially in parasitic inflammatory responses. In general, the causative agent often is not cytologically apparent. Neoplastic cells are seldom observed in CSF.

◆ **Protein Concentration**

Normal CSF (from all species) has a low protein concentration, generally 10 to 50 mg/dl, almost all of which is albumin. Any condition that disrupts the normal

A

B

Figure 12-4
Cytocentrifuge: used to concentrate cells in fluids of low cellularity for cytologic evaluation.

Figure 12-5
Cerebrospinal fluid from a dog. Note the several small mononuclear cells (lymphocytes) and a large mononuclear cell (nonphagocytic macrophage). (May Grünwald Giemsa stain, 1000×)

blood-brain barrier, such as hemorrhage, inflammation, or neoplasia, results in an increased CSF protein concentration as a result of increases in albumin and globulin. The protein concentration of CSF may be measured qualitatively or quantitatively.

The Pandy test and the Nonne-Apelt test commonly are used as qualitative screening procedures for CSF protein. They detect high-molecular-weight globulins (basically immunoglobulins) but are relatively insensitive tests. The Biuret procedure, used to quantitate total protein concentration in plasma or serum specimens, is not sensitive enough for use with CSF. Two simple quantitative procedures have been described, using either sulfosalicylic acid or trichloroacetic acid reactions; however, these are not available in kit form and are therefore unlikely to be used in the general practice laboratory. Therefore actual quantitative determination of protein concentration usually is performed only at a referral laboratory, often using procedures designed for determination of urinary protein concentration.

Pandy Test

For the Pandy test, 1 drop of CSF is added to 1 ml of saturated aqueous phenol. Turbidity is observed before and after the mixture is shaken. Phenol and CSF are immiscible; therefore after shaking, the CSF disperses as small droplets in the phenol, which should not be confused with a positive reaction (i.e., development of turbidity). If the sample is normal, no appreciable immunoglobulin is present and the solution remains clear (at most, slightly turbid), which is considered a negative result. If immunoglobulin is present at a concentration of 25 mg/dl or more, the solution becomes cloudy white. The degree of turbidity may be subjectively graded from 1+ to 4+, corresponding to increasing immunoglobulin concentration.

Nonne-Apelt Test

For the Nonne-Apelt test, 1 ml of saturated ammonium sulfate solution is overlaid carefully with 1 ml of CSF and allowed to stand undisturbed for 3 minutes. The junc-

ds remains clear with normal CSF. However, if CSF im-
on is increased, a white-gray zone forms at the junction.
ded subjectively from 1+ to 4+, reflecting increasing im-
tion.

st

acid procedure, 0.5 ml of CSF is added to 4.5 ml of 1.5% sulfo-
and allowed to stand for 10 minutes at room temperature. The op-
esuspended mixture is read at 420 nm and compared with a pro-
d in the same manner. (If the protein standard for blood protein
surement is used, it must be diluted 1:100 with distilled water.)

Acid Test

roacetic acid procedure, 0.5 ml of CSF is added to 1.5 ml of 5%
acid, mixed, and allowed to stand for 5 minutes at room temperature.
ensity of the resuspended mixture is read at 420 nm and compared with
eated likewise.

lectrophoresis

plex procedure may be performed on CSF; however, it is performed rarely
e clinical cases.

pretation

ipheral blood contamination of a sample may increase its protein concentration.
eally, an uncontaminated sample should be obtained (possibly by subsequent re-
eat collection). However, if this is impossible, the amount of protein contributed by
peripheral blood may be crudely approximated by considering that every 1000 erythrocytes present are accompanied by about 1 mg of protein. The equation used to
correct the CSF nucleated cell count (see previous discussion) may be modified by
replacing observed and corrected nucleated cell counts by protein concentrations
and peripheral blood WBC count (WBC blood) by the blood protein concentration.
The reservations concerning such "correction factors," expressed earlier, are equally
valid for corrections of protein concentration.

Fibrinogen Concentration

CSF contains no appreciable quantity of fibrinogen and therefore does not
ation, hemorrhage, or gross blood contamination increases the CSF fi-
ation. Sample clotting is possible in these circumstances unless the
a tube containing an anticoagulant, such as EDTA.

◆ Specific Gravity

The specific gravity can be measured using a refractometer (see Chapter 5). A eralization, normal CSF has a specific gravity between 1.004 and 1.008. Its clin fulness is not well established.

◆ Glucose Concentration

Normal CSF glucose concentration varies directly with blood glucose concentr such that it is generally about 60% to 80% of the blood value. Thus animals with h glycemia and normal CSF usually have higher CSF glucose concentrations than t with normoglycemia, whereas animals with hypoglycemia and normal CSF usually lower CSF glucose concentrations than those with normoglycemia. Consequently meaningful interpretation, concurrent CSF and blood glucose concentrations shoul measured. Methodology is the same as for blood glucose determinations.

Measurement of CSF glucose concentration is most useful as an aid to diagnosis acute septic suppurative inflammation involving CSF. In this situation, CSF glucc concentration is often much less than 60% of the blood value because of glucose m tabolism by bacteria and neutrophils. With successful treatment, the CSF glucose co centration returns to normal.

◆ Lactate Concentration

Lactate (lactic acid) is produced by anaerobic cellular metabolism. (For a more de-tailed consideration of lactate, see Peritoneal Fluid Analysis.) The value of CSF lactate measurement in animals has not been reported. Increased CSF lactate concentration has been used to assist in diagnosis of septic meningitis in people, although it is not specific for such conditions. Paired blood and CSF lactate values may augment simi-lar glucose measurements.

◆ Electrolyte Concentrations

Paired blood and CSF sodium, potassium, chloride, calcium, and magnesium concen-trations have been measured but are generally of little practical value. Measurement techniques are the same as for blood samples.

◆ Creatine Kinase Concentration

Creatine kinase (CK), previously referred to as *creatine phosphokinase* (CPK), is prob-ably the enzyme most frequently measured in CSF. Like most other enzymes, CK has a high molecular weight; therefore its movement between blood and CSF is limited by the normal blood-brain barrier. Normal CSF CK activity is low and values vary with the measurement technique. Methodology is the same as that for blood CK determination

Because CK activity in nervous tissue is relatively high, its measurement in CSF ha been suggested as an ancillary diagnostic test for nonspecific damage to neural tiss (e.g., neural hypoxia, trauma, inflammation, or compression by a space-occupying sion, such as a tumor). The CSF CK value therefore may be a useful guide to progno sis in canine neurologic cases and in premature foals. Increased values also may be observed after seizures.

AQUEOUS HUMOR ANALYSIS

Samples of fluid may be aspirated from the eye of an anesthetized animal. Such fluid is similar to CSF in that it has low cellularity, being composed mostly of small mononuclear cells, essentially no erythrocytes, and a low protein concentration. Interpretation of changes in aqueous humor is similar to that for CSF.

Aqueous (and vitreous) humor may be collected from a dead animal to investigate the concentration of urea and electrolytes before death. The concentration of urea, calcium, and magnesium in these fluids is related closely to that in blood. Consequently, if an animal is thought to have died from renal failure, hypocalcemia ("eclampsia" in dogs, "milk fever" in ruminants) or hypomagnesemia ("grass tetany" in ruminants), collection of aqueous humor may help confirm the diagnosis.

PERITONEAL FLUID ANALYSIS

The normal peritoneal cavity contains only sufficient fluid to ensure lubrication of the surfaces of the intraabdominal organs and the cavity wall. This fluid may be sampled by abdominocentesis. The procedure is performed on many species and usually is performed in the standing animal.

An area at the most dependent point in the ventral midline of the abdomen is prepared aseptically. *Abdominocentesis* (abdominal paracentesis) is performed using a sterile needle or cannula. Peritoneal fluid is collected into an EDTA blood tube for a total nucleated cell count, cytologic examination, and refractometric protein measurement. It also may be collected into a fluoride oxalate blood tube for glucose and lactate measurement and a plain tube for other laboratory tests, including measurement of protein concentration.

Indications for abdominocentesis in all species include investigation of an effusion (increased amount of fluid), and differentiation of causes, such as ascites, inflammatory exudation, and neoplasia. In horses, peritoneal fluid frequently is examined in cases of colic and chronic weight loss.

◆ Volume

Subjective estimation of the volume of peritoneal fluid in the abdominal cavity should be attempted at collection. Such an estimate is based on the ease of fluid collection (volume obtained/unit of time) and therefore requires familiarity with the technique of abdominocentesis in a given species. Useful categories are normal, slightly to moderately increased, and plentiful (markedly increased). The small volume of peritoneal fluid in clinically normal animals sometimes makes collection impossible. In fact, the collection of any fluid from the peritoneal cavity of dogs or cats is indicative of an effusion, which is also usually the case in cattle. Several milliliters of fluid usually may be collected from a normal horse. In all species, especially horses, several abdominocenteses should be attempted before the procedure is considered nonproductive.

◆ Color and Turbidity

Normal peritoneal fluid is colorless to straw-yellow and transparent to slightly turbid. Gross discoloration and increased turbidity may be due to increased cell numbers and/or protein concentration. Interpretation of such findings is discussed earlier in this chapter. Discoloration also could be due to free ingesta in the sample, which may be the result of bowel rupture or accidental bowel perforation during abdominocentesis (*enterocentesis*). These conditions may be distinguishable cytologically and by reference to other clinical findings.

◆ Odor

Normal peritoneal fluid has no odor. Collection of malodorous peritoneal fluid at abdominocentesis may indicate a necrotic segment of bowel within the peritoneal cavity, a ruptured segment of bowel with free gut contents in the cavity, or accidental enterocentesis. These conditions may be distinguishable cytologically and by reference to other clinical findings.

◆ Cell Counts

A total nucleated cell count is performed manually by the same method as for a CBC (see Chapter 2). As a cross-species generalization, normal peritoneal fluid has less than 10,000 nucleated cells/μl, usually 2000 to 6000/μl. Mononuclear cells may be visible as clusters of cells, which can make counting individual cells difficult.

◆ Cytologic Examination

Smears of peritoneal fluid are made as outlined earlier. The technique varies with the total nucleated cell count and fluid viscosity. Romanowsky stains usually are used. As previously discussed, the smear should be examined at 100×, 400×, and 1000× magnification.

A differential count of at least 100 nucleated cells should be performed, noting cell type and morphology. Nucleated cells are categorized as neutrophils, large mononuclear cells (a collective grouping of mesothelial cells and macrophages), lymphocytes, eosinophils, and any other nucleated cells. Notes on cell morphology should include comments on nuclear and cytoplasmic appearance. If bacteria are present, their morphology (bacilli, coccobacilli, cocci) and location (free or intracellular, i.e., phagocytosed) must be recorded. In such cases, another smear can be stained with Gram stain and the fluid cultured.

Normal peritoneal fluid contains few erythrocytes. The number present on a smear should be estimated. Suitable categories include rare, few, many, and large numbers. The number present varies with the method of sample preparation. Iatrogenic contamination and acute and chronic hemorrhage are distinguished grossly as outlined earlier (see Exfoliative Cytology). If erythrocytes have been present in the fluid for several hours, they may be phagocytosed by macrophages (erythrophagocytosis).

Published normal values for peritoneal fluid cytology of dogs and cats are scarce. Normal horses generally have an average of about 55% to 60% neutrophils, 25% to 30% large mononuclear cells, 10% to 20% lymphocytes, and an occasional eosinophil (below 1%). Values for cattle are somewhat similar, but normal animals often have comparable numbers of neutrophils and lymphocytes.

Exudates are fluids with increased cellularity and protein concentration because of inflammation. The following cross-species generalization may be made. Acute inflammatory reactions increase the total cell count, the percentage, and absolute numbers of neutrophils to greater than 95% of the nucleated cells. Subacute to chronic inflammatory reactions usually cause high-normal to elevated total nucleated cell counts, with elevated neutrophil percentages and numerous mesothelial cells and/or macrophages. Many of the latter cells may phagocytize degenerate cells or cellular debris (Figure 12-6). When an effusion is present, some mesothelial cells may be present as clusters or rafts of cells (see Figure 12-6). These clusters result from proliferation and exfoliation of cells from the peritoneal lining, or mesothelium, in response to a decrease in contact inhibition between cells on opposing surfaces of the peritoneum, because of the effusion. Migrating parasite larvae can cause increased neutrophil and eosinophil percentages, with or without an elevated total nucleated cell count.

Septic (bacterial) peritonitis generally causes a marked increase in the total cell count, predominantly resulting from neutrophils. Cellular morphology depends on the microorganism(s) present and may vary from cytoplasmic vacuolation with few nuclear changes evident to marked cytoplasmic vacuolation, marked nuclear swelling and disruption (*karyolysis*), and general cellular degeneration or fragmentation (Figure 12-7). Cases of simple peritonitis may have a single type of bacterium evident, whereas the bacterial population is frequently mixed in peritonitis resulting from

Figure 12-6
Raft of mesothelial cells (*R*) in peritoneal fluid from a horse with resolving peritonitis. Several neutrophils and erythrocytes, a phagocytic macrophage, and a mesothelial cell (*M*) are also present. (Wright's stain, 810×)

Figure 12-7
Septic peritonitis. Note the markedly degenerate cells (karyolytic neutrophils), bacilli *(B)*, and cocci *(C)*. (May Grünwald Giemsa stain, 1000×)

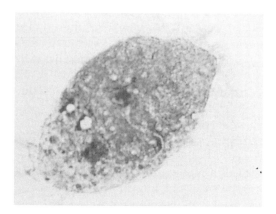

Figure 12-8
This sample collected by accidental enterocentesis in a horse contains a ciliated protozoal organism from the large bowel. A mixed population of bacteria also is usually present, with little evidence of inflammation. (May Grünwald Giemsa stain, 1000×)

devitalization or rupture of the bowel. Accidental penetration of the bowel during abdominocentesis may result in a mixed population of bacteria in the smear. However, in the latter case, leukocyte numbers and morphology are usually normal, and the bacteria are frequently not phagocytosed. Large ciliated organisms also may be noted in large-bowel enterocentesis in horses (Figure 12-8).

Transudates (ascitic effusions) typically have low total nucleated cell counts (less than 500/μl), with fairly normal differential counts or possibly an increase in the percentage of large mononuclear cells and low protein concentrations. The mononuclear cells are principally mesothelial cells, which may be in clusters or rafts and may be quite reactive in appearance (i.e., multinucleate, with variable nucleus and cell size, prominent nucleoli, and basophilic cytoplasm; see Figure 12-6). Reactive mesothelial cells may be difficult to distinguish from some tumor cells. Transudates are frequently secondary to congestive heart failure or may occur in animals with low blood albumin concentration.

Intraabdominal tumors may exfoliate cells into the peritoneal fluid. Cytologic diagnosis of such neoplasia may be difficult and is often a task for a specialist cy-

Figure 12-9
Effusion resulting from lymphosarcoma in a dog. Note the variation in the size of lymphocytes from "normal" small cells *(S)*, through to large cells with prominent nucleoli *(L)*. (May Grünwald Giemsa stain, 1000×)

Figure 12-10
Effusion resulting from an adenocarcinoma. Note the cluster of cells and the marked variation in nuclear size, cell size, and nuclear to cytoplasmic ratio (N:C). Nucleoli are sometimes apparent and are somewhat pleomorphic. A multinucleated cell is also present at right. (May Grünwald Giemsa stain, 1000×)

Figure 12-11
Effusion resulting from a mast cell tumor. (Wright's stain, 1000×)

tologist. However, the technician should be able to recognize abnormal lymphocytes (Figure 12-9) using the hallmarks of malignancy outlined in Chapter 11 and should be suspicious of clusters of pleomorphic, secretory-type cells (Figure 12-10). The presence of unexpected cells, such as mast cells (Figure 12-11), also should arouse comment.

◆ Total Protein Concentration

The total protein concentration (of the peritoneal fluid supernatant) may be measured by refractometry or by the Biuret procedure (both as for blood samples). Normal peritoneal fluid has a total protein concentration of less than 2.5 g/dl.

The most common causes of increased protein values in peritoneal fluid are inflammation and hemorrhage. Cats with peritoneal effusion because of feline infectious peritonitis (FIP) virus infection frequently have high peritoneal fluid protein concentrations (up to 8 g/dl), mainly resulting from gamma globulins. Fluid viscosity is also increased considerably in many cats with FIP.

◆ Fibrinogen Concentration

Normal peritoneal fluid has little fibrinogen (less than 50 mg/dl in horses) and consequently does not clot. Fibrinogen concentration increases with inflammation and/or hemorrhage. Collection into an EDTA tube prevents clotting in such situations. Fibrinogen concentration is not routinely measured, but if the total protein concentration in peritoneal fluid is greater than 2.5 g/dl, fibrinogen concentration may be determined as outlined for blood fibrinogen measurement, using the EDTA supernatant.

◆ Lactate Concentration

Use of paired blood and peritoneal fluid lactate (lactic acid) measurements has been advocated as a diagnostic aid in equine colic cases. The normal resting blood lactate concentration of horses is about 8 to 12 mg/dl. Regardless of the actual values, the blood lactate concentration of normal horses is always greater than that of peritoneal fluid. Horses with gastrointestinal disorders generally have peritoneal fluid lactate concentrations greater than corresponding blood values. Lactate is produced by anaerobic glycolysis, especially in ischemic tissues. Hypoxia of a section of bowel wall results in increased lactate production, much of which diffuses into the peritoneal cavity before entering the circulation to be removed by the liver. Less severe gastrointestinal disorders, such as impactions, tend to cause a smaller difference between peritoneal fluid and blood lactate concentrations than do serious ones, such as intestinal torsion (a twisted section of bowel). Peritonitis also increases peritoneal fluid lactate values.

The sample for lactate measurement (blood or peritoneal fluid) should be collected in a fluoride oxalate tube unless it is deproteinized immediately, in which case no preservative/anticoagulant is required. The fluoride stops cellular metabolism of glucose and consequent production of lactate, and the oxalate prevents sample clotting. Whole blood or peritoneal fluid, or their centrifuged supernatants, can be used for lactate measurements. (Fluoride oxalate plasma samples are stable for several days at 4° C.) The usefulness of paired blood and peritoneal fluid lactate measurement in other species has not yet been reported.

◆ Glucose Concentration

The glucose concentration in peritoneal fluid of normal horses is slightly higher (usually 1 to 10 mg/dl higher) than corresponding blood values. Measurement of paired blood and peritoneal fluid glucose concentrations may have diagnostic value in equine colic cases, especially those associated with peritonitis. Leukocyte and (possibly) bacterial metabolism of peritoneal fluid glucose in such cases lowers its concentration, occasionally to undetectable levels. Repeated measurement of peritoneal fluid glucose levels may help monitor the effectiveness of treatment. Successful therapy typically is associated with increasing peritoneal fluid glucose values, possibly before peritoneal fluid leukocyte numbers decrease markedly. The method of peritoneal fluid glucose measurement is the same as for a blood specimen. The merit of paired blood and peritoneal fluid glucose determination in other species has not been reported.

◆ Urea Nitrogen Concentration

The concentration of urea nitrogen in peritoneal fluid can be determined by the same method as blood urea nitrogen measurement. It is normally slightly higher than the blood urea nitrogen level (by 0.5 to 4.0 mg/dl in horses). An animal with a ruptured bladder usually has a markedly elevated urea nitrogen concentration in peritoneal fluid. The more long-standing the rupture, the greater the concurrent blood urea nitrogen value, because the urea nitrogen diffuses from the peritoneal cavity into the blood. However, the peritoneal fluid value always exceeds the blood value in this condition. Diagnosis of a ruptured bladder may be confirmed by injecting a dye, such as methylene blue, into the bladder through a urethral catheter and subsequently visualizing its presence in the peritoneal fluid.

PLEURAL FLUID ANALYSIS

As in the peritoneal cavity, the normal pleural, or thoracic, cavity contains only enough fluid to adequately lubricate the surfaces of the intrathoracic organs and the cavity wall. Techniques for thoracic fluid collection, or thoracocentesis, are well described for many species. Fluid is collected in EDTA tubes for total nucleated cell counts, cytologic examination, and refractometric protein measurements, and in a plain tube for determination of the total protein concentration. Other clinical chemistry determinations are performed infrequently on pleural fluid.

The main indication for thoracocentesis in all species is evaluation of increased thoracic fluid volume, or thoracic effusion. This condition may be due to transudation, hemorrhage, ruptured thoracic lymphatic duct (chylothorax), inflammation, or neoplasia.

◆ Volume

The volume may be subjectively judged, as when performing abdominocentesis.

◆ Color, Turbidity, and Odor

Normal pleural fluid is colorless to straw-yellow and transparent to slightly turbid. It has no odor. Interpretation of most pleural fluid discolorations is as presented earlier (see Exfoliative Cytology). An exception is chylothorax, which, although infrequently seen, is most common in cats and dogs.

Chylothorax usually produces a "milky" fluid, especially if the animal has recently eaten, because of the chylous effusion's high fat content and large number of lymphocytes. In fasted animals, the fluid may be tan. Unlike fluids with high leukocyte counts (which also may have a whitish color), chylous fluid does not have a clear supernatant after centrifugation. The fat in chylous fluid is present as small droplets (*chylomicrons*), which can be stained with Sudan III or IV. The fat in chylous fluid may be dissolved with ether, after the fluid has been alkalinized with sodium hydroxide or sodium bicarbonate. If significant numbers of erythrocytes are present, the fluid may have a reddish color.

◆ Cell Counts

A total nucleated cell count is performed by the same technique as for peritoneal fluid. Few published normal values exist for most species. However, as a cross-species generalization, normal pleural fluid has less than 10,000 nucleated cells/μl, usually 2000 to 6000/μl. Many normal animals may have fewer than 1000 cells/μl. Mononuclear cells may be present in clusters, making the counting of individual cells difficult.

◆ Cytologic Examination

Most of the comments concerning cytologic evaluation of peritoneal fluid can be extrapolated to pleural fluid. Normal pleural fluid may contain a slightly higher percentage of neutrophils (about 75%).

Chylothorax is characterized cytologically by a predominance of small lymphocytes with normal morphology. Fat droplets may be visible in smears stained with Sudan III or IV.

◆ Total Protein and Fibrinogen Concentrations

Procedures and normal values are the same as for peritoneal fluid. Chylomicron fat increases the pleural fluid refractive index. Consequently, in chylothorax, refractometric "protein" values are usually 2.0 to 6.0 g/dl.

◉ SYNOVIAL FLUID ANALYSIS

Synovial fluid is collected aseptically by insertion of a needle into the joint space, or *arthrocentesis,* from the unanesthetized or anesthetized animal, generally using a syringe. Arthrocentesis usually is performed as part of a lameness evaluation. Approaches to particular joints vary and have been well described for several species. When in doubt, the reader should refer to an anatomy book.

Simple tests on synovial fluid can yield much useful information. The volume of fluid collected influences the tests that can be run. If only one or two drops can be obtained, as in some normal joints of cats and dogs, gross assessment of fluid color and turbidity and cytologic examination of a direct smear, possibly with concurrent subjective assessment of viscosity, may be all that is practical. If 0.5 to 1 ml is collected, a total nucleated cell count and refractometric protein measurement (on EDTA-preserved fluid) may be added to the list of tests. Collection of larger volumes permits additional tests, such as the mucin clot test.

◆ Volume

The volume should be subjectively assessed at collection and compared with the expected (normal) volume. The volume varies tremendously among joints and species. Experience is the best guide. Generally, the volume of fluid is not increased in normal joints and those with degenerative joint disease, whereas it often is increased in inflamed joints. The volume of fluid actually collected also should be recorded, with a comment on the ease of collection.

◆ Color and Turbidity

Normal synovial fluid is clear to straw-yellow and nonturbid. Yellow synovial fluid is common in large animals, especially horses. Turbidity, when present, is due to cells, protein (or fibrin), or cartilage.

Normal synovial fluid contains few erythrocytes. Iatrogenic contamination at arthrocentesis is common. Differentiation of contamination and recent or old hemorrhage is as previously described (see Exfoliative Cytology).

◆ Viscosity

Viscosity reflects the quality and concentration of hyaluronic acid, which is part of the synovial fluid mucin complex. The function of mucin is joint lubrication. Viscosity may be quantitated with a viscometer; however, subjective assessment is most often used.

Normal synovial fluid is sticky. If a drop is placed between thumb and forefinger, as the digits are separated, it forms a 1- to 2-inch strand before breaking (Figure 12-12). Similarly, when gently expressed through a needle on a horizontally held syringe, it hangs in a 1- to 2-inch strand before separating from the needle tip.

Figure 12-12
Crude assessment of synovial fluid viscosity.

In general, viscosity is not decreased in normal joints and those with degenerative problems. It frequently is decreased in joints with bacterial inflammation as a result of mucin degradation by bacterial hyaluronidase, and in joints with a significant effusion (including hydrarthrosis) as a result of dilution of mucin (and hyaluronic acid).

Because EDTA may degrade hyaluronic acid, both viscosity and mucin clot formation usually are assessed on fluid to which no anticoagulant has been added. If anticoagulation is necessary, because of a high fluid fibrinogen concentration, heparin is the preferred anticoagulant.

◆ Mucin Clot Test

Synovial fluid mucin forms a clot when added to acetic acid. The nature of the resultant clot reflects the quality and concentration of hyaluronic acid. The following is one method.

Initially, 0.1 ml of 7-N glacial acetic acid is diluted with 4 ml of distilled water. Then 1 ml of synovial fluid (not EDTA preserved) is added, without touching the sides of the test tube. For smaller volumes of fluid, proportionately less dilute acetic acid is used. The solution is gently mixed and allowed to stand at room temperature for 1 hour. The mucin clot generally is graded as good (large, compact, ropy clot in a clear solution); fair (soft clot in a slightly turbid solution); poor (friable clot in a cloudy solution); or poor (no actual clot, but some large flecks in a turbid solution). Clot assessment is enhanced by gently shaking the tube. Good clots remain ropy, whereas poor clots fragment (Figure 12-13).

If only a few drops of synovial fluid are obtained at arthrocentesis, an abbreviated mucin clot test may be performed. If available after preparation of a cytologic smear (and possibly total nucleated cell count), a drop of non–EDTA-preserved fluid is placed on a clean microscope slide. Three drops of diluted acetic acid are added and mixed. The resultant clot is graded after about 1 minute. Assessment may be easier against a dark background.

◆ Protein Concentration

The protein concentration of synovial fluid may be determined by the Biuret method or by refractometry (as for a peritoneal fluid sample). In most species, synovial fluid

Figure 12-13
Mucin clot tests. Reading from left to right, these tests are graded as good (normal), good, fair, poor, and poor.

protein concentration is less than 2.5 g/dl. The pig is an exception, with normal values of 3 to 5 g/dl.

Normal synovial fluid contains no appreciable quantity of fibrinogen and consequently does not clot. However, the fluid may gel if left undisturbed for a few hours. This gelling, called *thixotropy*, is reversible, with normal fluidity restored simply by agitating the specimen.

Samples from traumatized or inflamed joints generally contain increased fibrinogen and clot rapidly, possibly even in the syringe at collection. Such samples should be immediately transferred into EDTA for cell counts and cytologic examination and into heparin for the mucin clot test.

◆ Cell Counts

Cell counts are performed on EDTA-preserved synovial fluid. Normal synovial fluid contains very few erythrocytes; however, iatrogenic contamination at collection is not uncommon. Erythrocytes also may be present in the synovial fluid of traumatized and inflamed joints. If erythrocytes have been present for several hours, erythrophagocytosis may be evident. Erythrocyte counts usually are not performed.

Numbers of nucleated cells vary considerably among joints and species. As a broad generalization, normal joints of all species contain less than 3000 nucleated cells/μl, with horses usually below about 500/μl, cattle usually below about 1000/μl, and dogs and cats usually below about 1500/μl. A WBC pipette, or a diluting system such as the Unopette, and a Neubauer hemacytometer are suitable for counting nucleated cells. The diluent used must not be acetic acid, because it causes the synovial fluid mucin to clot, invalidating results. The sample is diluted and counted as for a blood WBC count (see Chapter 2). Very viscous samples may be made more fluid by diluting 1:1 with saline-reconstituted hyaluronidase (150 μ/m). In general, total nucleated cell counts are mildly elevated in traumatic and degenerative joint diseases and moderately or markedly elevated in nonseptic and septic inflammation.

◆ Cytologic Examination (Cell Counts)

Slides for cytologic examination may be prepared on EDTA-preserved fluid or fluid without anticoagulant, the latter especially if only a few drops are obtained and the smear is made immediately. Thin smears are made by slowly advancing the spreader slide. Because of the high viscosity of normal synovial fluid, cells usually do not accumulate at the feathered edge of the smear. Margination of cells increases as viscosity of the fluid decreases. At low cell counts, especially below 500/μl, concentration of cells by centrifugational sedimentation and subsequent resuspension of cells in a small volume of supernatant fluid produces a more cellular smear. Slides usually are stained with a Romanowsky stain.

Cells in synovial fluid with good viscosity tend to align in a linear fashion in the direction of the smear, giving a "windrow" appearance (Figure 12-14). Mucin precipitation produces an eosinophilic granular background in Romanowsky-stained smears, the density of which reflects smear thickness. Cells in smears from viscous fluid may not spread out well on the slide, which can make their identification difficult. Such fluid may be diluted 1:1 with saline-reconstituted hyaluronidase (150 U/ml). This decreases sample viscosity after a few minutes, allowing more accurate cell morphology when smeared.

Normal synovial fluid generally contains at least 90% mononuclear cells and less than 10% neutrophils. Eosinophils are rarely observed. Mononuclear cells comprise about equal numbers of lymphocytes and monocytic/macrophage-type cells, which are nonvacuolated and nonphagocytic. Large vacuolated or phagocytic mononuclear cells comprise less than 10% of the differential count of normal synovial fluid (Figure 12-15). Macrophages become vacuolated in normal synovial fluid that is not processed soon after collection; therefore prompt preparation of smears is important to prevent this artificial finding.

As a generalization, mononuclear cells predominate in traumatic and degenerative arthropathies, usually with increased numbers of large vacuolated or phagocytic cells. Occasionally when joint erosion has progressed through to subchondral bone, osteoclasts may be observed (Figure 12-16). In contrast, neutrophils predominate in infectious arthropathies (because of bacteria, viruses, and mycoplasmas, for example) and many noninfectious conditions, such as rheumatoid arthritis and systemic lupus erythematosus (Figure 12-17). When cells are clumped together in a smear, new methylene blue stain may demonstrate interlocking fibrin strands. Rarely, the causative organism in

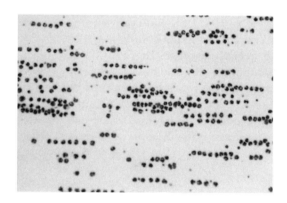

Figure 12-14
Smear of synovial fluid from a dog with acute, suppurative arthritis. Note the linear arrangement of cells ("wind rowing"), suggesting good fluid viscosity. (Wright's stain, 140×)

Figure 12-15
Synovial fluid from a dog. Normal synovial fluid mononuclear cells predominate. (From Baker R, Lumsden JH: *Color atlas of cytology of the dog and cat*, St Louis, 2000, Mosby.)

septic joint fluid may be observed cytologically, especially when phagocytosed. Culture is recommended when an infectious process is suspected. A chronic-active type of arthropathy is suggested when neutrophils and vacuolated/phagocytic macrophages are both increased in number. Lupus erythematosus cells, which are neutrophils containing phagocytosed nuclear chromatin, are seen occasionally in the synovial fluid of animals with systemic lupus erythematosus.

◆ Glucose Concentration

The glucose concentration of normal synovial fluid is measured infrequently and is about the same as that of blood. Interpretation of findings is similar to that for CSF and peritoneal fluid.

◆ Miscellaneous Tests

Particulate analysis may be performed on synovial fluid to assess the degree of cartilage damage. Synovial fluid aldehyde concentrations also reflect the degree of carti-

Figure 12-16
Synovial fluid from a dog. The large multi-nucleated cell is an osteoclast. Its presence suggests erosion of joint cartilage through to underlying subchondral bone. (May Grünwald Giemsa stain, 400×)

Figure 12-17
Smear of synovial fluid from a dog with acute, suppurative arthritis. Cell types present are neutrophils (*N*), erythrocytes (*E*), lymphocytes (*L*), and a large, slightly vacuolated macrophage (*M*). Note the normal (eosinophilic), granular, proteinaceous background. (Wright's stain, 780×)

lage damage. Both tests have been done in horses and require submission of samples to a laboratory specializing in these techniques.

TRACHEAL WASH

Cytologic evaluation of samples obtained from the trachea, bronchi, or bronchioles may assist with diagnosis of pulmonary disease in animals. Tracheal washes may be performed by passage of a catheter through an endotracheal tube in an anesthetized animal (orotracheal approach), or via the nasal passages (nasotracheal approach), or through the skin and trachea (transtracheal approach) in a conscious, sedated animal. The transtracheal route minimizes pharyngeal contamination of the specimen, but it is an invasive procedure and consequently requires aseptic technique. These procedures are commonly used in both small and large animals.

Sterile physiologic saline is used as the wash fluid. Several milliliters are infused (the quantity varies with the animal's size) and immediately withdrawn into the same syringe. Depending on the level within the respiratory tract at which the catheter tip is located, a tracheal, bronchial, or bronchoalveolar wash is obtained. The aspirated fluid may be transported to the laboratory in the collection syringe, a plain blood tube, or an EDTA blood tube. The last is preferable if a delay is anticipated before smears are made. However, because cells in tracheal washes often are poorly preserved and delayed sample processing causes artifactual degeneration, delays should be avoided.

Samples with little mucus (generally corresponding to small numbers of cells) should be centrifuged at low speed, and smears prepared from the sediment. Samples containing much mucus (and usually numerous cells) may not need to be centrifuge-concentrated before a smear is made. A gentle squash preparation is usually the best procedure, especially when mucus is present (see Chapter 11). Romanowsky stains are generally satisfactory.

Total nucleated cell counts are usually not performed on tracheal wash fluids. Cell numbers are subjectively recorded from evaluation of the smear. A tracheal wash smear from a normal animal contains few cells, usually with a small amount of mucus (Figure 12-18). The mucus often appears microscopically as eosinophilic to purple strands that may enmesh the cells. Epithelial cells are the principal cell type.

If the sample is collected from the level of the trachea, ciliated epithelial cells predominate. These cells are columnar to cuboidal, with a polar nucleus on the border opposite the cilia (see Figure 12-18). If the specimen is collected from the bronchi, bronchoalveolar epithelial cells are also fairly common. They are round, nonciliated cells with basophilic cytoplasm and may occur in clumps (Figure 12-19). A few goblet cells (secretory epithelial cells) also may be observed.

If the sample is a bronchoalveolar wash, alveolar macrophages may predominate. These are large individual cells with a large round to oval nucleus and a moderate amount of basophilic cytoplasm. If they become reactive or activated, the cytoplasm increases in volume and becomes more granular and vacuolated (Figure 12-20). Neutrophils, lymphocytes, eosinophils, plasma cells, mast cells, and erythrocytes are seen rarely in specimens from normal animals.

Figure 12-18
Transtracheal wash from a normal horse.
Note the ciliated columnar epithelial cell
and small amount of mucus (*M*) in the
background. (Wright's stain, 1050×)

Figure 12-19
Transtracheal wash from a normal horse.
Note the bronchoalveolar cells (*B*) and
free cilia (*C*) from ciliated epithelial cells.
(Wright's stain, 1050×)

Figure 12-20
Transtracheal wash from a horse with a
chronic-active inflammatory problem.
Note the neutrophil and two vacuolated
alveolar macrophages. (Wright's stain,
780×)

Abnormal tracheal washes are generally exudates. These samples contain numerous mucus strands and are cellular (Figure 12-21). Eosinophilic, spiral casts from small bronchioles (*Curschmann's spirals*) suggest a chronic bronchiolar problem (Figure 12-22). Cell morphology is highly variable among and within samples. Many cells may be unidentifiable. Neutrophils and macrophages are numerous. In acute inflammation, neutrophils are the predominant cell type and may represent more than 95% of nucleated cells. As the process becomes more chronic, mononuclear macrophages increase in number. The causative agent, possibly bacterial or fungal, may be noted, free and/or phagocytosed, in the smear. Tracheal wash samples can be cultured by routine microbiologic procedures.

The presence of bacteria or fungi in a tracheal wash does not necessarily mean the organism is pathogenic. Plant or fungal spores sometimes contaminate tracheal washes from herbivores (inhaled from feed) and may be phagocytosed by macrophages (Figure 12-23). Oral or pharyngeal contamination of the collection apparatus, or increased inspiratory effort with contamination of the upper tracheal mucosa by pharyngeal microflora, may cause inclusion of bacteria in a tracheal wash specimen. Such bacteria frequently are associated with or adherent to squamous epithelial cells of the pharyngeal mucosa (Figure 12-24).

Eosinophils are prominent (possibly more than 10% of nucleated cells) in inflammatory reactions with an allergic or parasitic component (Figure 12-25). Because cell preservation is often only fair, free eosinophil granules rather than intact eosinophils may be noted. Rarely, parasite eggs or larvae may be noted in the smear.

Figure 12-21
Transtracheal wash from a horse with an acute, septic suppurative, inflammatory reaction. Note the marked cellularity and high mucus content. (Wright's stain, 140×)

Figure 12-22
Transtracheal wash from a dog with a chronic inflammation. Note the alveolar macrophages (*M*) and Curschmann's spiral (*C*). (Wright's stain, 345×)

Erythrocytes rarely are seen in normal tracheal wash specimens. Recent hemorrhage may be evidenced by numerous intact erythrocytes in the smear. In contrast, with old hemorrhage, few erythrocytes may be noted and many of the macrophages may contain hemosiderin granules (dark-blue or red cytoplasmic granules) (see Figure 12-3 for such cells).

Figure 12-23
This tracheal wash from a horse contains reactive, vacuolated macrophages, one of which has ingested pollen (large, dark, elliptic structure). (May Grünwald Giemsa stain, 1000×)

Figure 12-24
Bovine tracheal wash containing squamous epithelial cells, with adherent bacteria. These bacteria represent nasopharyngeal contamination of the sample. (Wright's stain, 780×)

Figure 12-25
Tracheal wash from a dog. Large numbers of eosinophils suggest an allergic or hypersensitivity reaction, or possibly parasitism. (May Grünwald Giemsa stain, 1000×)

Neoplastic cells may be detected in tracheal wash specimens. Criteria for malignancy are as outlined in Chapter 11. Neoplastic cells are frequently in clusters (Figure 12-26), generally epithelial in origin, and frequently "secretory" in appearance (i.e., their cytoplasm is basophilic and vacuolated).

◆ Nasal Flush

Cytologic evaluation of samples obtained from the nasal cavity may be useful in investigation of diseases affecting the upper airway. Fluid (normal saline) may be infused into the nasal cavity via the nose, using a syringe and tubing, and then aspirated. This procedure is referred to as a *nasal flush*. Such specimens are processed as for a tracheal wash. A nasal flush from a normal animal contains cornified and noncornified squamous epithelial cells, often with adherent bacteria, and negligible evidence of hemorrhage or inflammation (Figure 12-27).

Various abnormalities may be demonstrated with this procedure, such as inflammation secondary to sepsis, fungi and yeasts, and neoplasia (Figure 12-28). These should not be confused with glove powder, which may be present in some specimens (Figure 12-29).

Figure 12-26
Tracheal wash from a dog with a bronchogenic carcinoma. Note the clusters of large mononuclear cells, with moderate variation in cell size, nucleus size, shape, number, and nucleus-to-cytoplasm ratio. Several cells also have prominent nucleoli of varying size, shape, and number. These findings are typical of malignancy. (May Grünwald Giemsa stain, 1000×)

Figure 12-27
This nasal flush from a dog shows a cornified squamous epithelial cell with adherent bacteria (*Simonsiella* species). These bacteria are part of the normal microflora of the upper airways. (May Grünwald Giemsa stain, 1000×)

◆ Ear Swabs

Cotton-tipped swabs may be used to collect a specimen from the ear canal for cytologic and microbiologic examination. The swab should be rolled gently along a clean glass slide to allow cells and organisms to adhere. The slide is then stained with a Romanowsky stain or Gram's stain. "Normal" specimens contain cornified squamous epithelial cells, with negligible evidence of inflammation and few microorganisms. Common abnormal findings are bacteria and yeasts, with or without inflammation (Figure 12-30).

Figure 12-28
Nasal flush from a dog. Note the numerous cryptococcal organisms with surrounding (clear) capsule. Some organisms show typical "budding" divisions. (May Grünwald Giemsa stain, 1000×)

Figure 12-29
Glove powder granules. Note the central "dimple." (May Grünwald Giemsa stain, 1000×)

Figure 12-30
This ear swab from a dog shows cornified squamous epithelial cells, with large numbers of bacterial cocci and *Malassezia pachydermatis* organisms. The latter are dark "peanut"-shape structures (larger than the cocci). (May Grünwald Giemsa stain, 1000×)

◆ Lymph Node Aspirate Biopsy

Fine-needle aspiration is a useful diagnostic procedure when investigating enlarged lymph nodes. Cytologic evaluation of lymph node aspirates is usually a task for a specialist. However, technicians should know how to prepare good-quality smears. General principles of the technique are described in Chapter 11. Causes of lymph node enlargement include the following:

- *Hyperplasia:* The increased lymphoid cell numbers are associated with inflammation and/or infection in adjacent tissues or surfaces. The numbers of lymphocytes in the node increase, but their morphology and relative proportions appear normal.
- *Inflammation of the lymph node (lymphadenitis):* The lymph node is inflamed and numbers of neutrophils and macrophages are increased. Lymphadenitis usually occurs when bacteria or other microorganisms are present in the node.
- *Lymphoid neoplasia (lymphosarcoma):* This may involve one or more nodes. It also may involve other organs (e.g., spleen, kidney, bone marrow) and possibly leukemia (see Chapter 2).
- *Plasma-cell myeloma:* This special type of lymphoid tumor involves antibody-producing cells (plasma cells or B-lymphocytes). These cells usually are present in relatively low numbers in normal and hyperplastic nodes. Plasma-cell myeloma also is called *multiple myeloma* or *plasmacytoma.*
- *Metastatic neoplasia:* If the lymph node is "draining" an area in which a tumor develops, the tumor may spread to the node, causing it to enlarge (Figure 12-31).

◆ Other Aspirates and Impressions

Other organs and palpable masses may be aspirated and smears prepared as is done for lymph nodes. Impressions may be prepared from excision biopsies or from swabs of mucosal and cutaneous surfaces. Basic evaluation involves differentiating inflammation from hyperplasia and neoplasia. Differentiation of the latter possibilities is done often by a specialist; however, as with lymph node aspirates, the technician should be familiar with preparation of smears from these areas, including evaluating

Figure 12-31
Lymph node aspirate from a dog. Note the group of large mononuclear cells among the lymphocytes. This is evidence of metastatic squamous-cell carcinoma. (May Grünwald Giemsa stain, 1000×)

the quality of the smear before submission to the laboratory. General principles are described in Chapter 11.

VAGINAL CYTOLOGY

Exfoliative vaginal cytology is a useful adjunct to the history and clinical examination in determining the stage of the estrous cycle in bitches and queens. It assists with optimal timing of mating or artificial insemination in small animals but is not of practical value for these purposes in mares, cows, does, ewes, or sows.

◆ Bitch

The sample is collected with the animal restrained in a standing position and the tail elevated. The vulva is cleansed and rinsed. A lubricated speculum or smooth plastic tube is inserted to a point just cranial to the urethral orifice in the vagina. A sterile swab (which may be moistened with sterile saline) is introduced and gently rotated against the vaginal wall. The swab is removed and carefully rolled along two or three clean microscope slides. After air drying, the smears are stained, generally with a Romanowsky stain. The cells collected are those exfoliated, or shed, from the vaginal wall (epithelial cells and neutrophils) and those passing through the vagina from the uterus, especially erythrocytes in proestrus and estrus in the bitch.

Cytologic findings must be interpreted in conjunction with the history and clinical signs. The findings at each stage of the canine estrous cycle are detailed below. These stages are convenient divisions in a continuum of change, brought about by variations in blood estrogen and progesterone concentrations. Because determination of the stage of the estrous cycle may be difficult based on a single examination, repeat examinations every few days may be necessary.

Anestrus

The anestrual bitch has no vulvar swelling and does not attract male dogs. A vaginal smear reveals predominantly noncornified squamous epithelial cells (large cells with a rounded border, abundant basophilic cytoplasm, and a large, round nucleus; Figure 12-32). Based on size, these cells may be categorized as intermediate (larger) or parabasal (smaller) squamous epithelial cells. The smear also may contain some neutrophils but no erythrocytes. Anestrus is variable in length but generally lasts less than 4.5 months.

Proestrus

A bitch in proestrus has a swollen vulva, with a reddish vulvar discharge. The bitch attracts but does not accept male dogs attempting to breed. As proestrus progresses toward estrus, the noncornified squamous epithelial cells of anestrus are replaced by cornified squamous epithelial cells. These cells are angular and fairly homogeneous and have jagged borders, an eosinophilic cytoplasm, and a pyknotic

Figure 12-32
Canine anestrual vaginal smear. Note the noncornified squamous epithelial cells, which are predominantly intermediate-type cells (*I*) with a parabasal cell (*P*). Neutrophils and bacteria are also present. (Wright's stain, 345×)

Figure 12-33
Canine estrual vaginal smear. Note the cornified squamous epithelial cells. Bacteria are also present. (Wright's stain, 345×)

nucleus; they also are called *superficial cells.* Concurrently, neutrophil numbers in the smear decrease and erythrocyte numbers increase. Proestrus may last 4 to 13 days, with an average of about 9 days.

Estrus

The estrual bitch has a history of recent proestrus and a swollen vulva, with possibly a pinkish to straw-color discharge, becoming whiter as metestrus approaches. Bitches in estrus accept male dogs attempting to mate. A vaginal smear reveals that all squamous epithelial cells are cornified (many appear to have no nucleus), neutrophils are absent, and erythrocytes are present (Figure 12-33). Erythrocyte numbers decrease and neutrophil numbers increase as diestrus approaches. Estrus generally lasts 4 to 13 days, with an average of about 9 days.

Metestrus

A bitch in metestrus has a history of recent estrus. The vulvar swelling and discharge have decreased, and she no longer attracts or is receptive to male dogs. Cornified squamous epithelial cells are replaced by noncornified squamous epithelial cells and abundant cytologic debris. By about the tenth day after estrus, all epithelial cells are noncornified. Neutrophils increase in number until about the third day of metestrus and then decrease to few by about the tenth day. Erythrocytes are generally absent throughout metestrus. Metestrus may last about 2 to 3 months. Cytologically, metestrus and anestrus are often difficult to differentiate.

Pregnancy

Pregnancy is not cytologically distinguishable from metestrus or anestrus.

Vaginitis and Metritis

Inflammation of the vagina or uterus results in a pinkish-white vulvar discharge, usually without vulvar swelling or clinical signs of proestrus or estrus. A vaginal swab reveals noncornified squamous epithelial cells and massive numbers of neutrophils, possibly with free and/or phagocytosed bacteria.

Bacteria

Bacteria may be present in vaginal smears at any stage of the estrous cycle (but especially during estrus) and usually have no pathologic significance (i.e., they are part of the normal vaginal microflora).

◆ Queen

Unlike the bitch, the queen (female cat) ovulates after coital stimulation. Cytologic findings at different stages of the estrous cycle are similar to those of the bitch for epithelial cells and neutrophils; however, erythrocytes are not present at any stage.

SEMEN EVALUATION

The American Society of Theriogenologists has published some guidelines for examination of male animals for breeding soundness. Evaluation of semen is an important part of such an assessment. Techniques for semen collection in common domestic animals are described in standard theriogenology texts.

When handling semen samples, veterinary technicians must avoid exposure to marked changes in temperature (especially cold), water, disinfectants, or variations in pH. Consequently, all laboratory equipment used in semen collection and examination should be clean and dry and warmed to about 37° C (98.6° F). This equipment includes microscope slides, coverslips, and pipettes. Stains and diluents also should be warmed to about 37°C. Samples should be processed in a warm room as soon as possible after collection.

The following characteristics are determined readily in the laboratory: volume of ejaculate, gross appearance, wave motion, microscopic motility, spermatozoal concentration, ratio of live:dead spermatozoa, assessment of morphology, and presence of foreign cells or material. Recording the animal's species, breed, age, brief history with salient clinical findings, suspected abnormalities, and the method of semen collection (e.g., artificial vagina, electroejaculation, massage) is important.

◆ Volume of Ejaculate

The volume of ejaculate is measured easily with a volumetric flask, which may be incorporated into the collection receptacle. Marked species variations occur and the method of collection greatly influences the volume obtained, its gross appearance, and spermatozoal concentration. As a generalization, ejaculate volume is larger but spermatozoal concentration lower (and the specimen apparently more dilute) when collected by electroejaculation than when collected by artificial vagina. Further, repeated ejaculation, whether associated with semen collection or sexual activity, decreases the volume and concentration of semen obtained at subsequent collections. Semen volume tends to be greater if collection is preceded by a period of sexual arousal ("teasing").

The ejaculate comprises three portions: a sperm-free watery secretion, a sperm-rich fraction, and a sperm-poor fraction. The first and third fractions are derived from accessory sex glands. In bucks, bulls, rams, and toms, all three fractions are collected together. However, with boars, dogs, and stallions, the third fraction conveniently may be collected separately, which is advisable because the third fraction is voluminous in these three animals and is therefore an unnecessary encumbrance in subsequent evaluation of the semen sample. In these three species, the first two fractions (collected together) are used in the other procedures that follow.

Approximate average total ejaculate volumes (all three fractions) are boar, 250 ml; buck and ram, 1 ml; bull, 5 ml; dog, 10 ml; stallion, 65 ml; and tom, 0.04 ml. Ejaculate volume does not necessarily correlate with fertility. In general, spermatozoal number, motility, and morphology are better guides to fertility. Obviously, however, small ejaculates may give cause for concern in species, which should have voluminous ejaculates. Knowledge of the ejaculate volume is necessary for determination of total spermatozoal numbers if the sample is to be divided (and possibly diluted) for artificial insemination procedures.

◆ Gross Appearance of Ejaculate

The opacity and color of the sample should be recorded. Opacity subjectively reflects the concentration of spermatozoa. Categories used include thick, creamy, opaque; milky opaque; opalescent milky; and watery white. This rule of thumb works best for semen from bucks, bulls, and rams, which normally have opaque, creamy-white semen because of high spermatozoal concentration. As the density of spermatozoa decreases, the specimen becomes more translucent and "milkier" in appearance. Semen from boars, dogs, and stallions is normally fairly translucent and white to gray. Contaminants, especially intact or degenerate erythrocytes, cause discoloration of semen.

◆ Sperm Motility

Sperm motility (movement) is assessed subjectively and depends on careful handling of the sample for meaningful results. Variations in temperature and exposure to non-isotonic fluids or destructive chemicals (including detergents) must be avoided. Motility is correlated with fertility; however, improper specimen handling adversely affects its assessment. If other tests, especially sperm morphology, suggest the semen is normal but sperm motility is poor, another sample should be examined to ensure that technical errors were not responsible for the poor motility. Motility may be conveniently assessed in two ways.

Wave Motion

Wave motion is a subjective assessment of the gross motility of sperm. Four general classifications are used: very good, good, fair, and poor, based on the amount of "swirling" activity observed in a drop of semen on a microscope slide at low-power (40×) magnification. These categories respectively correspond to distinct vigorous swirling, moderate slow swirling, barely discernible swirling, and lack of actual swirling but with motile sperm present, which may cause the sample to have an irregular oscillating appearance. Wave motion depends on high sperm density and is therefore best in samples from bucks, bulls, and rams, which normally have high sperm concentrations. Wave motion decreases as sperm concentration decreases. Consequently, normal boars, dogs, stallions and toms may have fair or poor wave motion. As a guide, if wave motion is very good or good, the sample should be diluted for evaluation of the percentage of motile sperm and their rate of motility.

Motility

Progressive motility of individual spermatozoa is determined on a relatively dilute drop of coverslipped semen, examined at 100× magnification. Because the motility of individual spermatozoa is difficult to appreciate in dense samples, such concentrated samples should be diluted before examination. Warm physiologic saline or fresh, buffered 2.9% sodium citrate solutions are suitable diluents.

A drop of semen is placed on a slide and diluted until a satisfactory concentration of spermatozoa is observed. The sample is then coverslipped to produce a monolayer of cells. Excessive dilution of the sample makes evaluation of motility difficult. The rate of motility is generally subjectively classified as very good, good, fair, or poor, corresponding to rapid linear activity, moderate linear activity, slow linear or erratic activity, and very slow erratic activity, respectively. The percentage of motile spermatozoa is broadly categorized as very good, good, fair, or poor, corresponding to about 80% to 100%, 60% to 80%, 40% to 60%, and 20% to 40% motile cells, respectively. As a generalization, to be considered satisfactory, a sample should have at least 60% moderately active spermatozoa. The importance of careful specimen processing cannot be overemphasized.

◆ Sperm Concentration

Several solutions are satisfactory for semen dilution before counting sperm numbers, including 5 g of sodium bicarbonate or 9 g of sodium chloride with 1 ml of formalin in 1 L of distilled water; 3% chlorazene; or 12.5 g of sodium sulfate with 33.3 ml of glacial acetic acid in 200 ml of distilled water (Gower's solution). The sample is diluted using an erythrocyte dilution pipette. Semen is drawn to the 0.5 mark, then diluent is drawn to the 101 mark, giving a 1:200 dilution. After thorough mixing, several drops are discarded from the pipette and a Neubauer hemacytometer is charged with fluid. The sample is allowed to settle for a few minutes and then checked for homogeneous distribution of spermatozoa. If this is not present, the sample in the pipette should be mixed thoroughly again and the cleaned hemacytometer recharged.

The number of spermatozoa in the central grid area (erythrocyte counting area) of one side of the chamber is counted at $400\times$ magnification. The number of spermatozoa/ml of semen is calculated by multiplying the number observed by 2 million. If spermatozoal concentration is high (e.g., in bucks, bulls, and toms), fewer squares may be counted and the multiplication factor adjusted accordingly. Spermatozoal concentration also may be determined by colorimetric and electronic particle counter techniques.

As outlined earlier, sperm concentration varies with the method of collection. As a generalization, average sperm concentrations (in millions/ml) are about 150 for boars and stallions, 3000 for bucks and rams, 1200 for bulls, 300 for dogs, and 1700 for toms.

◆ Live:Dead Sperm Ratio

Staining with a vital dye permits discrimination between live and dead spermatozoa. An eosin/nigrosin mixture is popular for this purpose and also permits examination of sperm morphology. The stain is prepared by adding 1 g of eosin B and 5 g of nigrosin to a 3% solution of sodium citrate dihydrate. This solution is stable for at least a year.

A small drop of warm stain is mixed gently with a small drop of semen on a warm microscope slide. After several seconds of contact between specimen and dye, the mixture is smeared as when making a blood smear and then rapidly dried. Once the smear is dried, microscopic examination may be delayed. Live sperm resist staining and appear white (clear) against the blue-black nigrosin background. In contrast, dead sperm passively take up the eosin and are stained a pinkish red (Figure 12-34). The ratio of live:dead sperm, expressed as a percentage, is determined by examination at $400\times$ or $1000\times$ magnification, preferably by observation of 200 cells.

Unfortunately, this procedure is susceptible to technical problems. Conditions that kill sperm, especially temperature changes, produce misleading results. Findings always should be interpreted with regard to other results, such as sperm concentration, motility, and morphology.

◆ Sperm Morphology

Sperm morphology is assessed readily on a nigrosin and eosin stained smear, prepared as outlined above. Other stains, such as India ink, hematoxylin and eosin, Wright's, Giemsa, and Cavarett's (a mixture of eosin B and phenol), have been used but offer no distinct advantages over nigrosin and eosin.

Species differences exist with respect to the fine points of sperm morphology, but all sperm have the same basic structure (Figure 12-35). The percentage of abnormal spermatozoa and their types are recorded after observing 100 to 500 cells. Counting the lower number of cells (100) is usually adequate once the technician has become proficient. Abnormalities conveniently are divided into head, midpiece, and tail problems. Abnormalities often are categorized as primary or secondary.

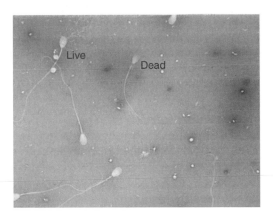

Figure 12-34
Live:dead staining of spermatozoa. (Nigrosin-Eosin stain 1000×) (Courtesy Dr. P.J. Wright, University of Melbourne.)

Figure 12-35
Diagrammatic representation of a normal spermatozoon, showing its three main components: head, midpiece, and tail.

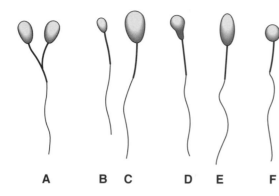

Figure 12-36
Diagrammatic representation of primary spermatozoal abnormalities involving the head. Abnormalities depicted are double head (bicephaly) **(A)**, small head (microcephaly) **(B)**, large head (macrocephaly) **(C)**, pear-shape head (pyriform) **(D)**, elongated head **(E)**, and round head **(F)**.

A   B   C   D   E   F

Figure 12-37
Diagrammatic representation of primary spermatozoal abnormalities involving the midpiece and tail. Abnormalities depicted are swollen midpiece **(A)**, coiled midpiece and coiled tail **(B)**, bent midpiece **(C)**, double midpiece **(D)**, and abaxial midpiece **(E)**.

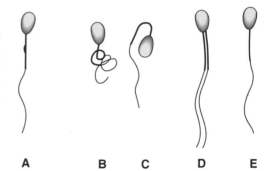

A   B   C   D   E

Primary defects occur during spermatozoal production and include the following: heads that are double, too large, too small, or oddly shaped (e.g., pearlike, round, twisted, knobby) (Figure 12-36); midpieces that are swollen, kinked, twisted, double, or eccentrically attached to a head (abaxial) (Figure 12-37); and tails that are coiled (see Figure 12-37). Primary abnormalities generally are considered more serious than secondary ones. Their percentage is fairly consistent if another semen sample is collected within several days. Slightly abaxial midpiece attachment in boars is probably not as significant as in other species because it may be found in numerous spermatozoa of apparently normal boars.

Secondary defects may occur at any time, from storage in the epididymis until the smear is made. Therefore because secondary abnormalities may be artifactual, careful specimen handling, as outlined earlier, is mandatory. Minimization of technique-induced secondary abnormalities permits easier sample interpretation. Secondary defects include tailless heads, protoplasmic droplets on the midpiece, and bent or broken tails (Figure 12-38). Obviously, for every tailless head is a headless tail, so the latter need not be counted. Protoplasmic droplets are distinct from swollen midpieces. Protoplasmic droplets are normally present while spermatozoa are in the epididymis. The droplets migrate caudally along the midpiece while the sperm cells mature in the epididymis. The droplets usually are shed before the spermatozoa leave the epididymis.

Figure 12-38
Diagrammatic representation of secondary spermatozoal abnormalities involving the midpiece and tail. Abnormalities depicted are tailless head **(A)**, headless tail **(B)**, distal protoplasmic droplets **(C)**, proximal protoplasmic droplets **(D)**, and bent tail **(E)**.

As a broad generalization, less than 20% of spermatozoa are abnormal in a normal animal and usually less than 10%. Higher percentages of abnormal spermatozoa may compromise fertility. Obviously, however, the total number of normal spermatozoa is important, not the percentage of abnormal sperm.

◆ Other Cells in Semen

Normal semen contains few (if any) leukocytes, erythrocytes, or epithelial cells, and no bacteria or fungi. If present, their approximate quantity should be noted. If bacteria or fungi are observed without an inflammatory response, sample contamination by the normal preputial microflora should be suspected. Attention to preputial sanitation before sample collection should remedy the problem. If indicated, a semen sample may be submitted for microbiologic examination.

Cells from the germinal layers of the testis are an unusual finding in semen and represent severe testicular damage. Such cells include spermatids, spermatocytes, and large ciliated cells (often called *medusa heads*). Precise categorization is unimportant, as long as these cells are classified as immature sperm cells.

EVALUATION OF PROSTATIC SECRETIONS

Disorders of the prostate are not uncommon in dogs but are rare in other domestic animals. Cells of prostatic origin may be collected by urethral catheterization, combined with prostatic massage (or penile massage) performed per rectum to stimulate prostatic secretion. Prostatic tissue may be aspirated by transcutaneous needle biopsy. Cytologic smears are prepared as outlined earlier in this chapter.

An enlarged prostate may be the result of prostatic hypertrophy, hyperplasia, metaplasia, neoplasia, or inflammation. Cytologic characteristics of these conditions are considered briefly below. Prostatic cells may occur singly or in clusters. Spermatozoa may be present in some fluid samples, especially those collected by penile massage.

carded because such milk is generally considered to reflect the bacterial and nucle-ated cell population of the teat canal rather than the mammary gland itself. If the sam-ple cannot be tested immediately or also is being collected for bacteriologic examination and/or direct cell counts, it should be collected in a clean, dry, sterile bot-tle with an airtight seal.

Care must be exercised to avoid contamination of the bottle by debris and bacte-ria. As a precaution, the bottle may be held almost horizontally and the lid held with its inside facing down, while the milk is squirted in. About 2 ml are required for the California mastitis test and about 5 ml often are collected for bacteriologic examina-tion. Accurate identification of each sample with respect to quarter and cow is criti-cal so that results can be recorded properly. The bottled specimen is refrigerated until used, preferably on the same day, but certainly within 36 hours. Heating, freezing, preservatives that denature protein (e.g., formalin), aging, and bacterial contamina-tion of the sample must be avoided because they decrease the mastitis test reaction by destroying DNA.

Small amounts of milk and reagent are mixed by gentle swirling in the cups of a special plastic paddle (one cup is used for each quarter of the udder). The reaction is graded immediately. The intensity of the reaction is proportional to the number of neutrophils present.

Other "cowside" mastitis tests, similar to the California mastitis test, include the field Whiteside test, the milk quality test, and the Michigan mastitis test. Laboratory procedures, usually for bulk milk specimens, to evaluate milk viscosity include the Brabant test and the Wisconsin mastitis test. As with the California mastitis test, all of these tests indirectly measure the concentration of "inflammatory products" (specifi-cally DNA), which do not necessarily correspond to the sample's bacterial content.

◆ Microbiologic Examination

Sample collection has been outlined previously, and microbiologic principles are de-tailed elsewhere (see Chapter 4). Numerous bacterial species have been implicated as causes of mastitis in cattle, including *Staphylococcus aureus, Escherichia coli,* and various species of *Streptococcus, Corynebacterium, Klebsiella, Mycobacterium,* and *Nocardia.*

Bacteria may be seen on direct smears of milk samples. Nucleated cell counts (in-direct or direct) do not necessarily parallel bacterial numbers. For example, if nucle-ated cells are numerous and fairly effectively combating the infection, bacterial numbers may be low. In contrast, early in the course of an infection, bacterial num-bers may be high while the neutrophil count is low (but increasing).

◆ Miscellaneous Tests

Other procedures for detection of bovine mastitis in general veterinary practice have been superceded by such tests as the California mastitis test because of the latter's simplicity and reliability. Some of these procedures are detailed in the sec-tions that follow.

pH

Normal milk has a pH of 6.4 to 6.8. Abnormal milk may be more acidic, more alkaline, or normal in pH. Refrigerated or, preferably, freshly collected samples are added to a pH-sensitive dye, such as bromthymol blue or bromcresol purple. Measurement of pH is incorporated into the California mastitis test.

Catalase Test

The catalase activity of normal milk is low. It increases in proportion to the elevation in cell numbers of the sample. The catalase test is not a "cowside" test.

Direct Microscopic (Somatic) Cell Count

Nucleated cell counts (also called *somatic cell counts*) may be performed on fresh, well-mixed milk samples. A simple technique is to spread evenly 0.01 ml of milk over exactly 1 cm^2 of a clean microscope slide. (A card with 1 cm^2 borders marked on it may be placed under the slide.) The slide is air dried, placed into modified Newman-Lampert stain for 2 minutes, drained, and air dried, then gently washed in warm water to remove excess stain. The modified Newman-Lampert stain is made by adding 0.6 g of methylene blue chloride to a mixture of 52 ml of 95% ethanol and 44 ml of tetra-chloroethane, which is stored at 4° to 7° C for 12 to 24 hours, then mixed with 4 ml of glacial acetic acid, filtered, and stored. This stain fixes and removes lipids from the smear while staining nucleated cells and bacteria. Cells and bacteria tend to be more numerous at the center of the smear.

Such manual counts are really estimates of cell numbers. However, rigid standardization of procedures and use of an optical lens micrometer to measure microscopic field size increases accuracy. Such considerations are well reviewed elsewhere. Microscopic field area may vary among technicians because of differences in interpupillary distance and eyepiece focal adjustment. Consequently, the field area at 1000× magnification can be measured with an ocular eyepiece micrometer. The equation to calculate microscopic field area at 1000× is:

Area $= d^2/4$

At 1000× magnification, field diameter (d) is often about 0.16 mm. Therefore field area is about 2×10^{-4} cm^2 (1/5000 cm^2). The number of cells/ml of milk equals the average number of cells per 1000×-magnification field multiplied by the microscope factor. The microscope factor is calculated as:

$$\text{Microscope factor} = \frac{1}{\text{Field area} \times \text{sample volume}}$$

In this example, the microscope factor is 500,000. Random examination of 20 to 50 fields is recommended to determine the average cell number per field.

Automated techniques are available for nucleated cell counts, including an electronic particle counter method (Coulter Milk Cell Counter: Coulter Electronics, Hialeah, FL) and a fluorescent dye technique (Fossomatic: Foss Electric, Hillerod, Denmark). However, equipment cost precludes their use in general veterinary practice.

Nucleated cell counts of normal milk are generally less than 300,000 to 500,000 cells/ml. Counts above 500,000 cells/ml indicate mastitis.

Differential cell counts sometimes are performed. Nucleated cells are categorized as neutrophils or mononuclear cells. Normal milk in midlactation generally has less than 10% neutrophils, whereas in severe acute mastitis, the milk may have up to 95% neutrophils.

EXAMINATION OF FECES FOR OCCULT BLOOD

A direct fecal smear, stained with Wright's stain, may be microscopically examined to look for intact erythrocytes in feces. However, unless the hemorrhage occurs in the terminal segments of the intestinal tract, erythrocytes are destroyed before passage in the feces. Reagent tablet tests (e.g., Hematest: Ames, Elkhart, IN) are available for detection of erythrocytes and/or hemoglobin in feces. The procedure relies on the peroxidase-like activity of hemoglobin to enhance the oxidation of a chromagen in the tablet to orthotoluidine, which has a blue color.

◆ Technique

A small quantity of fresh feces is smeared onto a filter paper square (provided with the kit) and placed on a clean, impermeable surface. A reagent tablet is placed on top of the center of the fecal smear and a drop of water is placed on top of the tablet. After 5 to 10 seconds, another drop of water is added and allowed to run down the side of the tablet. Blue discoloration of the filter paper at 2 minutes constitutes a positive reaction (Figure 12-41). Because blood or hemoglobin may not be distributed evenly in the feces, testing of more than one portion of a sample may be advisable. Obviously, hands and equipment must be free of blood contamination to avoid a false-positive result. A quality control can be run by using a 1:20,000 dilution of blood, instead of feces, in the test.

Figure 12-41
Fecal occult blood test.

Because the test reagent cross-reacts with myoglobin of muscle, the carnivores should be fed a diet free of raw meat beginning at least 3 days before testing. Any meat in the diet must be well cooked to minimize the likelihood of a false-positive result. False positives also may result if the diet is supplemented with iron or if compounds with peroxidase activity are present in the diet or are produced by intestinal bacteria.

Similar tests are available to examine vomitus (or gastric contents) for blood. These procedures are best used on specimens with a low pH.

TOXICOLOGY

The clinical signs and treatments of common poisonings of dogs, cats, horses, and food animals have been well reviewed in reference texts. Numerous agents may be involved, including herbicides, fungicides, insecticides, rodenticides, heavy metals (especially lead), household products (including phenols), automotive products (especially ethylene glycol), drugs (including medication), and various poisonous plants and animals. Often a presumptive diagnosis may be attained from an accurate history, including environmental factors, and a thorough clinical examination, followed by response to therapy or by necropsy. However, establishing a specific etiologic diagnosis may be difficult in some cases.

A few simple tests may be performed in the veterinary practice laboratory. In such situations, personnel must be familiar and competent with the test procedure, reagents must not be outdated, and special equipment may be required. These requirements, together with a sporadic demand for such tests, frequently dictate that practitioners send all toxicologic specimens to a specially equipped laboratory for analysis.

◆ Toxicologic Specimens

Suggestions on appropriate specimens and preferred methods of handling, packaging, and transport can be obtained by consultation with the toxicology laboratory. Such contact also ensures that the laboratory offers the procedures requested.

Submitted specimens should be free from contamination by extraneous environmental compounds or debris. Specimens should not be washed, which may remove toxic residues. Samples of different fluids, tissues, and feeds must be submitted in separate leak-proof (airtight), clean, plastic or glass containers. All containers should be individually identified by the owner's and veterinarian's names, animal's name or identification number, and the nature of the specimen before packaging into a large container for submission to the laboratory.

Samples of whole blood (at least 10 ml, usually heparinized), serum (at least 10 ml), vomitus, gastric lavage fluid, feces, and urine (about 50 ml) may be submitted from live animals. Samples of feed (portions of at least 200 g), water, and suspected baits also may be helpful in some cases. In fatal poisoning, samples collected during a thorough necropsy should include whole blood or serum, urine, gut (especially stomach) contents (at least 200 g, noting site of collection), and organ or tissue samples, especially liver and kidney, but sometimes brain, bone, spleen, or fat (generally, where practical, at least 100 g of each tissue). Chapter 10 contains a detailed description of necropsy procedures. Sending too large a sample is always better than not sending enough because excess can be discarded.

In general, serum or blood samples are best submitted refrigerated, whereas gut contents and tissues are best frozen. Preservatives are usually not required. An exception would be tissue samples submitted for histopathologic examination, which require fixation in 10% formalin and must not be frozen. If a preservative is used on a specimen submitted for chemical analysis, it is probably worthwhile also to submit an aliquot of preservative for reference analysis. Frozen samples should be insulated from other specimens and should arrive at the laboratory while still frozen. Dispatch to the laboratory by courier is recommended.

As litigation may result from poisoning cases, accurate and detailed records should be kept from the outset of the case. Establishment of a good working relationship with the toxicology laboratory, including provision of a good case history (and necropsy findings in fatal poisonings) when samples are submitted, helps ensure the best results.

The main advantages of the following tests are that they can be performed reasonably quickly in the practice laboratory. Results are therefore available more rapidly than if the sample was sent to a toxicology laboratory. However, they are best viewed as screening procedures, suggesting appropriate avenues of investigation and treatment. Verification of findings (especially positive ones) by a reputable toxicology laboratory is advisable, especially if subsequent legal action by the client is a possibility.

◆ Lead Poisoning

Lead is a fairly common environmental pollutant, in the air of cities and in old lead-based paints, lead shot (ammunition), linoleum, car batteries, solder, roofing materials, and petroleum products. Lead poisoning (plumbism) can occur in all species. Clinical signs vary with the species and are related chiefly to the gastrointestinal tract and nervous system. Hematologic examination of blood from an animal with lead poisoning may reveal basophilic stippling of some erythrocytes and increased numbers of circulating nucleated red blood cells (metarubricytosis) (see Chapter 2). Such findings in an animal that is not anemic and has clinical signs consistent with lead poisoning strongly suggest plumbism.

No simple, reliable in-house tests exist to detect lead in blood, feces, urine, milk, or tissues. Blood lead levels can be determined readily (by atomic absorption spectrophotometry) at a toxicology laboratory on whole blood, collected in EDTA, heparin, or citrate blood tubes. Tissue samples (especially liver and kidney) and feces also may be tested. Histopathologic examination of liver, kidney, or bone, stained by the Ziehl-Neelsen technique, may reveal characteristic eosinophilic, acid-fast intranuclear inclusion bodies in hepatocytes, renal tubular cells, and osteoclasts, respectively.

◆ Nitrate or Nitrite Poisoning

Nitrate or nitrite poisoning may occur in ruminants, pigs, and horses ingesting feeds with high concentrations of these compounds. Such may be the case in cereals, grasses, and root crops heavily fertilized with nitrogenous compounds. Water, especially from deep wells filled with seepage from heavily fertilized ground, may contain large quantities of nitrate. Nitrates are converted to nitrites in the feed or within the intestinal tract. Nitrites, absorbed from the gut, decrease the oxygen-carrying capacity of the blood by degrading hemoglobin to methemoglobin in erythrocytes. Consequently, the animal's blood becomes dark-red to brown. The severity of clinical signs is related to the quantity ingested. Death can be acute and many animals can be affected.

A rapid, fairly specific, semiqualitative test uses diphenylamine, which is converted to quinodial compounds with an intensely blue color, by nitrates and nitrites. Diphenylamine (0.5 g) is dissolved in 20 ml of distilled water and the solution made up to 100 ml with concentrated sulfuric acid. This stock solution may be used undiluted or diluted 1:1 with 80% sulfuric acid. The solution is applied to the inner portion of the plant's stem. An intense blue color within 10 seconds of application of the undiluted solution suggests greater than 1% nitrate is present (and the feed is potentially toxic). False positives may occur with numerous substances, the most significant of which is iron. Such iron is generally on the outside of the stalk; therefore careful application circumvents this problem.

A more dilute diphenylamine solution (the previous stock solution diluted 1:7 with concentrated sulfuric acid) may be used to test for nitrates/nitrites in serum or plasma, other body fluids, and urine. Three drops of the diluted diphenylamine are added to 1 drop of the sample on a glass slide over a white background. Nitrate/nitrite produces an intense blue color immediately. Hemolysis may mask the color change.

◆ Anticoagulant Rodenticides

Anticoagulant rodenticides (e.g., warfarin, diphacinone, pindone) act by inhibiting metabolism of vitamin K in the body. The latter is required for production of factors II, VII, IX, and X in the liver. Anticoagulant rodenticide poisoning initially prolongs the prothrombin time (PT) because factor VII is the first to be depleted. Subsequently, the partial thromboplastin time (PTT) and activated coagulation time (ACT) are prolonged as the other factors also become depleted. When an animal is bleeding as a result of such poisoning, both the PT and PTT (or ACT) are usually prolonged. Diagnosis of anticoagulant rodenticide poisoning is commonly based on these "screening tests" and the response to treatment with vitamin K.

◆ Chemicals That Denature Hemoglobin

A variety of compounds, when ingested, may result in damage to (oxidative denaturation of) hemoglobin in erythrocytes, with the formation of Heinz bodies (see Chapter 2). Such substances include paracetamol and methylene blue (cats), onions (dogs), red maple leaves (horses), and onions and brassicas (ruminants). Demonstration of Heinz bodies on a blood film is diagnostic of such poisoning.

Selenium-deficient animals are more prone to such oxidative injury because of a deficiency of glutathione peroxidase (an enzyme in erythrocytes that helps protect them against such damage).

Figure 12-42
Calcium oxalate monohydrate crystals ("hippurate-like" crystals) in the urine sediment of a dog with ethylene glycol (antifreeze) poisoning. (Unstained, 345×) (Courtesy Dr. R.L. Cowell, Oklahoma State University.)

◆ Ethylene Glycol

Ethylene glycol is the major constituent of most antifreeze solutions. Accidental ingestion can cause serious or fatal toxicosis, usually in dogs and cats.

Ethylene glycol and its metabolites can be detected in whole blood or serum samples by a toxicology laboratory. Its presence is strongly suggested when urine sediments from poisoned dogs or cats contain masses of calcium oxalate monohydrate crystals (Figure 12-42) and/or possibly calcium oxalate dihydrate crystals (see Chapter 5). The former were previously thought to have been hippuric acid crystals. Histopathologic examination of the kidney of fatally affected animals reveals renal tubular nephrosis and numerous oxalate crystals. The latter are most readily seen under polarizing light.

◉ SKIN BIOPSY

◆ P.J. Ihrke

Skin biopsy is a valuable tool in diagnosis of skin diseases. In addition, skin biopsy may have benefits other than offering a diagnosis. Ruling out such serious diseases as neoplasia may be of equal or greater importance. Skin biopsy also may be valuable in evaluation of the prognosis and response to therapy.

In general, skin biopsies are not performed as often as they should be in veterinary practice. The potential usefulness of a skin biopsy, unfortunately, often is reduced by poor timing, poor selection of biopsy sites, and poor biopsy technique. If basic guidelines are followed as to when, what, and how to biopsy, the chances of deriving beneficial information from a skin biopsy are greatly increased.

◆ Indications for Skin Biopsy

The most important reason for performing a skin biopsy is to establish a definitive diagnosis. A biopsy may be useful if a disease is not visually identifiable, other laboratory tests have not been diagnostic, or a disease has not responded to apparently rational therapy. Diseases that are clinically subtle or unusual also warrant biopsy. Most suspected or obviously neoplastic lesions should be biopsied. In addition, any severe or persistently ulcerated or eroded skin lesion should be sampled. In difficult cases, a biopsy may help rule out other diseases even though the suspected disease may not have definitive histopathologic characteristics.

Skin biopsy also may be used to formulate a prognosis. Biopsy may be helpful in assessing the degree of chronicity, determining the permanency of changes, or determining response to therapy.

Once an animal becomes a possible candidate for skin biopsy, the biopsy should be performed as soon as possible because chronicity, self-trauma, and topical or systemic therapy can potentially obscure a diagnosis. Lesions biopsied within 2 to 3 weeks after their development are much more likely to yield diagnostic results than those sampled long after they first appeared.

◆ What to Biopsy

If multiple lesions are present, those most representative should be sampled. Fully developed lesions usually are preferred to either very early or chronic lesions. An exception would be if a bullous autoimmune disease is suspected because early lesions are more likely to be useful. Because the stage of the lesion may be important in biopsy site selection, both the animal's owner and the veterinarian should be consulted when a site is selected. Traumatized lesions, acute ulcerations, or chronic lesions often do not yield worthwhile results. Smaller lesions should be resected in their entirety, or the advancing edge of a larger lesion should be biopsied.

Biopsy of ulcers or progressive ulcerative skin disease represents a special circumstance. Focal or indolent ulceration commonly reflects extensive preceding dermal changes (infectious, neoplastic, or collagenolytic diseases) underlying the ulcer. Consequently, diagnosis is accomplished by biopsy of the ulcer. Areas immediately adjacent to ulcers, in addition to the ulcerated area, should be sampled in progressive ulcerative skin disease. The diagnostic lesion usually is present at the junction of the epidermis and dermis. The area at the margin of the ulcer with intact epithelium is critical to establishing a diagnosis because sampling the ulcer provides the pathologist with a specimen of the dermis lacking the overlying epidermis.

If different stages of a disease are present, it may be beneficial to obtain multiple biopsy specimens. Often two or three tissue samples provide an answer, whereas a single sample may not. Most laboratories charge no more for processing and evaluating two or three samples than for a single sample. Consequently, multiple biopsies usually are indicated.

Ordinarily, the biopsy site should include abnormal skin only, particularly when the punch technique is used (see following). Identification of histopathologic lesions usually does not require comparison with normal skin. If hair loss is the primary clinical sign, the area of most complete hair loss should be selected. In addition, a separate specimen of normal skin should be sampled and identified for the pathologist. In this way, changes that might not be obvious in an isolated abnormal specimen may be clarified by comparison with a normal specimen.

Specimen selection for direct immunofluorescent testing or immunohistochemical testing is slightly different in that areas directly adjacent to well-developed new lesions (bullae or vesicles) should be sampled. The erythematous zone adjacent to a bulla or ulcer should be obtained for direct immunofluorescent testing if a bullous autoimmune disease is suspected. Lesional skin may yield false-negative immunofluorescent results because deposited immunoglobulins and complement may be swept away by inflammation.

◆ Necessary Instruments

A separate cold-sterilization tray containing the necessary instruments for performing a skin biopsy should be dedicated to this procedure. Because delicate handling of fragile biopsy specimens is imperative, the tray should include a small pair of curved iris scissors and several pairs of very fine eye forceps of various types. Small curved hemostats, a small needleholder, and suture scissors also should be available. The only necessary specialized instruments are Keyes cutaneous biopsy punches (4-, 6-, and 8-mm disposable skin biopsy punches: Accuderm, Fort Lauderdale, FL). Used punches may be placed in the sterilization tray and reused until dull. Most disposable punches may be reused at least three or four times.

◆ Methods of Skin Biopsy

Wedge Biopsy

Elliptic wedge biopsy specimens are commonly obtained with a scalpel. The wedge biopsy offers the advantages of a large, variably sized specimen that is easily oriented by the pathology technician. Solitary lesions are often best removed using this technique.

When a wedge biopsy specimen is taken, a sharp scalpel blade is used to totally excise the entire lesion, or the wedge is taken from an area of the lesion, through a transition zone, to normal tissue (Figure 12-43). The pathology technician then can trim the specimen on its long axis to provide the pathologist with a slide showing abnormal tissue, a transition zone, and normal tissue.

Excisional skin biopsy by the wedge method is indicated for solitary lesions. In addition, wedge biopsy is the method of choice if bullae or vesicles are present because it is potentially less traumatic to fragile tissues. A wedge biopsy is also recommended if diseases of the subcutaneous fat are suspected, as the subcutaneous fat often is lost when punch biopsy specimens are obtained.

The major disadvantage of the wedge biopsy technique is the time required to obtain the specimen. Because wedge biopsy procedures require substantially more

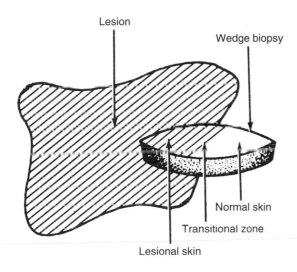

Figure 12-43
A wedge biopsy should include areas of the lesion, the transitional zone, and some normal skin.

time, may require general anesthesia, and require more sutures, wedge biopsy specimens are taken less frequently than warranted in many veterinary hospitals.

Punch Biopsy

The punch biopsy technique has a number of advantages over wedge biopsy. Of greatest importance, the ease and speed of the procedure encourage more frequent use of skin biopsy. Using the biopsy punch, 4-mm specimens require no sutures and 6- or 8-mm biopsy specimens require only one or two sutures.

Sample selection is different for performing a punch biopsy than for obtaining wedge biopsy specimens. Only abnormal tissue is sampled by punch biopsy. If a significant portion of normal skin is obtained, rotation of the sample in the wrong direction during processing could result in histopathologic examination of only normal skin. Consequently, the plug of tissue is taken entirely within the boundary of the lesion. Ideally, two or three punch biopsy specimens of various lesions should be submitted.

◆ Size of the Specimen

Large specimens may not be adequately fixed in formalin. Therefore individual wedge biopsy specimens should never be more than 2 cm wide or long, regardless of the size of the lesion removed.

Disposable skin biopsy punches of 4-mm, 6-mm, and 8-mm diameter are used most commonly (Figure 12-44). The 4-mm biopsy punches usually are reserved for difficult sites, such as the planum nasale and the skin surrounding the eye. The 6-mm punch specimens generally are the minimal acceptable size because specimens obtained from larger punches have more tissue to examine and less procurement artifact and thus are more likely to yield diagnostic lesions.

Figure 12-44
Materials needed for punch biopsy include a disposable biopsy punch, lidocaine, and a container of fixative.

Michel's fixative and transport medium, used for direct immunofluorescence testing, does not penetrate tissue as readily as formalin. Consequently, specimens should not be thicker than 4 mm in diameter. A 4-mm punch biopsy specimen or tissue trimmed from a larger specimen may be used.

◆ Technique

Most biopsies are accomplished with local anesthesia and restraint. Occasionally, anesthesia or tranquilization is necessary for a fractious animal or cases involving biopsy of difficult body regions, such as the planum nasale, periorbital region, or footpads, where total restraint is crucial. General or dissociative anesthesia is required more often for feline skin biopsy.

Haired prospective skin biopsy sites are clipped carefully to avoid skin irritation and inducement of an inflammatory artifact. Cleansing of the site is neither recommended nor necessary. The lesion must not be scrubbed or any scales, crusts, or surface debris disturbed because they may offer valuable diagnostic clues.

After clipping, the site is marked with an indelible marker (Sharpie: Sanford, Bellwood, IL) and undermined with 1 to 2 ml of 2% lidocaine deposited subcutaneously using a 25- or 26-gauge needle. Rinsing the syringe barrel with epinephrine before filling it with lidocaine restricts spread of the anesthetic and aids hemostasis. Approximately 1 ml of lidocaine generally is sufficient for each skin biopsy site. Proper anesthesia is enhanced by gently repositioning the needle several times and depositing the anesthetic in a fanlike pattern. Because sensory nerves radiate peripherally from the spine, the recommended site of injection is the side of the biopsy site closest to the spinal column so that needle repositioning does not cause additional discomfort to the patient.

Local anesthesia with subcutaneous lidocaine should not be used if a disease of the subcutaneous fat (panniculitis) is suspected because subcutaneous injection damages the tissue to be evaluated. "Ring block" regional anesthesia or general anesthesia is recommended to obtain subcutaneous tissue without artifacts.

The biopsy specimen can be obtained about 5 minutes after injection of the local anesthetic. The indelible marker dots prevent inadvertent sampling of unanesthetized regions because the bleb of local anesthetic may no longer be visible.

If a disposable biopsy punch is used, the punch is gently rotated in one direction until the punch blade has entered the subcutaneous tissue. The punch is rotated only in one direction because back-and-forth rotation increases the likelihood of specimen damage from shearing forces. With practice, a sudden easing of pressure is noted when the punch has successfully entered the subcutaneous tissue.

Once the specimen has been cut free from the surrounding skin, either by the wedge or punch method, the specimen should be removed gently by grasping the margin or the underlying subcutaneous fat with a pair of fine forceps. If necessary, iris scissors can be used to detach the subcutis. Fresh, unfixed tissue is extremely fragile. The specimen then is blotted gently on a paper towel to remove excess blood and placed with the subcutaneous side down on a small piece of wooden tongue depressor or cardboard. Gently pressing the biopsy specimen flat facilitates adherence and allows proper anatomic orientation of the specimen in the laboratory.

Specimens with the attached "splint" are then immersed or floated specimen-side down in the fixative. Timely placement of the specimen in the fixative is critical because artifactual changes may occur within 1 minute after the biopsy specimen is obtained. After these steps are accomplished, the biopsy site may be sutured. Postbiopsy complications, such as infection or dehiscence, are rare.

◆ Specimen Handling

Under most circumstances, 10% neutral phosphate-buffered formalin is the preferred fixative. When in doubt, the pathology laboratory should be consulted. The volume of fixative always should be at least 10 times that of the specimen. Adequate specimen fixation requires at least 24 hours before processing. Formalin freezes at $-11°$ C ($-24°$ F), and this freezing may cause substantial artifactual damage in unfixed specimens. Therefore to ensure proper fixation without freezing artifact, specimens should remain at room temperature for at least 6 hours before exposure to possible extreme cold.

Michel's transport medium and fixative is required for specimens to be processed for immunofluorescence studies. Specimens fixed in Michel's medium cannot be used for routine histopathologic examination. Properly buffered Michel's medium maintains its preservative properties over long periods in airtight containers.

Specimen mailers frequently are provided by pathology laboratories. Formalin-filled specimen containers should be sealed tightly and wrapped with tape to prevent leakage during transport. Because formalin can dissolve water-soluble ink, an indelible ballpoint pen should be used to write the history. Shipment of skin biopsy specimens in the same container with samples stored on ice is not recommended because freezing artifact may result.

Skin biopsy specimens for immunofluorescence or immunoperoxidase testing should be submitted concurrently with specimens for routine histopathologic examination. The pathologist can be requested to hold the specimen and to process it only if necessary for the diagnosis. In this way, time is saved in cases in which immunologic studies are indicated, and money is saved in circumstances in which these tests are not required to establish a diagnosis.

◆ Submitting the Specimen

The final step in the skin biopsy procedure is as important as the intermediate steps. The specimen should be sent to a laboratory most likely to arrive at the appropriate diagnosis. The first choice should be a laboratory with a veterinary pathologist with special expertise and an interest in dermatohistopathology. Because of the major differences between species, submission to a human medical pathologist is not recommended.

All biopsy specimens should be accompanied by the animal's breed, age and sex, clinical history, a physical description of the lesions, and clinical observations to aid the pathologist in histopathologic interpretation. Clinical findings, in fact, constitute the gross pathologic observations of the case and hence are critical. Useful, legible information provides better diagnostic results.

References

Baker R, Lumsden JH: *Color atlas of cytology of the dog and cat,* St Louis, 1999, Mosby.

Cowell RL, Tyler RD: *Diagnostic cytology and hematology of the horse,* ed 2, St Louis, 2002, Mosby.

Cowell RL, Tyler RD, Meinkoth JH: *Diagnostic cytology and hematology of the dog and cat,* ed 2, St Louis, 1999, Mosby.

DeNicola DB: Diagnostic cytology, collection techniques and sample handling, *Proc 4th Ann Mtg ACVIM,* 1987, pp 15-25.

Else RW, Lumsden JH, Davidson MG: *BSAVA manual of small animal clinical pathology,* Shurdington, Cheltenham, United Kingdom, 1998, British Small Animal Veterinary Association.

Gross TL, Ihrke PJ, Walder E: *Veterinary dermatopathology,* St Louis, 1992, Mosby, pp 3-7.

Littlewood JD: Investigative and laboratory techniques. In Harvey RG, Mason IS, editors: *Manual of small animal dermatology,* Shurdington, United Kingdom, 1993, BSAVA Publications, pp 33-44.

Moriello KA, Galbreath EJ: In Moriello KA, Mason IS, editors: *Handbook of small animal dermatology,* Oxford, United Kingdom, 1995, Pergamon Press, pp 45-8.

Index

A

Abdominal cavity parasites
  in cattle and other ruminants, 286
  in horses, 289
Abdominal worm, 289
Abortion, 108
  dilute carbol fuchsin stain for, 152t
Abscess
  bacterial staining for, 149, 150t-153t
  prostatic, 515
  specimens from, 110
Acanthocephalans, 261
  in swine, 291, 291f
Acanthocytes, 43, 43f
Acarina, 342-359
  mites in, 342-354, *See also* Mites
  ticks in, 354-359, 355f-357f, 359f
Accuracy of instruments, 19-21
Acid-alcohol
  in acid-fast stain, 143
  in fluorescent acid-fast stain, 144
Acid-fast granulomas, 150t-153t, 154
Acid-fast stain
  in fecal examination for coccidia, 307-308
  preparation of, 143
  procedure of, 147-148
Acid lipase deficiency, 54t
Acid production from glucose, 162
Acidic pH, 229
Acquired morphologic abnormalities of white
    blood cells, 52-53
Acromegaly, canine, 400
ACT, *See* Activated clotting time (ACT)
ACTH, *See* Adrenocorticotropic hormone (ACTH)
Actinobacillosis, 150t-153t, 154
Actinobacillus equuli, 113t
Actinobacillus ligniersii, 113t
Actinobacillus pleuropneumoniae, 113t
Actinobacillus salpingitis, 113t
Actinobacillus seminis, 113t
Actinobacillus species
  bacteriologic tests for, 113t
  identification of, 174, 175t
Actinobacillus suis, 113t
Actinomyces bovis, 113t
Actinomyces pyogenes
  bacteriologic tests for, 113t
  confirmatory tests for, 172
Actinomyces species
  bacteriologic tests for, 113t
  identification of, 174

Actinomyces suis, 113t
Actinomyces viscosus, 113t
Actinomycosis, 149-154, 150t-153t
Activated clotting time (ACT), 57
Activated partial thromboplastin time (APTT), 57
Addison's disease
  ACTH response test in, 389-390
  adrenal axis and, 388
  endogenous ACTH concentrations in, 391
Adenocarcinoma, 489, 489f
Adenohypophysis in adrenocortical function, 388
Adenovirus, 203t
  in dogs, 206
Adnexa, parasites of
  in cattle and other ruminants, 286, 286f
  in dogs and cats, 280
  in horses, 289
Adrenal axis in adrenocortical function tests,
    387-388
Adrenal-dependent hyperadrenocorticism, 390
Adrenocortical function tests, 387-392
  adrenal axis in, 387-388
  corticotropin-releasing hormone stimulation in,
    391-392
  corticotropin stimulation in, 389-390
  dexamethasone suppression in, 390-392
  endogenous ACTH concentrations in, 391
  urinary corticosteroids in, 388
Adrenocorticotropic hormone (ACTH)
  in adrenocortical function, 388
  endogenous concentrations of, 391
  response test of, 389-390
Aedes species, 332, 333f
Aelurostrongylus abstrusus, 277-278, 278f
Aerobic culture, 28t
Aeromonas hydrophila
  bacteriologic tests for, 114t
  identification of, 174
Aeromonas salmonicida, 114t
Aeromonas species, 114t
A:G, *See* Albumin-to-globulin (A:G) ratio
Agar
  bismuth sulfite, 135-136
  blood, 132-133
  chocolate, 134
  Hektoen enteric, 135
  lysine iron, 138
  MacConkey, 133-134
  mannitol salt, 134-135
  purple base, 135
  triple sugar-iron, 136-138, 137f